Living with Hereditary Cancer Risk

A JOHNS HOPKINS PRESS HEALTH BOOK

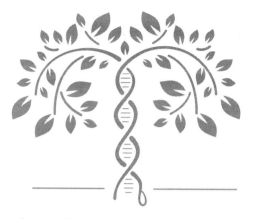

Living with Hereditary Cancer Risk

What You and Your Family Need to Know

Kathy Steligo, Sue Friedman, DVM, and Allison W. Kurian, MD

Foreword by Matthew Boland Yurgelun, MD

JOHNS HOPKINS UNIVERSITY PRESS

BALTIMORE

Note to the Reader: This book is not meant to substitute for medical care, and treatment should not be based solely on its contents. Instead, treatment must be developed in a dialogue between the individual and their physician. Our book has been written to help with that dialogue.

Drug dosage: The authors and publisher have made reasonable efforts to determine that the selection of drugs discussed in this text conform to the practices of the general medical community. The medications described do not necessarily have specific approval by the US Food and Drug Administration for use in the diseases for which they are recommended. In view of ongoing research, changes in governmental regulation, and the constant flow of information relating to drug therapy and drug reactions, the reader is urged to check the package insert of each drug for any change in indications and dosage and for warnings and precautions. This is particularly important when the recommended agent is a new and/or infrequently used drug.

Johns Hopkins University Press
2715 North Charles Street
Baltimore, Maryland 21218-4363
www.press.jhu.edu

Library of Congress Cataloging-in-Publication Data

Names: Steligo, Kathy, author. | Friedman, Sue, author. | Kurian, Allison, author.
Title: Living with hereditary cancer risk : what you and your family need to know /
    Kathy Steligo, Sue Friedman, DVM, Allison W. Kurian, MD ; foreword by
    Matthew Boland Yurgelun, MD.
Description: Baltimore : Johns Hopkins University Press, [2022] | Series: A Johns Hopkins
    Press health book | Includes bibliographical references and index.
Identifiers: LCCN 2021047176 | ISBN 9781421444253 (hardcover) | ISBN 9781421444260
    (paperback) | ISBN 9781421444277 (ebook)
Subjects: LCSH: Cancer—Genetic aspects—Popular works.
Classification: LCC RC268.4 .S74 2022 | DDC 616.99/4042—dc23/eng/20211106
LC record available at https://lccn.loc.gov/2021047176

A catalog record for this book is available from the British Library.

With the exception of figures 1.1, 1.2, and 8.1, all illustrations are courtesy of Facing Our Risk of Cancer Empowered.

Special discounts are available for bulk purchases of this book. For more information, please contact Special Sales at specialsales@jh.edu.

Contents

List of Tables   xi
Foreword, by Matthew Boland Yurgelun, MD   xiii

Introduction   1

Part I.
Understanding Cancer and Inherited Risk   6

1. The Link between Genetics and Cancer	**9**
The Basics of Genetics	10
Gene Wear and Tear and Repair	15
How Cancers Develop and Grow	16
Most Cancers Aren't Caused by Inherited Mutations	18
2. What's Swimming in Your Gene Pool?	**21**
Hidden Risk in the Family Tree	21
Plotting Your Genetic Pedigree	24
3. Signs of Hereditary Cancer	**30**
The Value of Genetic Counseling	32
Making Decisions about Testing	38
Insurance Coverage	43
Privacy and Protection	44
4. What Your Test Results Tell You	**46**
Positive, Negative, Maybe	46
Making Sense of Statistics	52
You Have a Mutation; Now What?	53

Part II.
Inherited Gene Mutations and the Cancers They Cause 62

5. Introducing *BRCA1* and *BRCA2*   65
Who Inherits a *BRCA* Mutation?   65
Signs of a *BRCA* Mutation   66
Levels of Risk   68

6. Lynch Syndrome: Five Genes, One Hereditary Syndrome   76
Signs of Lynch Syndrome in Families   76
Levels of Risk   78

7. Other Genes That Are Linked to Inherited Cancer Risk   87
Less Known, Less Studied Genes   89

8. Breast Cancer Basics   96
Signs and Symptoms   96
What Affects Breast Cancer Risk?   101
Types of Breast Cancer   105

9. Gynecologic Cancers   111
Ovarian, Fallopian Tube, and Primary Peritoneal Cancers   112
Endometrial Cancers   117

10. Gastrointestinal Cancers   123
Colorectal Cancer   125
Small Bowel Cancer   130
Pancreatic Cancer   130
Stomach Cancer   132
Anal Cancer   134

11. Genitourinary Cancers   136
Prostate Cancer   136
Bladder, Ureter, and Renal Pelvis Cancers   141

12. Melanoma   146
Melanoma of the Skin   147
Ocular Melanoma   155

Part III.
Strategies for Risk Reduction and Early Detection   158

13. Risk Management Guidelines   161
Guidelines for *BRCA1* or *BRCA2* Gene Mutations   162
Guidelines for Lynch Syndrome Gene Mutations   162
Guidelines for Mutations in Other Genes   162

14. Early Detection Strategies for High-Risk People   177
The Vocabulary of Screening   178
Surveillance for Breast Cancer   178
Surveillance for Gynecologic Cancers   184
Surveillance for Gastrointestinal Cancers   186
Surveillance for Prostate and Other Genitourinary Cancers   191
Surveillance for Melanoma   193
Screening for Other Hereditary Cancers   193

15. Medications That Reduce Cancer Risk   198
Risk-Reducing Medications for Breast Cancer   200
Risk-Reducing Medications for Gynecologic Cancers   203
Risk-Reducing Medications for Colorectal Cancers   204

16. Surgeries That Reduce Breast Cancer Risk   208
Mastectomy Procedures   209
Breast Reconstruction Choices   214
Side Effects, Risks, and Recovery   219

17. Surgeries That Reduce the Risk of
Gynecologic Cancers   222
Salpingo-Oophorectomy to Reduce the Risk of Ovarian Cancer   223
Hysterectomy to Reduce the Risk of Endometrial Cancer   230

18. Surgeries That Reduce the Risk of
Gastrointestinal Cancers   238
Total and Segmental Colectomy to Reduce the Risk of Colon Cancer   238
Total Gastrectomy to Reduce the Risk of Stomach Cancer   241

19. Factors That Affect Cancer Risk   249
Nutrition, Weight, and Physical Activity   250
Alcohol: An Unwise Choice   257
Smoking and Tobacco Products   257
Other Lifestyle and Behavioral Risk Factors   258

Part IV.
Treatment Choices for Hereditary Cancers 262

**20. Identifying Tumor Characteristics That Inform
Treatment Choices**   **267**

Staging and Grading Cancer   268

Targeted Approaches to Treatment   269

DNA Damage Repair Genes   271

21. Treating Breast Cancer   **277**

Cancer Type, Subtype, and Stage   278

Biomarker Testing   278

Genetic Testing   279

Options for Treatment   280

Follow-Up Care   287

22. Treating Gynecologic Cancers   **289**

Options for Ovarian, Fallopian Tube, and Primary Peritoneal Cancers   290

Options for Endometrial Cancer   297

23. Treating Gastrointestinal Cancers   **303**

Options for Colorectal Cancer   303

Options for Pancreatic Cancer   311

Options for Gastric Cancer   316

24. Treating Genitourinary Cancers   **321**

Options for Prostate Cancer   321

Options for Bladder, Renal Pelvis, and Ureter Cancers   331

25. Treating Melanoma   **339**

Options for Melanoma in the Skin   340

Options for Ocular Melanoma   347

Part V.
Living with Inherited High Risk 352

26. Regaining Sexual Health and Intimacy   **355**

Body Image   356

Coping with Pain   357

Reduced Sexual Desire   358

Erectile Dysfunction   360

Rebuilding Intimacy   362

27. Effects of Prevention and Treatment on Fertility   **365**
Preserving Fertility in Women   366
Preserving Fertility in Men   371
Other Parenting Alternatives   372

28. Managing Menopause   **377**
Symptoms of Early Menopause   378
Replacement Hormones   382
Long-Term Side Effects   384

29. Side Effects and Other Quality-of-Life Issues   **388**
Summarizing Side Effects by Treatment   389
Managing Immediate Side Effects   392
Long-Term Effects of Prevention and Treatment   402
Previvorship, Survivorship, and Follow-Up Care   406
End-of-Life Issues   406

30. Making Difficult Decisions   **410**
Start at the Beginning: Should You Be Tested?   410
Decisions about Your Cancer Risk   413
Decisions about Treatment   414
Prevention and Treatment Clinical Trials   416
Decision-Making in 15 Steps   418

31. You Are Not Alone   **421**
Create a Support System   421
Find Emotional Strength   424
Pursue Financial Resources   426
Look to the Horizon   427

Acknowledgments 429
Glossary 431
Notes 449
Resources 455
Index 457

Tables

Chapter	Table	Title	
1	1.1	Genetic Spelling Errors	15
2	2.1	Family Pedigree: Three Generations of Blood Relatives	27
5	5.1	Signs of a Possible *BRCA* Mutation in a Family	68
5	5.2	Average Probability of Developing Breast or Ovarian Cancer (%)	70
5	5.3	Estimated Lifetime Risk for Breast and Prostate Cancers in Men (%)	73
5	5.4	Estimated Lifetime Risk for Pancreatic Cancer (%)	75
6	6.1	Signs of a Possible Lynch Syndrome Mutation in a Family	77
6	6.2	Estimated Lifetime Risk of Lynch Syndrome Colorectal Cancer to Age 80	80
6	6.3	Estimated Lifetime Risk of Lynch Syndrome Cancers to Age 80 (%)	82
7	7.1	Genes with Inherited Mutations That Are Linked to Hereditary Cancer Risk	88
7	7.2	Estimated Lifetime Risk of Cowden Syndrome Cancers (%)	94
7	7.3	Estimated Lifetime Risk of Peutz-Jeghers Syndrome Cancers (%)	95
8	8.1	Estimated Lifetime Risk of Breast Cancer (%)	102
9	9.1	Estimated Lifetime Risk of Ovarian Cancer (%)	115
10	10.1	Genes with Inherited Mutations That Raise the Risk of Gastrointestinal Cancer	125
10	10.2	Common Gastrointestinal Cancer Symptoms and Risk Factors	126
11	11.1	Estimated Lifetime Risk for Prostate Cancer (%)	139
11	11.2	Estimated Lifetime Risk for Bladder, Renal Pelvis, and Ureter Cancers (%)	142
12	12.1	The ABCDE Rules: Common Differences between Moles and Melanomas	149
12	12.2	Estimated Lifetime Risk for Melanoma (%)	151
13	13.1	Summary of Guidelines for *BRCA1* and *BRCA2* Gene Mutations	163
13	13.2	Summary of Guidelines for Lynch Syndrome Gene Mutations	164
13	13.3	Summary of Guidelines for *APC* Gene Mutations	166
13	13.4	Summary of Guidelines for *ATM* Gene Mutations	167

13	13.5	Summary of Guidelines for *CDH1* Gene Mutations	168
13	13.6	Summary of Guidelines for *CHEK2* Gene Mutations	168
13	13.7	Summary of Guidelines for People with Two *MUTYH* Gene Mutations	169
13	13.8	Summary of Guidelines for *PALB2* Gene Mutations	170
13	13.9	Summary of Guidelines for *PTEN* Gene Mutations	172
13	13.10	Summary of Guidelines for *STK11* Gene Mutations	173
13	13.11	Summary of Guidelines for *TP53* Gene Mutations	174
13	13.12	Summary of Guidelines for Mutations in Other Genes	175
17	17.1	Benefits and Limitations of Risk-Reducing Gynecologic Surgeries	233

Foreword

Cancer genetics has always been deeply personal for me. My grandfather Clement Boland Sr. developed his first colon cancer at the age of 25 and later succumbed to a separate colon cancer in 1970 at the age of 49—nearly 10 years before I was born. Coincidentally, this was the same year that Henry Lynch and Anne Krush were completing their seminal work on the (unrelated) Cancer Family "G," now known as the first published family afflicted by the syndrome bearing Dr. Lynch's name. Like my grandfather, my great-grandfather developed his first colon cancer in his 20s and eventually died of a subsequent colon cancer at age 45. My grandfather was one of 13 children, 10 of whom were ultimately diagnosed with cancer, 6 of whom died prior to their fiftieth birthday. In spite of the pioneering work by Lynch, Krush, and others, the notion that such striking family histories indicated that cancer could be inherited was not widely accepted for some time, with familial clustering typically attributed to viral infection and other shared environmental exposures.

Family histories similar to that of my grandfather's family will seem all too familiar to some. For individuals from families who have experienced the anguish and uncertainty of such a history, it probably seems preposterous that the cause of these cancers could be anything other than hereditary genetics. By the 1990s, the scientific community finally began to pinpoint the genetic causes of many families' cancers. Dr. Mary-Claire King and colleagues discovered the *BRCA1* gene as a cause of hereditary breast and ovarian cancer, with the discovery of *BRCA2* following in short order. Mutations in both of these genes are now also linked to risks of prostate cancer, pancreatic cancer, and possibly other malignancies. Soon thereafter, *MLH1* and *MSH2* were identified by multiple investigators as the underlying basis for many Lynch syndrome families. (*MSH6*, *PMS2*, and *EPCAM* would later be identified as Lynch syndrome genes as well.) And in 1998, Dr. Parry Guilford and colleagues identified inherited variants in the *CDH1* gene as being the underlying cause of hereditary diffuse gastric cancer; these variants are now also linked to significant risk for lobular breast cancer. These pioneering discoveries were transformative for the families that had been rightly convinced for generations that there was an inherited basis to their cancer history. But in many ways, the discovery of these genes was the beginning of the story of cancer genetics rather than the definitive answer to these families' questions. As it turns out, inherited cancer genetics (not unlike family dynamics) can be quite complicated.

In *Living with Hereditary Cancer Risk*, the authors tackle the many layers of complexity and nuance that individuals face when confronted with inherited cancer risk: How did I get this? What can I do about it? Is cancer inevitable? How do I talk to my family about this? Is there hope? (Yes, there is!) The authors take the reader through a tour de force of inherited cancer risk syndromes, encompassing a nearly body-wide spectrum of cancer types, risk-reducing interventions, and strategies for surviving and thriving through the often-murky world of hereditary cancers. Perhaps most critically, this book goes beyond the "what" (as in "What does this mean for me?" and "What are my risks?") and takes the reader through the "how" (as in "How can I use this information to stay cancer-free?" "How does this change the treatment of my cancer?" "How can I have children if I might pass on inherited cancer risks?" and "How can I have a normal sex life?"). In doing so, this book and its lessons are an invaluable resource for those looking to transform the often-helpless sensation that accompanies an inherited cancer syndrome diagnosis into prevention, action, and empowerment.

For all of the groundbreaking advances that have occurred in the field of genetics, it remains imperative that health care providers remind our patients (and ourselves) that one's genes are not one's destiny. Plenty of questions and uncertainty remain in the field of inherited cancer risk, and much work remains to be done to continue addressing the many challenges faced by families living with such risk day in and day out. Thanks to the advocacy, education, and inspiration contained within these pages, however, the countless families out there like my own can now be equipped to deal with these adversities with immeasurably more knowledge, empowerment, and hope than the generations that preceded them.

Matthew Boland Yurgelun, MD
Director, Lynch Syndrome Center, Dana-Farber
Cancer Institute

Living with Hereditary Cancer Risk

Introduction

If cancer runs in your family or if you or a relative has tested positive for an inherited gene mutation that causes cancer, this book is for you. But why this book at this time?

In 2012, Johns Hopkins University Press published *Confronting Hereditary Breast and Ovarian Cancer*. At the time, it was the most comprehensive and up-to-date reference for people with inherited mutations in the *BRCA1* and *BRCA2* genes. The book was a compilation of the trusted information and support that the nonprofit organization Facing Our Risk of Cancer Empowered (FORCE) had been providing to the hereditary cancer community since 1999. But times have changed, and in the 10 years since that book's publication, an explosion of discoveries has broadened the scope of knowledge about hereditary cancers. Genetic testing has become more refined. There are more options for living with a high risk of cancer, and numerous personalized treatments have been engineered specifically to treat many hereditary cancers.

BRCA mutations have received plenty of press in the past several years, as many celebrities have openly shared their actions to reduce their high cancer risk and deal with hereditary cancer diagnoses. During this same period, the gene mutations that cause Lynch syndrome—an inherited high risk of developing colorectal, endometrial, and other cancers—have received less attention, despite being more prevalent than *BRCA* mutations. New research has also shed more light on mutations in lesser known genes, such as *ATM*, *PALB2*, *BRIP1*, *CHEK2*, and others, which also raise the risk for one or more cancers and affect many people. FORCE has expanded its mission to inform and support not only the *BRCA* community but also those who are predisposed to cancer due to these other high-risk genes. Today, we have much more information to share. In this book, we focus mainly on information about *BRCA* mutations and Lynch syndrome. To a lesser degree, we provide information on other, less common genetic mutations.

It's not unusual for more than one person in a family to have cancer. Although most cancers aren't hereditary, if you or your relatives have been diagnosed, you might wonder how you can learn if the cancers are due to an inherited predisposition. Should you be tested to determine whether you've inherited a mutation in a gene linked to cancer? Should someone else in your family be tested first? Genetic testing has come a long way from the early, cost-prohibitive, single-gene assays of a decade ago, and learning if you have a high-risk inherited mutation may now be only a blood or saliva test away. But testing is just one small part of the hereditary cancer journey. If a test reveals that you have a greater-than-average cancer risk, how do you cope with that knowledge? What can you do to remain cancer-free? If you develop cancer, how does knowledge of your inherited risk affect your treatment choices and your later life? You're not the first person to have these concerns or ask these questions. As professionals who deal with these medical and emotional issues daily, we help people who struggle with these concerns. We know that confronting hereditary cancer can be a complex, confusing, and highly individual journey. We also know that you can take actions to gain control of your health and your well-being.

Before we put fingers to keyboards to create this book, we considered how to develop the most comprehensive and objective resource possible for you and others who wonder what to do about their high cancer risk. We began with our existing base of information, writing about practical risk-reducing alternatives and treatment options with the goal of dispelling the myths and misinformation about hereditary cancer. Then we sprinkled meaningful extras throughout the text: personal stories from individuals who have dealt with these issues and confronted the same decisions you may face, views from the world's leading cancer and genetics experts, clarification about insurance coverage and discrimination protections, and perspectives from FORCE, including unique insights that we've acquired from serving our community. The result is *Living with Hereditary Cancer Risk: What You and Your Family Need to Know*, an up-to-date single source of research, insight, and inspiration, all bundled together to provide answers, whether you're well versed on or new to the subject.

Sorting through scientific terms, understanding risk management, and dealing with the emotions of it all can be overwhelming. Still, you deserve a normal life that isn't disrupted by fears about cancer. Decisions about hereditary cancer may be among the most difficult you'll ever make. But you needn't make them alone. This book is your road map through the maze of decisions that comes with living in a high-risk body, reducing your cancer risk, and, if necessary, choosing medical treatment. You needn't spend hours surfing the internet looking for information, trying to decipher studies on medical sites, defining terms, and attempting to distinguish between hype and fact. We've done that for you.

This book isn't meant to be a substitute for medical advice but rather is a trusty companion to help you understand your options and communicate with your health care team. The information we've included represents the best of what is now known about hereditary cancer risk. But since the field of cancer genetics is changing rapidly, you can always refer to the FORCE website (www.facingourrisk.org) and the other resources we include here for the results of new research and updated guidelines.

Living with Hereditary Cancer Risk was written to be inclusive of individuals of all sexual and gender identities. Whenever possible, gender-neutral language is used. When we use the terms "male" and "female" or "man" and "woman," we are referring to the gender assigned at birth. Many cancers that are associated with mutations in the genes discussed in this book occur in reproductive organs and are affected by reproductive hormones. The medical community doesn't yet know enough about how transitioning from one gender to another affects these cancer risks, and that is a priority for research.

You may be interested in some chapters more than others, especially if you already know that you have an inherited mutation or if you've been diagnosed with a hereditary cancer. We suggest that you start by reviewing the table of contents to see which chapters are most relevant to you. Page by page, you'll sort through and absorb all the information you need, gaining clarity to make the best decisions you can for yourself and your family. We've organized the book into five parts:

1. "Understanding Cancer and Inherited Risk" introduces the basics of genetics (how mutations are inherited, run in families, and lead to cancer over time); genetic counseling; and the implications of being tested for an inherited gene mutation.
2. "Inherited Gene Mutations and the Cancers They Cause" describes inherited gene mutations, hereditary cancer syndromes, and the cancers that are most associated with these mutations.
3. "Strategies for Risk Reduction and Early Detection" provides experts' guidelines for screening and early detection, as well as surgeries and medications that can reduce your high risk of hereditary cancer.

4. "Treatment Choices for Hereditary Cancers" walks you through options for the most common cancers associated with inherited gene mutations and cancer syndromes. This part also explains biomarker testing, which can identify unique tumor markers, and newer targeted and immunotherapies that are particularly effective for people with inherited gene mutations.

5. "Living with Inherited High Risk" discusses strategies for dealing with the day-to-day and long-term emotional and physical issues of cancer survivors and high-risk individuals. You'll read about fertility preservation, sexuality, coping with early menopause, managing the short- and long-term side effects of prevention or treatment, and tips for dealing with other quality-of-life issues.

Knowledge is both empowering and comforting. In many cases, it's life-saving. And although there is no single right answer for all readers—we're all individuals with unique concerns, circumstances, and priorities that affect our decisions—the practical, supportive information in these pages will demystify the complexity that surrounds so many issues related to hereditary cancer. It is our hope that this information will help to clarify your options and reduce your fear and anxiety about these issues, so that you can move forward confidently to make the decisions that are best for you and your family.

We don't have perfect medical solutions—no one does at this time—but you can potentially change your destiny by equipping yourself with resources, facts, and support.

Be informed. Be empowered. Be well.

Part I
Understanding
Cancer and
Inherited Risk

Our bodies are workaholics. Every minute of every day, even while we sleep, our nerves, muscles, blood, and other bodily support systems are busy keeping us in working order. In so many ways, the human body capably mends itself. Skin that gets scraped or cut regrows. Broken bones heal. The body's repair mechanisms are impressive, but they're not without limit; sometimes they're unable to correct physical damage. Digits or limbs that are lost can't regenerate, and the permanent loss of sight or hearing isn't something the body can restore.

When damage occurs in the human body, genes and cells can usually step up and fix it. When that's not possible, it's usually because an injury or disease is too powerful or too overwhelming or because our body's ability to heal or restore is impaired, and genes are unable to function as they should. This failure to fix can have dire consequences because unrepaired genetic damage can increase a person's susceptibility to cancer. Sometimes, that susceptibility can be passed from one generation to the next, leading to cancers that run in families.

How does a person go from being healthy to hearing "You have cancer"? This first part of the book explains how this happens and more, including

- how genes influence our chances of developing cancer,

- why some cancers run in families,

- how to learn whether your cancer or the cancers in your family are random or due to an inherited predisposition,

- what cancer statistics really mean, and

- how to talk with your family about an inherited predisposition for cancer.

Chapter 1

The Link between Genetics and Cancer

If the recipe you use to bake a cake includes a typo, your dessert might not turn out the way it should. The same thing happens when a genetic change called a mutation creates a "spelling error" that garbles a DNA recipe for a specific protein.

Few areas of science have changed the world of medicine more in the past 50 years than genetics, the study of how hereditary characteristics pass from parents to their children through DNA. Researchers now use advanced technology to gain genetic insights that were unimaginable just a few decades ago. Genetics allows them to trace a person's ancestry, study extinct species, and make crops more disease resistant. This science is also a key to understanding the origins of disease, because many diseases, including cancer, are caused at least in part by changes in our genes. A simple blood or saliva test can detect genetic changes that may make certain individuals more susceptible to cancer. Knowing that you have a predisposition to develop one or more cancers can be life changing, providing opportunities to reduce your likelihood of developing these diseases or to treat them early on. The more scientists understand how genetic changes lead to cancer, the closer we move toward better prevention, detection, treatment, and ultimately cure.

The Basics of Genetics

Genetics is a complex science with its own unique language. Cells. Chromosomes. DNA. Genes. We frequently hear or read of these genetic components, but what are they, how do they interact, and how do they influence our risk of cancer? With a basic understanding of these terms, we can better appreciate why cancer develops and how we might inherit a predisposition to one or more cancers. This understanding can help us to make informed choices about reducing our risk of developing these diseases.

We All Start with a Single Cell

Geraniums, spiders, poodles, and humans have the same fundamental microscopic cells that keep all organisms operating. Cells are the smallest unit of living things; all life begins as a single microscopic cell that grows and divides. One cell becomes two, two cells become four, four become eight, and so on until the entire plant, insect, animal, or human is formed. Humans have trillions of microscopic cells that grow and divide. This cellular life cycle—called cellular division—continues throughout our lives. Between conception and maturity, cells rapidly divide to spur tissue growth. Once we become adults, most cells divide primarily to replace older cells that are worn, damaged, or dying. This routine replacement occurs in billions of our cells every day, usually with order and precision: cells reproduce and die, and new cells take their place. Our bodies have more than 200 types of cells, which share the same basic structure but are programmed for specific tasks. Some cells distribute the oxygen we breathe, while others convert food into energy. Muscle cells enable movement, and nerve cells send messages between the brain and the rest of the body, allowing us to control muscle movement and receive sensations.

DNA

With the exception of red blood cells, all cells have a genetic control center called the nucleus (figure 1.1). Inside the nucleus are tightly twisted bundles of deoxyribonucleic acid (DNA), a chemical substance that stores and transmits the operating instructions we need to keep our bodies functioning. Compared to a computer, cells operate as the body's hardware, responsible for form and function, while DNA acts more like software, issuing instructions that tell cells

FIGURE 1.1 Our genetic structure

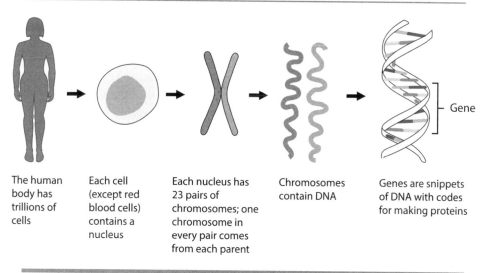

| The human body has trillions of cells | Each cell (except red blood cells) contains a nucleus | Each nucleus has 23 pairs of chromosomes; one chromosome in every pair comes from each parent | Chromosomes contain DNA | Genes are snippets of DNA with codes for making proteins |

what to do. Strands of DNA are organized into 23 pairs of chromosomes, one set from your mother and one set from your father. Most of our cells contain a complete set of our genetic material—the same DNA, chromosomes, and instructions—to create an exact copy of ourselves. (Egg and sperm cells are the exception; they have only one set of 23 chromosomes.)

All humans have about 99.9 percent of our DNA in common. Yet, except for identical twins, no two people are exactly alike. That's because our individual (one-tenth of a percent) variation determines our other inherited traits, like nose shape and hair texture. You and your sister may have inherited the same genes that determine your eye color, but your own variation of those genes resulted in your eyes being brown, while her unique genetic version gave her hazel eyes. Our individual DNA reflects our distinctive identities. A person's DNA can be used to link them to crime scenes or to screen for certain genetic abnormalities that lead to disease.

Genes: The Basic Units of Heredity

Everyone is unique—our individual genes make that possible. Genes are short segments of DNA that issue instructions for making thousands of proteins that build and support the body's critical functions: moving muscles, digesting food, and repairing damage to cells, tissue, and organs. Cells depend on these thousands of proteins to function correctly, to do their jobs in the right places at the right times. Proteins interact with each other and with other molecules to initiate these actions. They're the chemical building blocks of life; every bodily function depends on them. While cells make the proteins our bodies need, they do so in response to instructions issued by genes. Genes direct each cell to make specific proteins based on the type of cell and its needs. Genes are also the fundamental units of heredity; they hold DNA instructions that are passed from parent to child. Except for egg, sperm, and red blood cells, our cells contain two copies of each gene, one inherited from each of our biological parents. When someone says "It's in your genes," they're referring to a characteristic you share with your mother or your father. Some hereditary characteristics, such as height or eye color, don't affect your health or well-being. Other genes may cause traits like color blindness or a predisposition to develop diseases such as diabetes, asthma, or cancer.

Spelling Errors in DNA Recipes

Just as you follow a recipe to bake a cake, DNA functions as your body's cookbook, in which your genes are recipes for proteins made by your body. DNA recipes are written in a sort of biological shorthand that includes various combinations of a four-letter alphabet, each representing a different chemical base: A (adenine), C (cytosine), G (guanine), and T (thymine). Just as cookbook recipes use various combinations of the same ingredients to make different dishes, DNA issues instructions for all the proteins that our bodies need by combining different variations of these four "letters" into three-letter "words." The unique order of these letters spells out recipes for making everything from hormones to heart valves. Under a microscope, DNA molecules look like the rungs of a ladder made up of A-T and C-G pairs (figure 1.2).

If the recipe you use to bake a cake includes a typo, your dessert might not turn out the way it should. The same thing happens when a genetic change called a mutation (also known as a variant) creates a "spelling error" that garbles a DNA recipe for a specific protein. Mutations don't always cause a change in the protein, but some errors completely change the recipe and make it unreadable. Insertions and deletions cause words to shift, resulting in nonsense. Substitution errors can create sentences made up of real words that have different meanings: adding a "bug" egg instead of a "big" egg ruins

Unlocking the Human Genome

All living organisms have a unique genome, a complete set of the genetic information needed to create and grow that organism. (Genomics is the study of an organism's entire set of genes; it should not be confused with genetics, which studies only specific genes.) Using DNA samples from volunteers, the Human Genome Project discovered that humans have about 20,500 genes. This massive collaborative effort by thousands of scientists around the world was akin to translating every book ever written into a universal language: in this case, the genetic code that shows what each gene does and how abnormalities in genes cause disease. The information profoundly changed our understanding of human biology.

The project also produced a blueprint of our entire genetic code, showing the precise location of each gene on our chromosomes and indicating how our bodies work. Because genes appear in exactly the same order in all of us, knowing the location of a particular disease-causing gene was a game-changing medical discovery. Knowing where to look for changes in individual genes, scientists can now quickly analyze vast amounts of DNA—about 3 billion DNA units across all of a person's genes—to identify changes that may affect a person's health. This information is accelerating the pace of progress and discovery related to our knowledge of disease. Mapping the entire human genome has opened the door to advanced medicine that can be tailored for each individual.

FIGURE 1.2 The DNA ladder

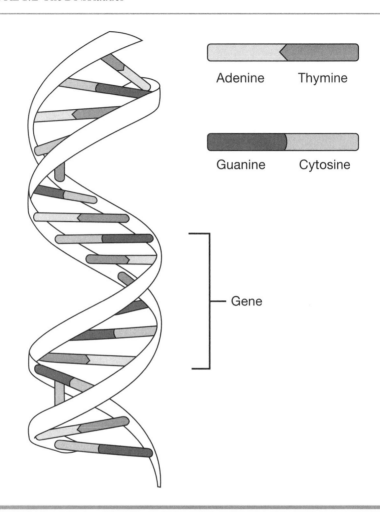

the recipe (table 1.1). Sometimes, even though all the right letters are there, they end up in the wrong place, or words become scrambled and create meaningless sentences, creating mutations called rearrangements. An error that occurs in egg or sperm cells can pass from parent to child.

Most of the time, the protein-making process proceeds flawlessly, because different protective genes are able to repair any damage that occurs. Gene damage that can't be repaired, however, changes the type and quantity of proteins that are made. This modifies how cells function, which can then lead to disease.

TABLE 1.1 Genetic Spelling Errors

INTENDED SENTENCE	MUTATION (SPELLING ERROR)	RESULT
Add one big egg	Deletion: If one letter gets dropped (in this case, the *A*), the entire sentence shifts and reads as nonsense.	Ddo neb ige gg
	Insertion: If an extra letter is added (in this case, a *d*), the entire sentence shifts and no longer makes sense.	Add don ebi geg g
	Substitution: If one letter is replaced with another (in this case, the *i* is replaced with a *u*), the sentence is legible, but it changes the meaning.	Add one bug egg
	Rearrangement: The words are still there but in the wrong order.	Egg add one big

Gene Wear and Tear and Repair

Our genes tend to accumulate—but then fix most—DNA damage throughout our lifetimes, usually without ill effect. This damage develops naturally as we grow older, as the wear and tear of living takes its toll on our ability to recuperate. The chance for a mutation increases as more cells divide and as our genetic repair mechanisms work less effectively than they once did. Mutations that occur in the cells that make egg and sperm are called germline mutations; these can be passed from parent to child.

Not all mutations are harmful. Many mutations are neutral and don't cause problems. The result of harmful inherited mutations, however, may be disease. That's why certain diseases and cancers tend to run in families, and why inheriting one or more of these gene changes can raise your risk for asthma, diabetes, and many other diseases. Parents who have a gene mutation that raises the risk for cancer can pass it to their children, even if the parents have never been diagnosed with cancer. Sickle cell anemia, cystic fibrosis, and Tay-Sachs disease are examples of inherited diseases that are caused by genetic mutations.

How Cancers Develop and Grow

Cancer is many different diseases—more than 200 cancers have been identified—that have one thing in common: they develop from mutations in cells that cause chemical or structural malfunctions that lead to uncontrolled growth. Mutations can develop when cells divide. Most, but not all, cells divide. (Brain and heart cells, for example, don't and thus are less likely to develop mutations.) We have two copies of each of our genes, a primary and a backup. If a mutation occurs in a gene that regulates cell growth or repairs cellular damage, the remaining healthy gene usually takes over the repair function so that the cells divide in a normal, orderly fashion without mishap. This prevents new acquired mutations and abnormal functions from being copied to the new cells. If the cell is beyond repair, other genes control the death of the abnormal cell. When you have a cut or burn in your skin, for example, your body responds by allowing the damaged cells to die and by creating new cells to replace the missing tissue—but only enough cells to do the job and no more. Having an inherited mutation leaves you with only one functioning copy of that gene, but this alone doesn't cause cancer. Cancer can develop if the remaining gene acquires a mutation or other abnormality and additional mutations accumulate in the cell. If you have an inherited *BRCA1* mutation and develop additional mutations in one of your breast cells, for example, you're more likely to develop breast cancer. If you have Lynch syndrome, new mutations that occur in one of your colon cells are likely to cause cancer there.

Cancer typically begins when neither copy of a protective gene is able to function normally. That starts a vicious cycle, as normal cells begin to change and grow unchecked. Damaged cells can quickly reproduce, passing on all their DNA code, including any unrepaired mutations, to the next generation of cells. Every subsequent division of unhealthy cells then perpetuates the existing errors. Instead of a well-managed process in which old cells die and new cells are created only when they're needed, cellular damage creates chaos in the body's otherwise orderly division process as malfunctioning cells ignore the body's signals to stop dividing. These rogue cells may form their own circulatory systems, evading the protective systems that are designed to kill them, and they keep replicating over and over again. Eventually, these flawed cells mass together to create a tumor (figure 1.3). Benign (noncancerous) tumors stay in place; malignant (cancerous) tumors can spread to other parts of the body. By the time a cancerous tumor is diagnosed, it holds billions of cells that behave irregularly:

- They grow when they aren't needed.
- They ignore genetic instructions to stop growing and die.
- They develop ways to evade the immune system and other processes that destroy abnormal cells.
- They clump together and form tumors.
- They may adapt to take advantage of other cells to better survive.
- They may break away from the primary tumor and invade other areas of the body.

FIGURE 1.3 A series of biological missteps must occur before healthy cells accumulate enough damage to eventually transition to cancer cells

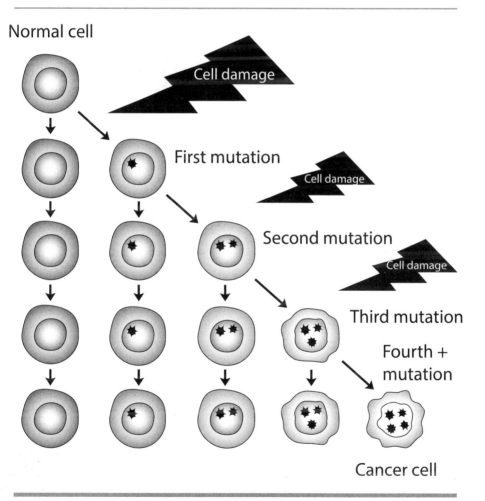

Adapted from "Understanding Gene Testing," National Institutes of Health, 1995

The Three Stages of Cancer Development

1. Initiation occurs when damaged DNA causes a cell to reproduce damaged copies of itself.

2. Promotion occurs when new cancer cells create a friendlier environment for themselves. They can grow larger and stronger as they recruit healthy cells to create blood vessels, which provide oxygen and nutrients. Cancer cells may also evade the immune system, the army of healthy cells that protects the body from infection and illness.

3. Progression occurs when unchecked cancer cells metastasize, meaning that they grow into the surrounding tissue, enter the blood or lymph system, and invade healthy tissue in other parts of the body. Left untreated or treated unsuccessfully, malignant tumors can overpopulate the body with cancer cells, which compete with healthy cells for space and nutrients.

Most Cancers Aren't Caused by Inherited Mutations

People who develop cancer are often surprised because they have no family history of cancer, but most cancers are sporadic. They develop over time from an accumulation of acquired (not inherited) mutations as we age and our DNA repair mechanisms become less effective. A smaller percentage of cancers are hereditary and tend to run in families. The same or related cancers that occur across several generations hint that hereditary factors may be the cause.

Exposure to carcinogens (substances that damage healthy tissue) can kick-start genetic changes that evolve into cancer. We're exposed to carcinogens every day: chemicals in the workplace and home; hepatitis, human papillomavirus, and similar viruses; pollution; hormones; ultraviolet rays; and some medical treatments, including radiation, chemotherapy, targeted therapy, and other medications. Numerous behavioral factors are also cancer culprits to varying degrees, including poor nutrition, alcohol use, smoking, obesity, and physical inactivity.

Acquired mutations are limited to the cells where the damage occurs. Too much sun exposure can impair your skin cells and cause an age spot, for example. When damaged skin cells divide, the new cells they create have the same genetic damage and produce the same age spot. This type of acquired genetic abnormality doesn't extend to all other cells in your body or to egg or sperm cells, so your children won't inherit your damaged skin cells, although they might acquire age spots of their own. Inherited mutations, on the other hand, exist in all cells, including egg and sperm cells, and can be passed to you from either parent—just like your mother's wavy hair and your father's brown eyes—and from you to any or all of your children.

Differences between Sporadic and Hereditary Cancers

Gene mutations, whether they're acquired or inherited, can cause cancer. There are some differences between the two, however.

- Hereditary cancers are caused in part by gene mutations that are passed from parents to their children. Other blood relatives may share the same gene changes. Sporadic cancers arise from gene damage that is acquired from aging, behavioral factors, environmental exposures, hormones, and other influences. Acquired gene changes aren't shared among relatives or passed on to children. About 10 percent of all cancers are thought to develop from inherited mutations; this percentage may be higher or lower, depending on the cancer type.
- Hereditary cancers often occur at an earlier age than the sporadic forms of the same cancers. People with inherited mutations may benefit from earlier or more frequent cancer screening.
- Hereditary cancers are sometimes more aggressive and more likely to metastasize than the sporadic forms of the same cancers.

- People with hereditary cancers are more likely to develop a second cancer.
- Inherited mutations may raise the risk for multiple types of cancers.
- Hereditary and sporadic cancers may respond differently to the same treatment.
- Hereditary cancers may affect multiple family members.
- Sporadic and hereditary cancers may affect health care decisions differently.

Inherited and Acquired Gene Mutations

Inherited or germline mutations are passed from the mother's egg cells or the father's sperm cells, which are called germ cells. If one of these cells carries a mutation, the damaged DNA transfers at conception to each of the child's cells. Parents who have a mutation that causes colon cancer, for example, can pass that susceptibility to any of their children, and each successive generation may also inherit the same damage.

Acquired or somatic mutations develop sometime after birth in cells other than egg and sperm cells. This can happen during cell division or as a result of exposure to toxic environmental factors. Acquired mutations cannot be inherited.

Chapter 2

What's Swimming in Your Gene Pool?

If your family has been affected by cancer, you've probably wondered about your own risk. A genetics expert can evaluate your pedigree—your family's medical history—to identify any patterns of disease that may indicate that an inherited mutation exists in your family and whether you or a relative should consider genetic testing.

M ost of your appearance results from traits that you inherit from your parents. You can thank them for your cute dimples, dark eyes, and height. These traits are written into your DNA, and you can pass them—and genetic mutations—to your children. Half of our genes come from each parent, so it's possible to inherit a genetic mutation from either your mother or your father. If either of your parents has a particular gene mutation, you and each of your siblings have a 50 percent chance of inheriting it. Likewise, each of your children has the same 50 percent chance of inheriting your mutation and high cancer risk (figure 2.1). Children who don't inherit your mutation don't have the same high risk for certain cancers.

Hidden Risk in the Family Tree

Knowing your family's medical history is one of the most important steps you can take to understand your own cancer risk. Patterns of cancer and other diseases on both sides of the family hold clues that can help you make the

FIGURE 2.1 Each child has a 50 percent chance of inheriting a parent's gene mutation

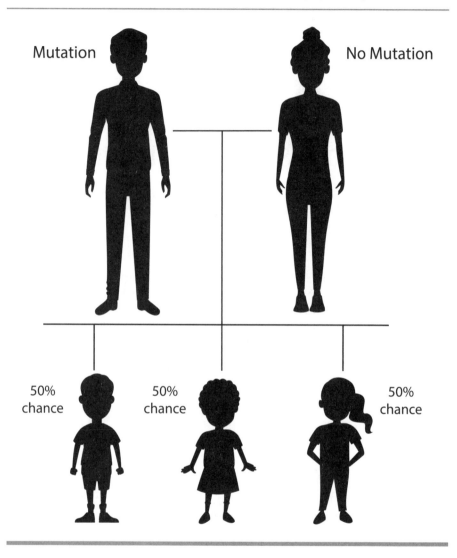

best decisions about your own health. Because either parent can pass a mutation to their children, ignoring one or the other side of the family can hide potential risk. This is especially important for gene mutations that are predominantly linked to women's cancers. With so much attention paid to *BRCA* gene mutations and breast and ovarian cancer, for example, the link to prostate cancer may be overlooked. Knowing which side of the family has your

Finding Genetic Answers in Pea Plants

In 1866, Austrian monk Gregor Mendel, considered the father of genetics, made a stunning declaration based on his experiments in crossbreeding pea plants: "factors" (now called genes) determine traits that are passed unchanged to descendants, and for each trait, individuals inherit a pair of genes, one from each parent. Mendel's work proved why the offspring of plants, animals, and people so often resemble their parents. His work was mostly ignored until 1900, when independent experiments by three other scientists proved Mendel to be correct, and the scientific world began to take notice. His conclusions became the foundation of modern genetics: genes pass from parent to child, as do abnormalities within the genes that raise a person's risk for disease.

mutation can help determine whether relatives on that side may have the same mutation and associated high risk. By reviewing your family history, a genetics expert may be able to determine whether a family mutation came from your mother's or father's side.

Sometimes, it can be difficult to determine whether a mutation runs in a family. Environmental exposures, lifestyle choices, having a small family or few female relatives, or having relatives who died early from other causes may obscure familial cancers. In some cases, a family's medical history may not be available. That's the case for many Ashkenazi Jewish families; they cannot trace their family history before the Holocaust. If you were adopted and don't know your family history, or if your relatives died before age 50 of unknown causes, a genetic counselor may still be able to help determine the likelihood that you inherited a mutation based on the information available. Even in families that don't have a known mutation, patterns of disease can indicate increased cancer risk. These familial cancer clusters may be caused by genes or combinations of genes that haven't yet been linked to increased cancer risk. Shared environmental or behavioral factors—like exposure to toxic chemicals or smoking—may also be contributing factors. Having several family members who have had breast, ovarian, uterine, colorectal, melanoma, pancreatic, or prostate cancer may indicate that you have an above-average risk for the same cancers. For example, nearly one in three people with colon cancer has family members who have been similarly diagnosed.[1]

— *My Story* —
My Mutation Came from My Dad

Diagnosed with breast cancer, I thought I had no relevant family history. My father's first cousins had the disease, but they were already in their 60s by then, and they seemed like such distant relatives. After my diagnosis, I met with a genetic counselor who realized from my small family tree that my cancer likely came from my father's first cousin—I don't recall a single health form ever asking about the health history of my father's side of the family. If my father had more women on his side of the family, we may have seen more breast cancer. Sure enough, like my two cousins, I tested positive for a *BRCA2* mutation.

—*Ellyn*

Plotting Your Genetic Pedigree

If your family has been affected by cancer, you've probably wondered about your own risk. A genetics expert can evaluate your pedigree—your family's medical history—to identify any patterns of disease that may indicate that an inherited mutation exists in your family and whether you or a relative should consider genetic testing. Even if you have no reason to suspect that you should be tested for an inherited mutation, creating a family pedigree and sharing it with your doctor is an important step in protecting your health (figure 2.2).

Your pedigree can help your doctor recognize a familial pattern of health issues that may be prevented or caught early, when treatment is more likely to be effective. This important document identifies your biological relatives, their relationship to you, and any diseases they've had. To develop your pedigree, investigate and document as many of the following items as possible for each of your relatives, both living and deceased:

FIGURE 2.2 A sample family pedigree

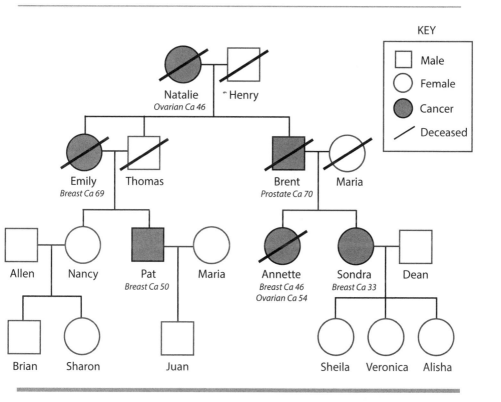

- Ethnicity or ancestral country (or region) of origin.
- Current ages of living relatives and ages at death of deceased relatives. If someone's exact age is unknown, estimate it as accurately as possible. If your maternal aunt died between 30 and 40, for example, but you don't know her exact age at the time, record "deceased in her 30s."
- Any chronic mental or physical disorder. For cancer, include where it began in the body, such as breast, prostate, kidney. If possible, distinctly note the type of cancer someone had. If Aunt Sarah says her mother had brain cancer, try to determine whether it was truly brain cancer or a different type of cancer that metastasized to the brain, if that information is available. Try to find out if a relative's "female disease" was cancer of the ovaries, uterus, cervix, or other reproductive organ.
- Age at onset of symptoms or diagnosis.

- Cause of death.
- Other family health information that may be important.

A genetics expert ideally needs these data from both sides of the family for three generations to determine whether a hereditary cancer pattern exists. So, if possible, collect information about your first-, second-, and third-degree biological relatives (table 2.1). Your first-degree relatives share half of your DNA, your second-degree relatives have a quarter of your DNA, and on average, third-degree family members share one-eighth of it. Generally, the closer the relationship between you and family members, the more DNA that you share. Cancer in a first-degree relative more substantially affects your risk than cancer in a second-degree relative, which is more significant than cancer in a third-degree relative. If possible, include information about all your blood relatives, including half siblings (with whom you share only one biological parent). Don't include step-relatives or in-laws in your pedigree. Although they're a part of your family as a result of marriage, they don't share your bloodlines.

Clarifying Your Clan

It can be confusing to figure out how to label your close relatives, particularly in very large families with several cousins. In many families, your first cousins are the children of your aunts and uncles (your parents' siblings). The children of your first cousins are your first cousins once removed. Your children and your cousins' children are second cousins to each other. But not all families or cultures use the same labels to describe relatives. So when you gather your family history, whenever possible you should try to clarify how that person is related to you.

TABLE 2.1 Family Pedigree: Three Generations of Blood Relatives

FIRST-DEGREE RELATIVES	SECOND-DEGREE RELATIVES	THIRD-DEGREE RELATIVES
siblings	half siblings	cousins
children	uncles, aunts	great-grandparents
parents	grandparents	great-aunts, great-uncles
	grandchildren	
	nieces, nephews	

Uncovering Your Medical Roots

The sooner you can collect your family history the better, because as each generation ages, the potential for information to become lost or forgotten increases. Asking your blood relatives whether a family tree or list of family members already exists is a good place to start. This type of information is sometimes recorded in family bibles and other genealogy materials. Start with your first-degree relatives—your parents and siblings—then include your grandparents, aunts, and uncles before moving on to cousins, nieces, and nephews. If you have great-grandparents who are living, ask them what information they can contribute. Or start with a relative who acts as the family historian. You might want to conduct your research with conversations, emails, or a survey. Family reunions or other gatherings can be the perfect opportunity to gather information. Emphasize how this information can help current and future family members manage their risk for disease. If individuals are uncomfortable talking about medical issues, ask if they're willing to provide you with written information.

In some families, discussing cancer is private or taboo. This can be particularly true when discussing breast, endometrial, colorectal, ovarian, and prostate cancer. It's important to respect the wishes of others. Some relatives may not know or want to talk about or share their medical histories. If you were adopted, ask your adoptive parents for information, and if possible, ask your birth parents about their medical history and yours. Accessing your adoption agency records may be another option. The more accurate the details, the more helpful the information will be. Share this information and your own medical information with all of your adult relatives, because it affects all of you.

You may gather all your details before creating your pedigree or add them to your chart as they become available. The Centers for Disease Control and

Prevention provides easy-to-use online tools for both methods (https://www .cdc.gov/genomics/famhistory). The section "Family Health History" produces your pedigree based on your input. Hop online, follow the prompts, and then print your chart. If someone in your family has already created a pedigree, most or all of the work will be done for you. Make sure it's up to date and reflects all the specific information you need. Make it as comprehensive as you can. Your pedigree is a valuable, living document. Keep a copy in a safety deposit box, and if the document is stored on your computer, be sure to make a backup copy. Update your pedigree whenever a birth, death, or diagnosis occurs in the family.

— *My Story* —
Breaking the Cycle of Silence

In the African American community, you don't talk about cancer very much. We are very secretive and private. Every month when I go to my hairdresser, I talk about being a colorectal, endometrial, and skin cancer survivor to break the cycle of silence and dispel myths.

—Wenora

— EXPERT VIEW —
Ignorance Isn't Bliss

BY MÓNICA ALVARADO, MS, CGC

Older relatives and those who were raised to believe that it isn't acceptable to discuss cancer and other serious illnesses may be reluctant to share details about the family's cancer history. If you can help your relatives understand that sharing information about the family's pedigree is an important legacy, they may be more likely to cooperate. Here are some tips:

- If you can win the support of your family matriarchs and patriarchs, the most influential people in your family, other relatives will help you.
- Elderly relatives, your parents, and older siblings are more likely to know about your ancestors.
- Generally, women are much better than men at remembering health information. If you can identify key female relatives, ask them to help.
- Use other relatives as intermediaries if you're trying to get information from someone you don't know well.

- If you have amateur genealogists in your family, they may have already collected the family history.
- Take advantage of family events, such as weddings, reunions, and funerals, to contact relatives.
- Use additional resources, like family diaries, newspaper clippings, public records, public libraries and archives, books, and pamphlets, for other suggestions.
- Be sensitive to the fact that adoption, divorce, drug abuse, suicide, and other topics may be difficult to discuss. Acknowledge that, but try to explain why it's important to have the most accurate history available.

Signs of a Family Mutation

- A relative who developed or died from any illness at an early age.
- Cancers that develop at a young age.
- Multiple relatives on the same side of the family with the same disorder.
- More than one type of cancer in the same relative.
- The same disease in multiple generations.
- Individuals who develop an uncommon cancer, including pancreatic cancer or male breast cancer.
- Specific combinations of diseases in a family—such as breast and ovarian cancer or colorectal and endometrial cancer—which may indicate the presence of a family mutation.

Chapter 3

Signs of Hereditary Cancer

On the beneficial side, testing clarifies cancer risk and empowers you to make decisions about current and future medical options. Your testing may help to inform others in your family about their hereditary cancer risk as well. On the other hand, testing can be complicated. It doesn't always provide a simple "Yes, you have increased risk" or "No, you don't."

If you could see into your future and change your potentially high-risk destiny, would you? Additionally, if you were considering cancer treatment and looking at your genes might help you select a more effective treatment, wouldn't you want that information? Genetic testing for an inherited mutation offers the opportunity to do both. Although it can't predict your health, genetic testing can give you insight your ancestors never had, a peek into your medical future, and the potential to change your fate.

Genetic testing includes hundreds of blood and tissue tests, which act as a kind of hereditary horoscope. Still, it isn't a true crystal ball. The glimpse it reveals doesn't guarantee that you will or won't get cancer, but if you've inherited a risk-increasing gene mutation, testing gives you and your family lifesaving information and a chance to reshape your future. It can serve to clarify which is the best option for managing your risk: wait and see what happens, screen to detect early-stage cancer, or preemptively act to reduce your odds of hearing "You have cancer." If you develop cancer, genetic testing can help you understand why it developed, identify your risk for another diagnosis, guide your treatment decisions, and help your relatives understand their risk. You may benefit from genetic testing if your family medical history shows the following signs of hereditary cancer:

- A blood relative has tested positive for an inherited gene mutation linked to cancer.

  or

- You or any of your family members have had
  - pancreatic, ovarian, fallopian tube, primary peritoneal, or male breast cancer at any age;
  - breast, colorectal, or endometrial cancer at age 50 or younger;
  - breast or prostate cancer at any age and Eastern European Jewish ancestry;
  - triple-negative breast cancer at any age;
  - prostate cancer at age 55 or younger or metastatic prostate cancer;
  - two separate cancer diagnoses;
  - rare or young-onset cancer (typically refers to cancers diagnosed before age 50);
  - more than 10 colon polyps;
  - colorectal or endometrial cancer at any age with tumor testing that suggests Lynch syndrome; or
  - tumor testing that shows a mutation in a gene associated with hereditary cancer.

  or

- More than one family member on the same side of the family has had a combination of the following:
  - colorectal cancer;
  - breast cancer;
  - ovarian, fallopian tube, or primary peritoneal cancer;
  - endometrial cancer;
  - prostate cancer;
  - pancreatic cancer;
  - stomach cancer;
  - melanoma;
  - a rare cancer; or
  - young-onset cancer.

— *My Story* —
A New Understanding

If I had a crystal ball, I'm not sure I'd want to know what the future might reveal. When I'm 18, I'll decide whether or not to be tested. No matter what my result, I'll always be a part of a family with hereditary cancer. My mom, grandmother, aunt, great-aunt, and two cousins have an inherited mutation and have had cancer. Cancer is the furthest thing from the minds of most people my age, but not for me. My family's genetic background has given me a new understanding that sets me apart from my peers. Even though it was frightening to watch my mother go through treatment, her courage comforted me. Now I see that ignoring my fears doesn't take away my risk, and none of us is invincible. Mom used to say that living with cancer risk was like having a dark cloud over her. My cloud might appear in that crystal ball. I'm pretty sure that someday, I'll have the strength to take a look.
—Arielle

The Value of Genetic Counseling

With advances in genetic science, doctors can now personalize cancer care. This is a giant leap forward from a one-size-fits-all approach to treatment, but it requires health care professionals who have expertise in genetics. Genetic counseling is a well-established field that continues to evolve as discoveries are made. Counseling is a critical first step before genetic testing, even if you eventually decide not to be tested. Although genetic counseling is important for anyone with a family history of cancer, not everyone benefits from genetic testing. The National Comprehensive Cancer Network (NCCN), a consortium of the nation's leading cancer experts who develop standard-of-care guidelines in oncology, and most other medical organizations recommend genetic counseling before genetic testing.

You Need an Expert to Unravel Your Genetic History

When a stubborn rash refuses to go away, you see a dermatologist. When cancer is diagnosed, you consult with an oncologist. Likewise, when you want to know if your family has a hereditary pattern of disease or learn about your risk for cancer, you need a genetics expert. Cancer risk assessment isn't always straightforward. Hereditary red flags aren't always obvious, and recognizing and interpreting them requires particular training and skill. While your primary doctor, gynecologist, and other clinicians may be knowledgeable and compassionate professionals, they might not have the advanced training, expertise, or time to provide the range of services you'll experience with a genetic counselor. Trained in disease-related genetics and psychosocial counseling, genetic counselors are skilled interpreters of risk who represent the human side of science. A counselor will help you navigate the entire counseling and testing process, answering and probably anticipating your questions while being sensitive to your concerns and fears. Your primary doctor can provide a referral to a genetic counselor. Or use the searchable online directory of the National Society of Genetic Counselors (www.nsgc .org). If you have difficulty finding a genetic counselor, the FORCE toll-free helpline (866-288-7475, ext. 704) will help you find an expert in your area or by phone.

Genetic counselors provide the following critical services:

- Identify patterns of inherited cancer that run in your family.
- Discuss the benefits and limitations of genetic testing to help you decide if it's right for you.
- Determine which family members, if any, should consider genetic testing, and in what order.
- Decide which genetic test is most appropriate.
- Help obtain insurance coverage if you decide to be tested.
- Interpret test results and explain what they mean for you and your family.
- Estimate your cancer risk whether or not you have an inherited mutation.
- Discuss options for early detection or reducing your cancer risk.
- Explain how a mutation affects your treatment options or the risk of another cancer (if you have a cancer diagnosis).

Questions for Your Genetic Counselor

- Does my family history show a pattern of inherited disease?
- Should I be tested to see if I have an inherited predisposition to cancer?
- For which mutations should I be tested?
- How reliable are the test results?
- What does the test mean for me and my family members?
- What are my options if I test positive?
- What are the implications of a negative test?
- How will my test results influence my cancer treatment?
- Will my insurance pay for testing? If not, what are my options for low-cost testing?

— THE **FORCE** PERSPECTIVE —

When Counseling Doesn't Happen

We've seen instances where a lack of genetic counseling led to harm. A FORCE member and two of her siblings received genetic testing through a doctor who had no specific training in genetics. None of them had genetic counseling before being tested. All three were told that their test for a *BRCA* mutation was positive. Considering herself at high risk for breast and ovarian cancer, the FORCE member had her healthy ovaries removed. When another relative was later tested for the same mutation, her genetic counselor determined that the FORCE member's test result was, in fact, not positive. The misinformation had resulted in her unnecessary, irreversible surgery, and pointless testing (along with related anxiety and cost) her siblings didn't need.

———————————

— *My Story* —
Don't Try This: Genetic Testing without Counseling

I received my genetic test results without the benefit of a genetic counselor because I didn't know there was such a thing! A nurse took my family history, read the options on the brochure, and told me I would probably test positive. No one ever asked me why I wanted to be tested or what I would do with the results. Without any preparation, I was informed that I was positive. I met with a group of doctors, who told me I needed to have a bilateral mastectomy right away. No one wanted to answer questions about my risk, my options, or what this test result meant for my family. It's cruel to receive results in this way, then be sent on your way and wished good luck. I never felt so alone in my life.

—*Alice*

What to Expect from the Process

After an in-depth assessment of your personal and family medical histories, your genetic counselor will use computer programs, national guidelines, and expertise to determine whether you or other relatives would likely benefit from genetic testing. She'll translate what may seem to be incomprehensible concepts into clear terms, put your test results into proper perspective, and then help you and your family cope with the information. A genetic counselor won't try to persuade you to be tested nor tell you what to do once you receive the results, but she will support the decision you feel is right for you. If you're undecided about testing, your counselor can put you in touch with individuals who are willing to share their own testing experience. A genetic counselor can ensure that your decision to be tested or not is based on facts and is in your best interest.

If you decide to be tested, your counselor will explain the process and arrange for a blood or mouth rinse sample. Your sample will be sent to a commercial testing laboratory, where a technician will separate the genes to be tested from the rest of your DNA and scan them for abnormalities (figure 3.1). After

FIGURE 3.1 The genetic counseling and testing process

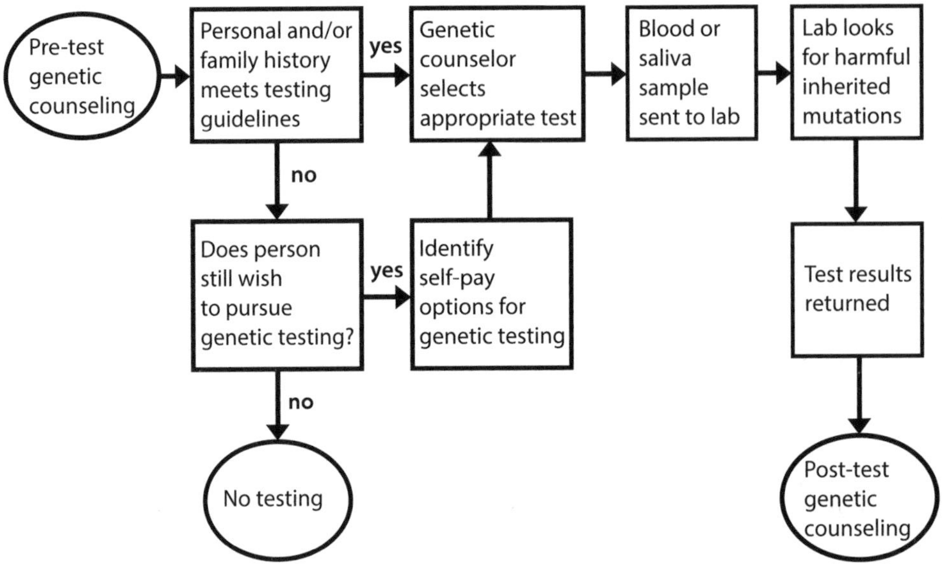

your test, the counselor will explain your result and how it affects your cancer risk. If your test is negative, she may recommend other genetic tests to help further define the cause of cancer in your family. If your test shows that you've inherited a mutation that puts you at high risk for cancer, your counselor will discuss risk management options and research studies for which you may be eligible. Based on your family medical history, she'll also identify other family members who might benefit from genetic counseling and testing.

As genetics research progresses, we're learning more about mutations and other causes of hereditary cancer. So it's a good idea to update your status each year or when any new case of cancer is diagnosed in your family with your genetic counselor, who'll continue to be an invaluable resource.

— My Story —

What's the Point of Knowing?

Talking with my father about genetic testing, he asked, "What is the point in knowing?" I think he believed the knowledge would just cause me suffering. Better to wait for your fate and be surprised by it than suffer with the knowledge that it is coming. Perhaps this was part of his pragmatism or part of his growing up in the Philippines, where resources were limited—you just played the cards you were dealt. At that time, my father didn't know there was something you could do if you had positive test results. Once he knew I could take actions to reduce my risk and that what I got in return was the opportunity to avoid cancer, he and my mother told me that testing was the bravest thing I'd ever done for myself and for those who love me.

—*Grace*

— **EXPERT VIEW** —

Experience Counts

BY JANA PRUSKI-CLARK, MPH, MS, CGC

Until people go through the process of genetic counseling with a trained genetics professional, they may consider genetic testing to be a clear-cut test that will tell them if they have an inherited mutation or not. Genetic testing is more than just a laboratory test. It offers many benefits, providing information about your medical options for cancer screening, risk reduction, and treatment. It also has limitations, including those related to cost, insurance coverage, privacy, and interpretation of results, especially when results are uncertain or uninformative.

Both positive and negative results can have a psychological impact. Despite all of our medical advances, it's never easy to hear that you're at increased risk for cancer. As genetic counselors, we know that testing involves individuals yet affects entire families. Who else should be tested? Do relatives want to know your results? What, how, and when do you tell your kids? Genetic counselors are trained to help you answer these questions as they support you and your family throughout the entire process. Although we may not have walked in your shoes, we've walked alongside others with cancer in the family, and we can share that knowledge with you.

Previvor or Survivor?

If you've ever been diagnosed with cancer, you're a survivor. You're a previvor if you have a family history of disease, an inherited mutation, or another factor that predisposes you to cancer and you've never been diagnosed.

Making Decisions about Testing

Genetic testing isn't perfect, and like most things in life, it has advantages and disadvantages. On the beneficial side, testing clarifies cancer risk and empowers you to make decisions about current and future medical options. Your testing may help to inform others in your family about their hereditary cancer risk as well. On the other hand, testing can be complicated. It doesn't always provide a simple "Yes, you have increased risk" or "No, you don't." Learning that you've inherited a predisposition to cancer can quickly change your world. You may feel helpless, uncertain about your future, overwhelmed, and even guilty about the chance of passing your mutation to your children. Before you're tested, consider that your results may or may not provide you with clear answers about your risk. A genetic counselor can help you sort through these issues.

— EXPERT VIEW —

Should Your Minor Children Be Tested for Mutations That Are Linked to Adult-Onset Cancers?

BY KENNETH TERCYAK, PHD

The question of testing children is common among parents who test positive for an inherited mutation, and sometimes children ask whether they can be tested. Experts recommend genetic testing for children under age 18 only if there are medical reasons to do so. Most inherited mutations cause adult-onset cancers, but some mutations are linked to increased cancer risk earlier in life. Very young children lack the capacity to make an informed choice about genetic testing. Even older children and adolescents may have difficulty appreciating the long-lasting reach of the information and the psychological implications of learning their carrier status. Some may come to regret their decision later on. This is why participating in patient education and counseling before genetic testing for hereditary cancer is so important.

Decisions about genetic testing are usually deferred until late adolescence or young adulthood and are made under medical supervision. For gene mutations linked to adult-onset cancer, no action is usually taken before age 18 even if testing shows that children have a mutation. Parents can, however, talk openly with their children about their own testing experiences, including why they made a particular choice, what it means for them and their health, and how other adults in the family might also be tested when the time is right. Be open and honest about what you know and how you feel. This can be an opportunity to teach about and support children in maintaining healthy lifestyles, to engage in conversations about ways to prevent cancer, and to help direct family members to information and support resources, such as FORCE. Even in the context of a parent's cancer diagnosis, it can be comforting for children, adolescents, and young adults to know that researchers are working hard to find ways to prevent cancer, and treatment breakthroughs can and do happen.

Who Should Be Tested First?

If no one in your family has had genetic testing or has tested positive for an inherited mutation, consideration might be given as to who should be tested first. Even though you might be anxious to find out if you have a mutation that causes cancer, it may make more sense for someone else in the family to be tested first, as determined by your family pedigree. If that family member tests positive, other relatives can then be tested for the same mutation.

- Genetic testing is most reliable when it begins with a family member who has been diagnosed with cancer and has the highest likelihood of testing positive for a mutation. If you've never had cancer, but your paternal aunt had ovarian cancer or young-onset breast cancer, for example, testing her first will be more informative. If she tests positive for an inherited mutation, your father could be tested for the same mutation. If he also has the mutation, then you and your siblings can be tested. If your father's test shows no known mutation, there's no point in testing you or your siblings for your aunt's mutation. Your father can't give you a mutation he doesn't have. If your father is no longer living, however, you might want to be tested for your aunt's mutation because there's no way to know if he had it.

- When multiple relatives have had the same type of cancer or cancers that are related, it's best to first test whoever was diagnosed at the earliest age or with the least common cancer. If your uncle Rinaldo had prostate cancer at age 62 (which is common) and your sister Jane had ovarian cancer at age 46 (which is uncommon), Jane should be tested first since Rinaldo's prostate cancer might have been sporadic. If Jane tests positive, other undiagnosed relatives can then be tested for her mutation.

- When it's not possible to begin testing with a cancer survivor in the family, a genetic counselor can determine whether other relatives should be tested, and in what order. The chance of having an inconclusive negative result is greater when family members who have never had cancer are tested first, which can lead to a false sense of security. If both sides of the family show a history of cancer, individuals on both sides should speak with a genetic counselor. If your mother tests negative and your father has a family history of cancer, his side of the family may benefit from genetic counseling.

- In families with no known mutation, a genetic counselor can identify who should be tested first or next. This might be you, or it could be another member of the family.

Which Test Is Right for You?
Genetic tests explore segments of specific genes where we can expect to find a mutation. Even though scientists know that other mutations exist, we can test only for those we know about. It's like space exploration. We know

Do-It-Yourself Testing:
Not a Good Idea

Increasingly, testing for inherited mutations is available without genetic counseling and, in some cases, without involving a health care professional at all. Genetic testing is subject to federal regulatory standards called the Clinical Laboratory Improvement Amendments (CLIA). While any result may be incorrect due to testing errors or misinterpretation, CLIA requirements dictate quality control, the qualifications of laboratory personnel, and proper testing procedures that promote accuracy and reliability.

Direct-to-consumer genetic tests that are available on the internet are often unregulated and may not be CLIA-certified or have the same standards or accuracy. Further, insurance may only cover genetic tests that are preceded by genetic counseling. Experts caution against making any medical decisions based on these services until you've spoken with a health care professional. Even though testing through an online service might seem appealing, an expert in cancer genetics is your best bet for an informative experience.

Asking a Relative to Be Tested

Before a mutation is identified in a family, genetic counselors determine who should be the first one tested. This might not be you, even if you're the only one who has had genetic counseling. Asking another relative to test first can be particularly challenging if you're not close to them or if they're uninterested or unwilling. They might be concerned, upset, or confused about genetic misinformation they've received from someone other than a genetics expert. Relatives are more likely to pursue testing when they understand how their results can benefit them and others in the family. The best way to ensure they receive balanced and credible information is to direct them to a genetics expert.

how to navigate to Mars, yet we haven't a clue about traveling to other solar systems—even though we know they're out there. Some hereditary cancers are caused by well-studied genes and mutations, and many commercial labs know exactly where to look for them. Less common gene mutations may require different testing procedures or other labs. Improved testing technology now detects more mutations than ever before. If you were tested before 2014, a genetic counselor can determine whether you should be retested for a mutation that may have been missed by earlier tests. Most genetic tests are one of three types.

- Multigene panel tests search for mutations in multiple genes in a single test. The genes included may vary, depending on the panel. These broad tests may be most useful when multiple genes are suspected or associated with the cancers in a family or when previous testing for a limited number of genes didn't find a mutation in the family.

- Full-sequencing tests look for abnormalities in many areas of a gene that is associated with the cancers in question. This is a logical approach for the first family member to be tested if the pattern of cancer in the family points to one specific gene.
- Single-site tests search one gene for a specific mutation that has already been identified in the family.

If You're Young and Undiagnosed

If you're a young previvor, you may be faced with decisions about genetic testing that differ from those of your older counterparts. If cancer runs in your family, will you benefit from being tested now? If you test positive, how do you balance concern about developing cancer with complex decisions to reduce your risk? Which approach is best for you, and when is the best time to consider testing? Your health care team can help you sort through these issues, even if you're not ready to be tested now.

Insurance Coverage

Most public and private health insurance plans cover the cost of genetic counseling and testing if you meet certain criteria and your doctor recommends the test. Some insurers may require that you have genetic counseling before being tested and that you provide a letter from your genetic counselor or referring physician stating the medical necessity of your genetic test.

Coverage and out-of-pocket costs vary, depending on your situation, the test involved, and the terms of your insurance plan. Medicare only pays for genetic testing for inherited mutations if you have been diagnosed with cancer. Medicaid coverage of genetic counseling and testing varies by state. Some Medicaid programs may cover testing fees if you meet the state's requirements. Under the Affordable Care Act, most health plans must pay for the entire cost of genetic counseling and testing for a *BRCA* mutation with no out-of-pocket cost to patients, but this coverage has limitations.

- It only applies to testing for a *BRCA1* or *BRCA2* mutation.
- It only applies to women with a personal or family history that suggests a *BRCA1* or *BRCA2* mutation.
- It only applies to women who aren't undergoing cancer treatment. (You may be covered if you've completed treatment.)

- It doesn't apply to testing for mutations in any other gene, to people in treatment, or to testing for men. Out-of-pocket costs may apply for these circumstances.

Testing can be costly, so it's important to know in advance what your health insurer will cover and under what terms. Your genetic counselor will review your coverage, help you obtain preauthorization, and if necessary, help you appeal if your insurance denies payment for counseling or testing. If you don't have insurance or you're denied coverage and can't afford to be tested, some labs offer discounted or no-cost testing if you meet certain medical and financial criteria. Your genetic counselor can determine your eligibility for these programs. Some research studies offer opportunities for genetic testing at no charge to people who meet certain criteria, although results may not be available for months.

Privacy and Protection

The Genetic Information Nondiscrimination Act (GINA) prohibits discrimination by health insurers and employers based on your test results, your family's history of disease, or because you have an inherited mutation. Health insurers may not deny coverage, define the terms of coverage, or set copayments or premiums based on genetic information. Employers may not use your genetic information to make decisions involving hiring, firing, promotions, or other aspects of your employment. GINA doesn't apply to

- Businesses with fewer than 15 employees.
- A previous disease or diagnosed condition, including cancer. GINA protections apply to your inherited risk for disease. Once you're diagnosed, GINA no longer applies. However, the Affordable Care Act prohibits group and individual health plans from denying coverage, excluding benefits, or charging higher premiums due to any preexisting condition, including a cancer diagnosis or a genetic test result.
- Life insurance, long-term care insurance, or disability insurance. Some people apply for these plans before they're tested. Several states have laws that protect against genetic discrimination with these types of insurance, offering more protection than GINA, but not all do.

- Active members of the military, veterans obtaining health care through the Veterans Health Administration, individuals using the Indian Health Service, or participants in the Federal Employees Health Benefits Program. Military members' and veterans' health care policies provide protections similar to those of GINA.

The Health Insurance Portability and Accountability Act (HIPAA) requires health care professionals to notify you of your privacy rights. In most instances, HIPAA requires your permission before anyone shares your health information. Your genetic test results are kept in confidence as part of your medical records.

Chapter 4

What Your Test Results Tell You

Being tested and then sharing your results with your family are actions that break the cycle of hereditary cancer. Other family members who do the same also help their loved ones protect themselves from cancer.

The wait is over. You've wondered, worried, and anxiously anticipated your genetic test results. Now you're about to find out whether you're indeed at high risk or if you can perhaps breathe a sigh of relief. But that piece of paper in your hand may not completely clarify your cancer risk. Your genetic counselor is the best resource for understanding your test results and explaining the implications for you and other family members. If your test wasn't ordered by a genetic counselor, it's a good idea to consult with one now so that you can fully understand your result before sharing it with your family and the rest of your health care team.

Positive, Negative, Maybe

Genetic testing doesn't always produce definitive answers about whether you have a mutation. A positive test doesn't guarantee that you'll develop cancer, and a negative test doesn't ensure that you won't. A test result may be positive, negative, or inconclusive.

Positive for a Deleterious Mutation

Testing labs use different terms to describe a positive result. The phrases "positive for a deleterious mutation," "positive for a pathogenic mutation," positive for a pathogenic variant," and "clinically significant mutation detected" confirm that you have a gene mutation that is known to be harmful. What this means:

- You almost certainly inherited the mutation from one of your parents.
- You have an increased risk for one or more cancers.
- Your biological siblings have a 50 percent chance of having the same mutation.
- Each of your biological children has a 50 percent chance of inheriting your mutation.
- Your blood relatives on the same side of the family from which you inherited the mutation may have the same mutation.

— THE FORCE PERSPECTIVE —

Keeping Up with Changing Terminology

Scientists and health care professionals don't always use the same terminology when discussing inherited gene changes, and they often use jargon that can be confusing to patients. For example, some experts typically refer to all DNA changes as "mutations." However, while mutations can be harmful, beneficial, or neutral, many people assume that a mutation is always a harmful gene change. Therefore, some experts now refer to genetic mutations as "variants." When referring to harmful mutations that cause disease, scientists favor the term "pathogenic." But in a survey conducted by multiple cancer advocacy groups, including FORCE, people indicated a dislike for the term "pathogenic variant" because it reminded them of "pathogen," another word for an infectious virus or bacteria. Throughout this book, we use the term "mutation" to refer to a harmful mutation (pathogenic variant) unless otherwise stated.

When you're unclear about what a term means, it's important to ask for clarification. When talking with health care professionals or reviewing test results, you may encounter different terms that mean the same thing.

- a gene change: mutation or variant
- a gene change that doesn't cause disease: harmless, benign, or nonpathogenic

- a gene change that may cause disease: harmful, deleterious, clinically significant, or pathogenic

------

No Mutation Detected

A result that says "no mutation detected" means that you show no evidence of any mutations in the genes included in the test. If a family member has already tested positive for a mutation, your test result is truly good news. It means that you didn't inherit the family mutation, and therefore you can't pass it on to your children. (It is remotely possible that you have a different mutation, but your genetic counselor can advise you about this.) Your cancer risk is likely

De Novo Mutations

Most mutations discussed in this book are inherited from one or both parents. However, some people develop a de novo or new mutation, which is occurring for the first time in a family. This happens if a mutation develops when egg or sperm cells are forming or during an embryo's early development in the womb. In this case, neither parent will have the same mutation. This may explain the positive genetic tests of people who have a mutation in all of their cells, even when their parents test negative. Like other inherited mutations, de novo mutations raise the risk for cancer and can be passed on to children, who have a 50 percent chance of inheriting their parent's new mutation. De novo mutations rarely happen for most genes, but some genes, including *APC*, *PTEN*, and *TP53*, are more likely to have a de novo mutation.

the same as that of anyone in the general population, and you should begin or continue routine screenings as recommended by your doctor.

Some people who test negative feel guilty if their sibling, parent, or other close relative tests positive for a mutation. Others may develop a false sense of security, feeling that their negative test exempts them from regular screenings, which, of course, it doesn't. Depending on your circumstances, a negative test doesn't guarantee that you don't have increased cancer risk. You should be screened closely and stay in touch with your genetics expert for new information and additional tests if any of the following circumstances apply:

- If several people in your family have had cancer but test negative for a specific mutation, the underlying cause may be a different or as yet unknown mutation, a combination of gene changes, or a common behavior or environmental exposure.

- If you're the first in your family to have genetic testing, and if you were tested for mutations in only one or a few genes (such as the three Ashkenazi founder mutations), "no mutation detected" means that you have none of them. However, you might have a different mutation that indicates a high cancer risk. A genetic counselor can explain if you or a family member might benefit from a more comprehensive full-sequence test or a multigene panel to broadly search for other inherited mutations.

- If your family has no known mutation and you haven't had cancer, the next step may be to test a relative who has been diagnosed with a cancer that runs in your family. You may still be at high risk for that cancer due to a mutation that is unknown or wasn't included in your test.

— My Story —
Why My Sister and Not Me?

When my sister and I were tested, I imagined that if we were both positive, even though our decisions might have been different, whatever route we took we would take it together. When I tested negative, after the initial tears of joy and feeling that I dodged a bullet, I wondered why my sister wasn't negative too. Why must she go through the unthinkable while I carry on with my life? It didn't seem fair. I remember thinking that for once, God seemed to be on our side, as I have two daughters and my sister has no children. If nothing else, this could be the end of the mutation in our family. Whenever I felt guilty about being negative, I used that thought as a way to feel better. Looking back, I don't think I would have had my sister's strength and courage. Given a choice, she too would have been negative, but if someone in our family had to be positive, she would have wanted it to be her.

—*Linda*

A Variant of Uncertain Significance

Small genetic changes aren't always significant. A slight variation that may be the difference between brown eyes and green eyes doesn't affect eye function. The same is true with gene mutations; some increase risk, while others don't. A test result of "genetic variant, favor polymorphism" means that you have a change that isn't known to raise cancer risk. "Genetic variant, favor deleterious" means that you have a gene change that is strongly suspected—but unproven— to increase cancer risk. When a test identifies a gene change of undetermined cancer risk, the result is known as a "variant of uncertain significance" (VUS). This is an uninformative result that doesn't provide a clear answer about cancer risk. VUS test results may have several possible explanations, even in a family that has a strong history of cancer.

- The VUS is harmful: not enough research exists to conclude that it's deleterious.
- The VUS isn't harmful: cancers that run in the family are caused by a mutation in a different gene or in an unknown gene for which there is no available test.
- The VUS isn't harmful: cancers that run in the family are due to environmental factors or a combination of genetic and environmental factors.

If your genetic test shows you have a VUS, your personal and family medical history will determine the recommended cancer screenings and risk management. These recommendations may differ from what is advised for people with a deleterious mutation or those in the general population. A VUS may be reclassified when more evidence becomes available, so it's a good idea to check with your genetics expert every year or two so that you'll know if more information has been discovered about your variant.

— EXPERT VIEW —

How Scientists Approach Classifying Variants of Uncertain Significance

BY BRIAN H. SHIRTS, MD, PHD

Scientists use many sources of information to help classify variants of unknown significance as benign (harmless) or pathogenic (harmful). They use public databases to see how frequently a variant shows up in different populations. More common variants are less likely to cause severe disease. Computer programs can predict the effect of new variants on the structure of the protein and compare them with those of known benign and pathogenic variants. Genetic testing laboratories, doctors, and scientists often share data that have been stripped of any identifying information about the patients, including how often a variant has been detected, how often that variant has been seen in patients with cancer, and how many relatives of those patients were reported to have cancer.

The more careful that health professionals are in gathering family histories, the more helpful this information becomes in classifying the variant. When multiple family members have the same VUS, identifying those who also develop cancer allows scientists to statistically determine if a variant and disease occur together more than would be expected by chance. To help classify variants, many laboratories offer free or reduced-cost testing for relatives of patients with VUS. Researchers then combine all of these sources of information.

The process of variant classification usually takes years. However, a single family with a carefully collected medical history may provide compelling information that can make classification go much faster. Patients are often notified if their variant becomes reclassified, but the message may be delayed or dropped if they have switched health care professionals or if their providers are not in contact with the testing laboratory.

Making Sense of Statistics

We often hear or read about foods, behaviors, or other factors that affect our chance of developing cancer, but it's not always clear what these reports mean. The concept of cancer risk can be confusing because it's often expressed in different ways. The National Cancer Institute calculates the "one-in-X" cancer figures we hear so often, which are based on the incidence of cancers in the United States. These statistics change as the rates for specific cancers increase or decrease. The well-known 1-in-8 breast cancer estimate, for example, is based on the rate of breast cancer among the entire US population of women, which is approximately 12 percent. Similarly, about 4 percent of people in the United States develop colorectal cancer in their lifetime. ("Lifetime" risk statistics throughout this book refer to risk up to age 80, unless otherwise stated.) That means that for every 25 people who live to be 80, one develops colorectal cancer at some point during their lifetime. It also means that 24 of 25 people won't develop colorectal cancer.

"One in 8" and "1 in 25" are broad estimates that don't define what you need to do to address your current cancer risk and how it will change as you grow older. For many reasons, your chance of developing cancer differs from someone else's. Therein lies the complexity, if not the impossibility, of pinpointing an individual's exact risk. Your risk of breast cancer probably isn't 1 in 8, and your risk of colorectal cancer probably isn't 1 in 25 because you're not average. Your chance of developing different cancers is a moving target that changes throughout your lifetime, depending on your ancestry, age, family medical history, lifestyle, and other factors. Your odds of developing cancer may be higher or lower than someone in the general population.

The Spectrum of Estimated Inherited Risk

Calculating someone's precise inherited risk for cancer is, at best, an estimate that is based on current research. Risk assessment is an evolving field. While it's becoming more precise as researchers learn about other influential genes and factors, much is still unknown. Estimates are usually based on calculations from early studies of large multicancer families, which are updated as more people are tested. It's still difficult to be sure how much of a family's cancer risk is related to an inherited mutation and how much to environmental influences shared by family members. In the absence of definitive predictions, genetics experts describe a person's odds of developing cancer with a range of numbers, and even those ranges vary.

Absolute and Relative Risk

When health care professionals speak about your cancer risk, it's important to know what type of risk they're talking about. Absolute risk is the chance of developing cancer over a certain period, such as a one-in-eight chance of breast cancer to age 80. Relative risk is a percentage of increase or decrease calculated by comparing people who have a particular risk factor with people who don't, like a smoker compared to a nonsmoker.

Knowing your lifetime risk for various cancers has limited value when you're considering ways to manage your current risk. If you have an inherited mutation, addressing your risk over a specific time frame is more useful. Considering your life plan and situation over the next 5–10 years, including employment, education, insurance, and family planning, may influence the risk management decisions that you make now.

— THE FORCE PERSPECTIVE —

Putting Media Reports into Context

Media stories about behaviors, foods, or other factors that raise or reduce cancer risk can be misleading if they aren't put into the proper context. Hearing that "exercise reduces breast cancer risk by 50 percent" doesn't necessarily mean that your risk is half that of your sedentary neighbor, even if you jog every day. Consider risk reports with caution, and talk to your doctor about how they may or may not affect you.

You Have a Mutation; Now What?

Learning that you have a high-risk gene mutation can be informative and unsettling at the same time. While it may be a relief to finally know why certain cancers run in your family, you probably have more questions than answers, and challenging decisions may lie ahead. Before you do anything, take a moment to breathe and gather your thoughts. Give yourself time to absorb what you've heard, process your feelings, and find out what else you need to know. Remember that your genes don't necessarily define your destiny and that you can take steps to manage your risk. Your genetic counselor can put your risk into perspective, help you sort out your feelings, and suggest how to consider your next steps. This book also can be a source of guidance. Chapter 31, for example, can help you cope with your feelings, whatever they may be, and build a supportive network that will be there when you need it.

Assemble Your Health Care Team

In addition to your primary physician and a genetic counselor, you'll need other specialists who will coordinate different facets of your care. The members of your medical team may change as you pursue recommended cancer screenings, prevention procedures, and treatment if you develop cancer. (Read more about putting your health care team together in chapter 31.)

— THE **FORCE** PERSPECTIVE —

Taking Time to Process, Grieve, and Adjust

Interactions with thousands of people who have inherited high risk for cancer have revealed a wide range of emotions:

- gratitude for the knowledge genetic testing provides
- fear, anxiety, or sadness at learning that they have a mutation
- relief to have tested negative
- guilt for testing negative, particularly when a close relative tests positive
- guilt about possibly passing a mutation to their children
- loss of their innocence or safety
- relief at finally understanding why they or their loved ones developed cancer
- feeling pressure from themselves or loved ones because they feel scared or sad instead of grateful for not having cancer
- concern about stopping intense cancer surveillance, even when a test is a true negative
- anger, frustration, or sadness because of ambiguous test results, which make risk management decisions more difficult

Sharing Information with Your Family

There's never a good time to learn that hereditary disease runs in your family or that you might be genetically predisposed to cancer. Being tested and then sharing your results with your family are actions that break the cycle of hereditary cancer. Other family members who do the same also help their loved ones protect themselves from cancer. Experts refer to this sequence of testing-sharing-testing-sharing as "cascade testing."

It's important to disclose your genetic test result, especially if it's positive, because close or distant relatives may share your mutation and high risk. Of course, you needn't share your complete medical records and details with everyone if you prefer not to. But it's helpful to disclose your exact gene mutation or provide a copy of your lab test result, so if relatives decide to be tested, their testing lab will know what to look for. Your genetic counselor can identify information that will be helpful to others and which relatives should be informed of your results.

Planning Ahead

Considering what to say and how to say it before you speak to family members can pave the way for a smooth and successful conversation.

- Download information from the FORCE website (www.facing ourrisk.org). "The Genes between Us" is a step-by-step guide that includes resources for sharing genetic information with relatives. The separate information-sharing worksheet will help you organize your thoughts about the best way to deliver your information.
- Assemble your medical pedigree and your genetic test results. Ask your genetic counselor to provide other relevant information.
- Gather information about the inherited mutation you have, the associated cancer risks, and risk management options.
- Prepare a list of support resources and genetics experts for your relatives (see the searchable database at www.nsgc.org).

Coping with Family Dynamics

The support of those close to you can help you shoulder the burden of hereditary risk, gain a new perspective, and forge stronger family bonds and improved communication. The subject is disturbing, however, and deeply personal, and it may generate conflict. Not everyone appreciates knowing that they may have an unusually high cancer risk. Some relatives may prefer to ignore what they perceive as bad news. The decision to address or ignore inherited risk should be their own. Family members who don't know as much as you do about hereditary cancer may be confused or put off by terms they don't understand.

Ideally, these issues are best approached as a family, with nonthreatening dialogue and the opportunity to voice concerns openly. That's not always easy or possible, especially if your relationships aren't cordial, and you may feel tense or unsure about approaching the subject. The most effective way to share medical information will depend on your relationship with your family and how well you communicate with each other. If a particular relative typically acts as the family organizer or conduit—the person who always seems to know and share what's going on with everyone—consider speaking with that person first. If your family has a preexisting conflict, consider involving a professional counselor, a trusted friend, or another neutral third party to facilitate productive communication.

You may need to approach family members in different ways, depending on your level of closeness or estrangement. When it isn't possible or desirable to speak face-to-face with physically distant or estranged family members, you can call, send a letter, or email them. Clarify how you're related, if necessary, and explain that you have medical information that may be relevant to their health. If you're unsure of what to say, start with "I just learned some medical information that affects our family's risk for disease. May I share it with you?" or "I was tested for a hereditary mutation, and I have my results. Are you interested?" If you wish, your genetic counselor can draft a family letter with basic information about the mutation found (including a copy of the test result, if desired), which you can give to your family members. It is helpful to provide the names of genetics specialists in their area so they can get credible information and make their own informed decisions about genetic testing.

Your family will need time to absorb your news, just as you did. Respect their right to gather information and make their own decisions. Be supportive without being insistent.

— *My Story* —

My Family's Decisions

At 32, my only sister developed early-stage breast cancer with no lymph node involvement. With no family history of breast cancer, we thought her diagnosis was an anomaly. Her medical team considered a double mastectomy to be too radical for someone so young, so she had lumpectomy, radiation, and chemotherapy. Nine months later, a new primary cancer appeared in her other breast; this time, it was also in her lymph nodes. Within months, her cancer spread to her lungs, bones, and brain. Her oncologist said genetic testing wouldn't change her treatment. He didn't consider whether it would affect me or other female relatives, and he never recommended a genetic counselor. My sister passed away, leaving her 4-year-old child without a mother.

Terrified about my health, I rejoiced when my *BRCA* test result was negative. My celebration was short-lived when I learned that a negative test means little when there is no known familial mutation. My anxiety soared out of control. I bruised myself looking for breast lumps, and I needed antidepressants to get through the days. Then I decided not to duplicate my sister's experience. I learned about prophylactic mastectomy and oophorectomy and contacted doctors. Finally, through FORCE, I was advised to see a genetic counselor. I insisted that we had no history of breast or ovarian cancer: my mother, her two sisters, and their mother were alive and well. My father's only sister and her daughters were too. The only cancer casualties were my paternal great-grandmother (unknown young-onset cancer) and grandmother ("stomach cancer"). My counselor explained that "stomach cancer" could have been ovarian cancer and showed how a mutation could have passed from my father to my sister without affecting other female relatives. She urged me to have my parents tested. I left feeling scared, yet also empowered that my uninformative test could be informative if either parent tested positive.

Approaching my parents about testing was one of the hardest things I've ever done. They had lost their oldest child and wanted to put cancer behind them. It was unbearable for them to think that one of them might have passed my sister the mutation that took her life. Eventually, they agreed, but only if I alone received their results and never told them. One of them did test positive for a *BRCA1* mutation, confirming me as a true negative.

—*Rhonda*

Before You Decide Not to Share

If you feel that sharing your test result will be a burden to your relatives, consider the potential risk of *not* disclosing the information. Don't assume that they're already informed about a genetic predisposition or that they might not want to know about your mutation. You won't change their cancer risk by keeping the information from them, and staying silent may limit their options for early detection or prevention. Although you may have valid reasons to delay telling your relatives, there is no perfect time for them to learn about their cancer risk, just as there is no convenient time to receive a diagnosis of cancer.

— *My Story* —

A Legacy of Silence

My mother never discussed her breast cancer, her radical mastectomy, or her feelings. Only when I was 44 and facing my breast cancer— 33 years later—did she share the details with me. As a child, I would sneak peeks at her satin prosthesis; it scared me to pieces. As a teenager, I wondered about my own risk, even then. I vowed to never keep my children in the dark about our family's cancer legacy. Now, it's my turn. I must find the right words to tell my children about others in our family who have developed cancers: my aunt, my cousin, my sister, and me.

—*Lauren*

— EXPERT VIEW —

What Should You Tell Your Children about Cancer and Risk?

BY KAREN HURLEY, PHD

It's natural to want to protect your kids from difficult topics, and it may feel less distressing in the short run to act like everything's fine.

Tips for Talking with Your Children

Adapted from the Parenting at a Challenging Time Program at
Massachusetts General Hospital (www.mghpact.org)

- Use simple, age-appropriate terms to explain concepts and answer your children's questions.

- Validate your children's concerns. Pushing your children's fears aside makes the situation appear too big and scary to talk about.

- Realize that your feelings are separate from your children's, and they may be different.

- Avoid unrealistic promises. Broken promises can diminish trust.

- Allow your children to tell you how little or how much they want to know. Some children are more curious, while others are more private.

- Respect your children's life paths and their decisions about being tested.

However, children can pick up on adult distress without understanding what's happening, and they can be sensitive to subtle changes in routine, such as hushed phone conversations, increased doctor appointments, or preoccupation with big decisions. In the long run, well-intentioned efforts to shield children can undermine their trust. Instead, provide simple, realistic information that matches your child's cognitive and coping abilities, realizing that each child might need a different approach, depending on age, maturity level, temperament, or other life stressors.

It's natural to put your child's well-being first, but make sure you tend to your own stress level as well. Communication about risk may be particularly complicated by guilt feelings about the possibility of passing on a mutation. Guilt is a common response to uncontrollable events, and you may blame yourself even though you know intellectually that genetic inheritance is completely random. A good antidote is to take control of teaching your children about coping with life's difficulties. You can pass on a legacy of resilience, empowerment, and love, which will help them deal not only with cancer risk in the family but with any challenge that life offers.

Part II
Inherited Gene Mutations and the Cancers They Cause

Cancer is common, so it's not surprising that many families have someone who has had a diagnosis. Some families, however, have a pattern of cancers, which may suggest that hereditary factors are at work. Cancers that are rare, affect multiple relatives or relatives in more than one generation, or are diagnosed at unusually young ages can be signs of a genetic susceptibility in the family. A small family or an incomplete sharing of medical history between family members may sometimes hide a pattern of cancer that suggests a mutation is present. Depending on the type of mutation and the gene involved, a person's lifetime risk for different cancers may be slightly, moderately, or significantly increased. Some inherited mutations increase the risk for a specific cancer. Others elevate risk for several cancers; these are sometimes referred to as hereditary cancer syndromes. Some mutations also cause other health issues, such as colon polyps, benign tumors, or developmental disorders, which require additional medical intervention.

This part of the book addresses inherited mutations and hereditary syndromes that predispose families to cancers. The associated levels of risk are based on National Comprehensive Cancer Network published guidelines unless otherwise stated. NCCN panels conduct annual reviews of available research data to estimate lifetime cancer risks. These estimates change as more people are tested and more information is discovered. With the exception of the *MUTYH* genes (see chapter 7), the inherited mutations discussed here are autosomal dominant. This means that inheriting a single copy of a damaged gene is sufficient to cause a specific trait, including a predisposition for disease. *MUTYH* is an autosomal recessive gene, which means that a related disease occurs when both copies are mutated, although a single gene mutation can somewhat increase risk.

Knowing that you have an increased risk for cancer can provide you with an opportunity that most people don't have. You can be screened more frequently than someone who doesn't have a harmful mutation, and you can take steps to reduce your risk. Increased screening makes it more likely to identify cancer early, when treatment is more often successful.

We don't know why some people with inherited mutations develop one or more related cancers, while others who have the same mutation don't develop any. Inheriting a harmful mutation or cancer syndrome doesn't guarantee that you'll develop cancer, but it does make it more probable. Whether your family has a mutation that heightens the chance for one or several cancers, a genetic counselor or other genetics expert can help you identify and understand your risk and make decisions about how to manage it.

In this part, we cover several cancer categories:

Adenocarcinomas begin in the glands that line the inside of an organ. Breast, colon, prostate, gastric, and pancreatic cancers are examples.

Squamous cell carcinomas begin in the cells that cover internal and external body surfaces. Skin, cervical, and mouth cancers are examples.

Sarcomas develop in bone, fat, muscle, and other supporting tissues of the body.

Leukemias develop in blood cells and grow in bone marrow.

Lymphomas occur primarily in white blood cells and lymph nodes.

Chapter 5

Introducing *BRCA1* and *BRCA2*

Although the lifetime risk for cancer is high in people with *BRCA* mutations, the level of risk varies widely, depending on your gender, the type of cancer, which mutation you have, and whether it's in *BRCA1* or *BRCA2*.

BRCA1 and *BRCA2* are genes with similar functions. When they work properly, these genes make proteins that help repair DNA damage in cells. Inherited mutations in *BRCA* genes may prevent the body from carrying out this critical function. Over time, more mutations can then develop in cells, leading to cancer. Compared to the general public, people with an inherited *BRCA1/2* mutation have higher risk for several cancers, including breast, ovarian, pancreatic, prostate, and a type of skin cancer known as melanoma.

Who Inherits a *BRCA* Mutation?

About 1 in 400 people in the United States—less than 1 percent of the population—has a mutation in *BRCA1* or *BRCA2*. Mutations in either gene tend to occur in families that have a history of breast or ovarian cancers on the same side of the family tree. (Relatives who have a *BRCA1/2* mutation usually share the same one.) The chance of having a *BRCA* mutation increases substantially in individuals who have ovarian, pancreatic, or triple-negative breast cancer; cancer at an early age; or multiple affected relatives. Yet not all families with multiple cases of breast and ovarian cancer have a *BRCA1/2* mutation. Although *BRCA1* and *BRCA2* are the best-studied genes linked to breast, ovarian, prostate, and pancreatic cancer, as well as melanoma, mutations in other genes can predispose individuals to the same cancers (see chapters 6 and 7). Cancers that run in a family can also be caused by shared environmental, lifestyle, or other factors.

Thousands of harmful mutations have been identified in the *BRCA1* and *BRCA2* genes, and some are common in certain populations. People of Ashkenazi (Eastern European Jewish) descent have the highest known incidence of inherited *BRCA* mutations, and they develop hereditary breast and ovarian cancer more frequently than people of other ancestry. One in 40 Ashkenazim are estimated to have a *BRCA1/2* gene mutation—10 times more than the general population.[1] At some point in history, Ashkenazi ancestors developed DNA defects in some of their genes, including *BRCA1* and *BRCA2*. These founder mutations were passed from generation to generation with greater frequency than in other populations because Ashkenazi Jews have maintained their shared gene pool by living in relative geographic and cultural isolation. The three most prevalent Ashkenazi founder mutations are 185delAG and 5382insC in *BRCA1* and 6174delT in *BRCA2*. Less often, members of this population have a different *BRCA1* or *BRCA2* mutation or a mutation in a different gene, such as *CHEK2*.

Although *BRCA1/2* mutations occur more frequently in people of Ashkenazi descent, they're found in varying degrees among all races and ethnicities in the United States. Some Hispanics—mostly those of Mexican heritage—carry the same mutations that are usually found in Ashkenazim, possibly due to a shared Spanish ancestry. *BRCA1/2* mutations occur more often (than in the general population) among families from the Bahamas, Barbados, French Canada, Iceland, the Netherlands, Norway, and Poland and among some ethnic groups with relatively small numbers of ancestors.[2]

Signs of a *BRCA* Mutation

If your family medical history shows any of the signs of a *BRCA1* or *BRCA2* mutation, a genetic counselor can determine if you or any of your relatives should be tested (table 5.1). A genetic counselor can also determine whether *BRCA* gene testing or a more extensive multigene panel is most appropriate.

Are You Ashkenazi?

Eighty percent of the world's Jewish population have roots in medieval Germany ("Ashkenaz" is the Hebrew word for Germany) and later dispersed throughout Hungary, Poland, Russia, and the rest of Eastern Europe. The remaining 20 percent are Sephardic Jews, whose ancestors are from Spain, Portugal, North Africa, and the Middle East. Sephardim don't usually carry Ashkenazi founder mutations. Most of the Jewish population in the United States is Ashkenazi.

— *My Story* —
My Age Was a Red Flag

I was shocked to be diagnosed at age 33 because I was the first in my family with breast cancer. The only other cancer I knew of was my dad's mother, who had died young of "kidney cancer" decades earlier. Eight months after completing treatment, I read an article about the family link between breast and ovarian cancer. It stated that *BRCA* mutations were more common in younger women with breast cancer and in people of Ashkenazi Jewish descent. That was me. I realized my grandmother's "kidney cancer" may have been advanced ovarian cancer. Genetic counseling and testing confirmed that I had a *BRCA2* mutation. I wish my doctors had referred me to a genetics expert when I was diagnosed. Had I known of my *BRCA* status then, I would have made different surgical choices.

—Sue

TABLE 5.1 Signs of a Possible *BRCA* Mutation in a Family

You or any blood relative has had	a positive test for a *BRCA* mutation
	breast cancer before age 50
	cancer in both breasts
	more than one diagnosis of breast cancer
	breast and ovarian cancer
	triple-negative breast cancer
	male breast cancer
	ovarian, fallopian tube, or primary peritoneal cancer
	metastatic prostate cancer
	pancreatic cancer
More than one relative on the same side of the family has had	breast cancer
	pancreatic cancer
	prostate cancer

Note: For people of Ashkenazi Jewish ethnicity, any family history of breast, ovarian, pancreatic, or prostate cancer may indicate a mutation in the family.

Levels of Risk

Although the lifetime risk for cancer is high in people with *BRCA* mutations, the level of risk varies widely, depending on your gender, the type of cancer, which mutation you have, and whether it's in *BRCA1* or *BRCA2*.

Breast and Ovarian Cancer Risk in Women

Compared to the general population of women, a mutation in either the *BRCA1* or *BRCA2* gene considerably raises breast and ovarian cancer risk. Knowing whether your mutation is in a *BRCA1* or *BRCA2* gene can help you make decisions about managing your risk and, if necessary, inform your treatment options. Estimates of lifetime cancer risks associated with *BRCA1/2* mutations are derived from studies of multicancer families. Expert guidelines for managing these risks are discussed in chapter 13.

Discovering and Naming
BRCA1 and *BRCA2*

In 1990, genetics researcher Mary-Claire King demonstrated that a single inherited gene mutation caused breast and ovarian cancer among several members in some families. Although the link between the two cancers had been suspected since the late 1800s, Dr. King's proof that breast cancers could be inherited paved the way for more investigation. A frenzy of subsequent research followed, and in 1994, scientists documented the precise location of the first *BRCA* gene on chromosome 17. A second *BRCA* gene was identified on chromosome 13 the following year. Researchers named the genes BReastCAncer1 (*BRCA1*) and BReastCAncer2 (*BRCA2*). With the exact location of the genes identified, a blood test was then developed to screen individuals for these cancer-causing mutations.

Doctors sometimes refer to inherited *BRCA1/2* mutations as hereditary breast and ovarian cancer (HBOC) syndrome. This was initially an appropriate term because these were the only cancers linked to these genes at the time. Since then, *BRCA1/2* gene mutations have been related to pancreatic and prostate cancers and melanoma. The terms "*BRCA*" and "HBOC" can be somewhat misleading, because they focus on women's cancer risks while giving the impression that men aren't affected.

TABLE 5.2 Average Probability of Developing Breast or Ovarian Cancer (%)

	BREAST CANCER RISK (*BRCA1* MUTATION)	BREAST CANCER RISK (*BRCA2* MUTATION)	OVARIAN CANCER RISK (*BRCA1* MUTATION)	OVARIAN CANCER RISK (*BRCA2* MUTATION)
by age 30	2.9	2.5	almost none	almost none
by age 40	19.2	13.5	2.5	1.3
by age 50	39.5	31.5	13.1	3.7
by age 60	52.5	47.5	30.4	10.6
by age 70	64.6	61.0	48.3	20.0

Source: Chen J, Bae E, Zhang L, et al. "Penetrance of breast and ovarian cancer in women who carry a BRCA1/2 mutation and do not use risk-reducing salpingo-oophorectomy: An updated meta-analysis," JNCI Cancer Spectrum 4, no. 4, 2020:pkaa029.

Knowing your lifetime risk for cancer is informative, but it has limited value when you're considering ways to manage your risk now. Addressing your risk over a specific time frame is more beneficial. This is particularly important if you have a *BRCA1/2* mutation, because you have a greater chance of being diagnosed before age 50 than someone who doesn't have a mutation (table 5.2).

— EXPERT VIEW —

Decade-by-Decade Risks for Breast and Ovarian Cancer in Women

BY TIMOTHY R. REBBECK, PHD

The figures in table 5.2 were derived from researchers who combined multiple studies that estimate cancer risks in *BRCA* mutation carriers. Combining studies to obtain composite risk estimates is a good way to provide more representative numbers when trying to understand risk variations across many small populations, as we see in *BRCA* carriers. Each study reported different risk results. These differences can be explained by which families and individuals were included, the total number of individuals who were included, how the studies were analyzed, and other factors. This is our best estimate of decade-by-decade risk for *BRCA1* and *BRCA2* mutation carriers based on the aggregate of these studies. As we study more people with *BRCA* mutations, we gain a better idea of risk. It is important to remember that risk varies considerably between people and that these estimates represent average risk across all populations. An individual's risk may be quite different from the average.

All women are at risk for ovarian cancer whether or not they have a mutation. The average lifetime risk for ovarian cancer in women without a mutation is 1.3 percent. But your risk is significantly higher if you have a *BRCA* mutation. You're also more likely to be diagnosed at a younger age. In both groups of women, risk increases as you grow older. Women with *BRCA* mutations, however, tend to fare better after a diagnosis. They often respond better to certain types of treatment and live longer than other women with ovarian cancer. Mutations in *BRCA1* also raise the chance of developing a rare form of aggressive uterine cancer, although that risk is less than 5 percent to age 70. In addition to a significant risk for a first cancer, women who have a *BRCA* mutation face other risks related to breast and ovarian cancer, including

- cancer that develops at an early age
- higher risk for cancer in the opposite breast (after an initial diagnosis)
- higher risk for triple-negative breast cancer (if the mutation is in *BRCA1*), which can be aggressive and difficult to treat
- a higher chance of having a second new cancer after an initial diagnosis

---

— *My Story* —
My Mom Changed Her Mind about Testing

When my mom was first diagnosed with ovarian cancer, she chose not to have genetic testing. Five years later, she experienced a recurrence. My sister's gynecologist and my midwife then raised the subject of our risk for ovarian cancer due to our mother's diagnosis. We asked our mother to reconsider genetic counseling and testing. Once it was clear that her genetic test results could directly affect her daughters' care, my mother was happy to look into it. She tested positive for a *BRCA1* gene mutation. My sister and I then had genetic testing. I tested positive, and she tested negative. We were lucky that our mom was alive to get the test first, so we know that my sister's test result is a true negative. This means that her breast and ovarian cancer risk is no higher than an average person's. I'm grateful that my mom decided to be tested. She did it for us, and it really changed our care. It's empowering to be able to have that information and to make the best decisions for your health.

—*Sheila*

Inheriting Multiple *BRCA* Mutations

While uncommon, it's possible to inherit a mutation in the *BRCA1* and *BRCA2* genes, especially for individuals who are Ashkenazi Jewish. People who have a mutation in both *BRCA* genes are believed to have similar risks for breast, ovarian, and fallopian cancer as individuals with *BRCA1* mutations. The risks for melanoma, pancreatic cancer, prostate cancer, and male breast cancer are thought to be equivalent to those of someone with a *BRCA2* mutation.

If you have mutations in both *BRCA* genes, or you and your spouse each have a mutation, the risk of passing one or both mutations to your children is 75 percent. Embryos can grow with a double mutation in the *BRCA2* gene, but experts believe that they must have at least one working copy of *BRCA1* to survive. Children who inherit a mutation in both copies of *BRCA2*—one mutation from each parent—develop Fanconi anemia (FA), a rare and serious childhood disorder characterized by bone marrow that doesn't produce enough blood cells. (Several other gene mutations also cause FA.) Some children with this disorder have altered skin pigmentation, deformed thumbs, a very small head size, or stunted growth. Abnormalities in the heart, kidneys, genitalia, or hearing may also develop. Blood abnormalities usually develop before age 12 and may include fatigue, paleness, bleeding, bruising, or a susceptibility to infections from a low level of white blood cells.

Breast and Prostate Cancer in Men

Men who inherit a *BRCA* mutation, especially a *BRCA2* mutation, have higher risk for breast and prostate cancers. The lifetime risk for breast cancer in men who have a *BRCA1* mutation is greater than the risk of men who don't have the same mutation, but it's much lower than the risk of women with the same mutation (table 5.3). To a lesser degree, mutations in *CHEK2*, *PALB2*, and other genes can also cause male breast cancer. Other factors that affect breast cancer risk in the general population may also raise the likelihood of breast cancer in men with *BRCA* mutations, including

TABLE 5.3 Estimated Lifetime Risk for Breast and Prostate Cancers in Men (%)

CANCER	GENERAL POPULATION	*BRCA1* MUTATION	*BRCA2* MUTATION
breast	0.1	2.0	7.0
prostate	12.0	20.0–30.0	30.0–60.0

Sources: Silvestri V, Leslie G, Barnes D, et al. "Characterization of the cancer spectrum in men with germline BRCA1 and BRCA2 pathogenic variants: Results from the Consortium of Investigators of Modifiers of BRCA1/2 (CIMBA)," Journal of the American Medical Association Oncology 6, no. 8, 2020:1218–30; Lecarpentier J, Silvestri V, Kuchenbaecker KB, et al. "Prediction of breast and prostate cancer risks in male BRCA1 and BRCA2 mutation carriers using polygenic risk scores," Journal of Clinical Oncology 35, no. 20, 2017:2240–50.

- Growing older.
- Having family members of either gender who have breast cancer.
- Being alcoholic, obese, or having a chronic liver disorder (conditions that increase estrogen levels).
- Having Klinefelter syndrome, a rare male genetic disorder that creates high estrogen levels. Men with this condition develop breast cancer 20–60 times more than other men.[3]
- Having gynecomastia (a benign condition characterized by enlargement of male breast tissue) or other factors that may raise a man's risk for breast cancer.

The lifetime risk for prostate cancer in men who have a *BRCA1* mutation is about 20–30 in 100, and it is about 30–60 in 100 for those with a mutation in *BRCA2* (table 5.3). The average lifetime risk for people without a mutation is about 12 in 100. Compared to those who don't have a mutation, those who do tend to have higher lifetime risk, diagnosis at a younger age, and more aggressive cancers.[4]

— EXPERT VIEW —

Men React Differently to Genetic Risk

BY MARY B. DALY, MD, PHD

Male members of families with a *BRCA1/2* or other breast cancer–associated mutations are less likely to be included in family conversations about cancer risk and are less likely to be informed of test results received by their female relatives. Reasons for the selective sharing of test results with predominantly female relatives include a closer bond with women than with men in the family, the desire to protect other female relatives from breast and ovarian cancer, and the hope of receiving emotional support from them.

Men more often use avoidance and denial strategies to cope with cancer risk in the family. Their socialization to value physical strength above all else and their reluctance to acknowledge vulnerability can challenge their recognition of genetic health threats and the need for preventive health behaviors. As a result, men may be unaware of the health implications for themselves and for other family members of carrying a *BRCA* mutation. People who choose not to undergo genetic testing not only may pass up the chance to take active steps to protect their own health, but also may miss the opportunity to provide valuable cancer risk information to their children and other relatives.

— *My Story* —
Thriving after *BRCA* and Breast Cancer

I'm an 81-year-old father of four and grandfather of six. None of these is an unusual accomplishment except that I'm also a seven-year survivor of breast cancer. I found the lump while showering. A mastectomy followed, as did a bout with bladder cancer. And prostate cancer. And skin cancer. After my breast cancer diagnosis and learning I was *BRCA2*-positive, my four children were also tested. True to the 50–50 chance of inheriting my mutation, two were positive and two were negative. I'm still here, surviving and thriving. It's entirely possible.

Most people don't know that men can get breast cancer. My advice to other men is to get in the shower and run your hands all over yourself. And if any family members have had breast cancer, go get the *BRCA* test. It's a simple blood test that may save your life or the life of someone you love.

—*Guy*

TABLE 5.4 Estimated Lifetime Risk for Pancreatic Cancer (%)

GENERAL POPULATION	*BRCA1* MUTATION	*BRCA2* MUTATION
1.6	3–6	5–10

Sources: American Cancer Society. "Key statistics for pancreatic cancer," https://www.cancer.org/cancer/pancreatic-cancer/about/key-statistics.html; Pilarski R. "The role of BRCA testing in hereditary pancreatic and prostate cancer families," American Society of Clinical Oncology Educational Book 39, 2019:79–86.

— *My Story* —
Living Optimistically with *BRCA*

I grew up thinking a lot about breast cancer, since my mom was diagnosed when she was 38. At 7 years old, I didn't understand what it meant that she had a mastectomy and then recovered. I thought nothing about her having only one breast. Ten years later, a pattern of early-onset breast cancer emerged from her father's side of the family. Mom had a recurrence and another mastectomy, and her uncle and cousin were also diagnosed. Their family tree showed breast, ovarian, and stomach cancers among men and women. Mom then learned that she had a *BRCA2* mutation. I was stunned when I also tested positive; I didn't know what my future held. Now I needed to consider my own risk for prostate cancer, pancreatic cancer, and breast cancer. I began living a very healthy lifestyle, eating 10 fruits and vegetables a day and running 35 miles a week. I'm now training for my sixth marathon. Combined with annual physicals and prostate exams, I'm in good stead for the future, and five years after receiving my test result, I'm more optimistic about what it means to live with a *BRCA2* mutation.
—*Richard*

Pancreatic Cancer and Melanoma

BRCA1/2 mutations also predispose people to pancreatic cancer (table 5.4) and melanoma, although to a much lower degree than the risk for breast, ovarian, and prostate cancer. A *BRCA2* mutation is believed to increase the risk for melanoma, but the exact risk is unclear. More research and evidence are also needed to establish a link between *BRCA1* and melanoma.

Chapter 6

Lynch Syndrome

Five Genes, One Hereditary Syndrome

Although Lynch syndrome affects nearly 1 in 300 individuals, 90–95 percent of people with this syndrome are estimated to be unaware of their high-risk status.

The *BRCA1/2* genes receive a lot of attention and publicity, but more people inherit mutations in *MLH1*, *MSH2*, *MSH6*, or *PMS2*. These are mismatch repair (MMR) genes, which ordinarily produce proteins to correct DNA damage that occurs when cells divide. Mutations in any of these genes can cause Lynch syndrome, which carries an extremely high predisposition for colorectal cancer (in the large intestine or rectum) and endometrial cancer (in the lining of the uterus) and a higher-than-average risk for several other cancers. Certain mutations in a fifth gene, *EPCAM*, can also cause Lynch syndrome by disabling the nearby *MSH2* gene.

Signs of Lynch Syndrome in Families

Lynch syndrome can run in families of any ancestry. About 1 in 300 people inherit a gene mutation for this syndrome, although many of them may be unaware because they haven't had genetic testing. Colorectal and endometrial cancer that runs in families, especially at younger ages, is a strong indicator of a possible Lynch syndrome diagnosis (table 6.1).

TABLE 6.1 Signs of a Possible Lynch Syndrome Mutation in a Family

You've been diagnosed with cancer, and testing of your tumor found an abnormality known as DNA mismatch repair deficiency (also known as microsatellite instability).*

or

You've been diagnosed with colorectal or endometrial cancer and any of these factors apply.	• cancer before age 50 • a second diagnosis of a Lynch syndrome–related cancer** • a first- or second-degree relative diagnosed with a Lynch syndrome–related cancer before age 50** • two or more first- or second-degree relatives on the same side of the family with a Lynch syndrome–related cancer at any age**

or

Your family history includes	• a blood relative who tested positive for a Lynch syndrome gene mutation • a first-degree relative diagnosed with a Lynch syndrome–related cancer before age 50** • a first-degree relative with colorectal or endometrial cancer and a second diagnosis of a Lynch syndrome–related cancer at any age** • two or more first- or second-degree relatives on the same side of the family with a Lynch syndrome–related cancer, at least one of which was diagnosed before age 50** • three or more first- or second-degree relatives on the same side of the family with a Lynch syndrome–related cancer at any age**

*See chapter 20.

**Colorectal, endometrial, stomach, ovarian, pancreatic, urothelial (bladder, ureter, renal pelvis), brain, biliary tract (liver, gallbladder, bile ducts), or small intestinal cancers, or rare skin tumors involving the sweat glands (known as sebaceous gland tumors or keratoacanthomas, described in this chapter).

Testing for Lynch Syndrome Mutations

If your family medical history raises concerns about Lynch syndrome, a genetic counselor can determine whether you or any of your relatives should be tested for a Lynch syndrome gene mutation or have a more extensive multi-gene panel. The appropriate test can confirm the presence of an inherited mutation in an *MLH1*, *MSH2*, *MSH6*, *PMS2*, or *EPCAM* gene. If the test result is positive for a mutation in one of these genes, other members of your family can then be tested for the same mutation. A genetic counselor can explain the meaning of a positive genetic test result or a negative result, which doesn't necessarily exclude the presence of an inherited cancer syndrome in you or your family members.

If you have Lynch syndrome and are diagnosed with cancer, your mutation status may change your treatment options. You'll find more information about tumor testing, postdiagnosis genetic testing, and treatment options in part IV of this book, "Treatment Choices for Hereditary Cancers."

Levels of Risk

Cancer risks linked to Lynch syndrome vary, depending on the gene involved, the organ affected, and your gender. In addition to an increased lifetime risk for several different cancers, people with Lynch syndrome have an increased risk for developing cancer more than once during their lifetime (often in the same organ) and for developing cancer at a younger-than-average age. The recommendations for diligent and lifelong screening provided in chapter 13 can help you to manage and reduce your cancer risk and detect Lynch cancers early, when treatment has the best chance of succeeding.

Colorectal Cancer

Lynch syndrome is the most common cause of hereditary colorectal cancer, which develops much earlier in life than sporadic colorectal cancer (table 6.2). The associated lifetime risk is very high—up to 60 percent—especially for those with a mutation in an *MLH1*, *MSH2*, or *EPCAM* gene (table 6.3). *MSH6* mutations confer up to 40 percent risk, while the risk linked to *PMS2* mutations is up to 20 percent. Lynch syndrome causes adenomatous polyps, which are growths in the lining of the large intestine that can change from benign to malignant more quickly than in people who don't have a mutation. Removing these polyps helps to prevent colorectal cancer, which is why people with Lynch syndrome require more frequent screening of their colons compared to people in the general population.

The Research Pioneer behind Lynch Syndrome

In the 1960s, long before genetic testing was available and before syndromes related to gene mutations were known, exposure to environmental toxins was believed to be the primary cause of most cancers. With an analytical mind and a doctorate in human genetics, Henry Lynch thought differently. He was convinced that a genetic link was the key to the colorectal cancers that ran through his patients' families. The medical community had already made the connection between polyposis (hundreds to thousands of polyps in the colon) and increased colon cancer risk. But as Dr. Lynch researched more and more colon cancer families, he noticed that many patients didn't have polyposis. This reinforced his hypothesis that the repeated patterns of some familial cancers were caused by an unknown nonpolyposis disorder.

In 1967, Dr. Lynch published data describing a "cancer family syndrome" in several families with clusters of gastrointestinal and gynecologic cancers. The children of affected parents tended to develop these same cancers at an early age. This, he said, was the work of a hereditary condition following an autosomal dominant inheritance pattern, which means that one copy of a gene has an inherited mutation. The medical community, however, was not ready to seriously consider the concept of hereditary cancer. Dr. Lynch continued his work, and in 1985, he introduced the term "hereditary nonpolyposis colorectal cancer" (HNPCC) to describe the pattern of cancer among families. Years later, other researchers identified *MLH1*, *MSH2*, *MSH6*, and *PMS2* as DNA mismatch repair genes.

While acknowledging the absence of the large numbers of polyps that characterize other hereditary colorectal cancer syndromes, the term "HNPCC" fails to recognize that other organs are often affected. HNPCC is now known as Lynch syndrome in honor of the "father of cancer genetics" whose pioneering research involved more than 3,000 families.

TABLE 6.2 Estimated Lifetime Risk of Lynch Syndrome Colorectal Cancer to Age 80

	GENERAL POPULATION	PEOPLE WITH LYNCH SYNDROME
estimated risk	4.2%	≤ 60.0%
average age at onset	67–71	mid-40s
evolution from polyp to cancer	10–15 years	3 years

Source: National Comprehensive Cancer Network. "Guidelines: Genetic/familial high-risk assessment: Colorectal." Version 1.2021, May 2021.

Gender-Related Cancers

The likelihood of endometrial cancer is significantly higher for women who have Lynch syndrome mutations compared to those who don't. The average woman's lifetime risk of endometrial cancer is about 3.1 percent, while the risk with Lynch syndrome can be as high as 60 percent, depending on which gene has the mutation (table 6.3). Women with mutations in *MLH1*, *MSH2*, *MSH6*, or *EPCAM* also have a higher risk of ovarian cancer (table 6.3). It is unclear whether women with a *PMS2* mutation have an increased risk for ovarian cancer; any increase over the general population is believed to be small. Nor is it clear whether women with Lynch syndrome have an increased chance of developing breast cancer.

Men who have a mutation in *MSH2* or *EPCAM* may be more likely to develop prostate cancer than men with average risk. However, current guidelines don't recommend any additional changes for screening of those with Lynch syndrome.

Individuals with Lynch syndrome, particularly men with mutations in the *MSH2* gene, have an elevated risk for developing cancer in the bladder or ureters (the ducts that move urine from the kidneys to the bladder).

Other Cancers and Benign Conditions

Individuals with Lynch syndrome are more prone to several other cancers as well. The risk of these cancers is generally higher than they are in the general public, but lower than Lynch syndrome–related risks for colorectal, endometrial, and ovarian cancers (table 6.3).

Sebaceous carcinoma is cancer that begins in the oil glands of the skin. It may first appear as a thickening of the skin or a painless bump on the eyelid

Signs of Hereditary Polyposis Colorectal Cancer Syndromes

Numerous genes can cause large numbers of precancerous colon polyps during a person's lifetime. Compared to the general population, individuals with a hereditary polyposis syndrome typically have many polyps, which appear at a younger age and often develop more quickly. Hereditary polyposis syndromes are different from Lynch syndrome, which tends to cause fewer polyps. (Lynch syndrome used to be referred to as hereditary nonpolyposis colorectal cancer, or HNPCC, to distinguish it from colorectal cancer syndromes that cause lots of polyps.)

Speak with a genetic counselor about testing for a polyposis syndrome if you or anyone in your family has a precursor to colorectal cancer: 10 or more adenomas, 5 or more serrated polyps, or 2 or more hamartomatous polyps. Many of these less common syndromes may cause cancers at a very young age. Familial adenomatous polyposis (FAP), for example, can cause an extraordinarily high risk for colorectal cancer, starting as early as adolescence. Many people with FAP have risk-reducing surgery that removes their large intestine and rectum to lower their lifetime risk for cancer.

TABLE 6.3 Estimated Lifetime Risk of Lynch Syndrome Cancers to Age 80 (%)

CANCER	GENERAL POPULATION	*MLH1* MUTATION	*MSH2* MUTATION	*MSH6* MUTATION	*PMS2* MUTATION	*EPCAM* MUTATION
colorectal	4.0	≤60	≤50	≤40	≤20	≤50
endometrial	3.1	≤55	≤60	≤50	≤25	≤60
prostate	12.0	≤15	≤25	≤15	unclear*	≤25
ovarian	1.3	≥10	≥10	≤10	unclear*	≥10
bladder	2.4	≤10	≤15	≤10	unclear*	≤15
gastric (stomach)	1.0	5–10	5–10	5–10	unclear*	5–10
renal pelvis and ureter	1.0	≤5	2–30	≤5.0	unclear*	2–30
small bowel**	0.3	≤5	≤5	≤5	unclear*	≤5
pancreas	1.6	≤5	≤5	≤5	unclear*	≤5
biliary tract**	0.2	1–3	1–3	1–3	unclear*	1–3
brain**	0.6	≤2	≤2	≤2	unclear*	≤2

Source: National Comprehensive Cancer Network. "Guidelines: Genetic/familial high-risk assessment: Colorectal." Version 1.2021, May 2021.

*Experts do not all agree that the risks for these cancers are increased with *PMS2*.

**These are rare cancers with little data on which to base these numbers. Experts believe the risk is increased, but the amount is unclear.

that discharges blood or fluid as it grows. It is usually removed to prevent the cancer from spreading to other parts of the body.

Some benign skin lesions (damaged areas of tissue) are associated with Lynch syndrome:

- Sebaceous adenomas are benign tumors of the sebaceous glands in the skin, which secrete a substance that lubricates the skin and hair. Most sebaceous adenomas grow wherever sebaceous glands are located: the nose, cheeks, and other parts of the head and face. Less frequently, they may appear on the neck, trunk, arms, and legs.
- Sebaceous epitheliomas are another form of benign skin tumor that usually appears on the neck or face. Appropriate screening is important because in many cases, people with this type of tumor have already developed an undiagnosed cancer.
- Keratocanthomas are small, benign skin lesions that may grow quickly over several weeks or months. These growths often appear when a person has some other type of cancer, particularly in the stomach, intestines, urinary tract, or male reproductive system, so it's important to be screened appropriately.

Inheriting Multiple Lynch Syndrome Mutations

Although rare, children may inherit a mutation from both parents in both copies of the *MLH1*, *MSH2*, *MSH6*, *PMS2*, or *EPCAM* genes. Having two mutations in the same gene (one from each parent) causes constitutional mismatch repair-deficiency (CMMRD) syndrome. When two people with Lynch syndrome mutations in the same gene have offspring, the chance of having a child with CMMRD is 25 percent. CMMRD can cause several serious health issues. Those affected often develop cancer before age 18 and have more than one cancer during their lifetime. Their risk is greater for childhood brain cancers, leukemia, and non-Hodgkin lymphoma.

CMMRD also raises the risk for gastrointestinal and colorectal polyps. People with CMMRD syndrome have changes in skin pigmentation, including freckles and café-au-lait spots (patches of skin that are darker than the surrounding skin). Individuals with CMMRD may develop cancers in the ovaries and uterus. Genetic testing can confirm the presence of this syndrome for those whose personal or family history shows a pattern of several cancers at a young age.

Assembling Your Team of Health Care Experts

If you have Lynch syndrome, your risk is high for several cancers, and you need a multidisciplinary health care team of physicians who understand and have experience with the specific screening, prevention, and treatment protocols for Lynch syndrome cancers. Your team may include a genetics expert, oncologist, gynecologist, gastroenterologist, urologist, dermatologist, surgeon, and other specialists. Clinical psychologists can help you and your family deal with the anxiety and emotional stress of living with elevated risk for multiple cancers.

— *My Story* —

Being Uninformed about a Tumor Test Left Us in the Dark

When my mother was diagnosed with small bowel cancer, I looked at her pathology report, which read: "Immunohistochemistry for mismatch repair gene products: MSH6 loss . . . suggesting MSI-H colorectal cancer, which is associated with Lynch syndrome." Her surgeon had never mentioned this piece of information. Two years later, my mother had genetic testing, which confirmed her Lynch syndrome *MSH6* mutation. Then I was tested, which confirmed that I too inherited the same mutation.

—*Aya*

— EXPERT VIEW —

Is Lynch Syndrome Underdiagnosed?

BY HEATHER HAMPEL, MS, LGC

Although Lynch syndrome affects nearly 1 in 300 individuals, 90–95 percent of people with this syndrome are estimated to be unaware of their high-risk status. This is a major public health problem, particularly because the cancers associated with Lynch syndrome are preventable as long as screening and prevention options begin early enough and occur frequently enough. While awareness that breast and ovarian cancers can run together in families has grown, there is still a general lack of awareness that colorectal and endometrial (uterine) cancers can also run together in a family. This causes Lynch syndrome to be overlooked by both families and health care providers.

The 2010 Michigan Behavioral Risk Factor Survey found that only 22 percent of Michigan adults with a personal and/or family history of colorectal cancer had heard of a genetic test for the disease. These respondents were primarily young and female. Of those who had heard of such genetic testing, only 3 percent knew if they or a family member had been tested for a mutation.

In the first major US study of universal tumor screening for Lynch syndrome, we screened 1,566 colorectal cancer patients and 565 endometrial cancer patients in Columbus, Ohio, and found 58 with Lynch syndrome. Only one of these families was aware of their Lynch syndrome status before our study.

The Healthy Nevada Project, which tested nearly 27,000 individuals, found that 1 in 75 had either hereditary breast and ovarian cancer syndrome, Lynch syndrome, or familial hypercholesterolemia (an inherited condition that causes very high cholesterol levels). A staggering 90 percent of these individuals were not aware of their genetic status before participating in the research study. We have a long way to go to help identify families with these common, actionable hereditary conditions so that they can benefit from potentially lifesaving interventions.

Outdated Terms Related to Lynch Syndrome

"Turcot syndrome" is an outdated term that was used to describe families with colorectal polyps, colorectal cancers, and brain tumors. Once the genes associated with hereditary colorectal cancer were discovered, it was learned that these families either had Lynch syndrome (usually associated with glioblastomas) or familial adenomatous polyposis (usually associated with medulloblastomas). It's now apparent that anyone with Lynch syndrome can develop a brain tumor, so the term "Turcot syndrome" is no longer used today.

"Muir-Torre syndrome" was once used to describe families with colorectal cancers and tumors of the sweat glands on the skin. Once the genes were discovered, it was learned that these families had Lynch syndrome. It's now known that anyone with Lynch syndrome can develop one of these skin tumors, and the term "Muir-Torre syndrome" is no longer used.

Chapter 7

Other Genes That Are Linked to Inherited Cancer Risk

The *PALB2* gene works with the *BRCA2* and *RAD51* genes to repair DNA damage. A mutation in *PALB2* increases the lifetime risk for female breast cancer to as much as 40–60 percent and also elevates the likelihood of ovarian cancer. The risk for male breast cancer and prostate cancer with this mutation hasn't been defined, but it's believed to be increased as well.

Cancer is common, yet only 5–10 percent are caused by inherited gene mutations. This small percentage, however, includes people diagnosed with many types of cancer that may have resulted from mutations in numerous different genes. While mutations in the *BRCA1*, *BRCA2*, and Lynch syndrome genes are the best-studied causes of hereditary cancers, mutations in other genes can also predispose individuals and families to cancer. These inherited mutations influence breast, ovarian, and prostate cancer risk. That risk is usually lower than for people with *BRCA* mutations but higher than the average person's risk. Similarly, several inherited mutations affect colorectal cancer risk, though not all of those gene mutations increase risk to the same degree as mutations related to Lynch syndrome.

Inherited mutations in lesser known genes cause cancers that often develop earlier than the same cancers in the general population. Some inherited mutations increase the risk for a specific cancer. Others elevate the risk for several cancers and are sometimes referred to as hereditary cancer syndromes. Most of the inherited mutations discussed in this chapter are rare. All of them carry heightened cancer risk, yet none have been studied as much as *BRCA* and Lynch syndrome genes. We'll better understand these less familiar mutations—and others that will be discovered—and the risks they carry as genetic research advances and more people are tested for mutations in these genes (table 7.1).

If you have a mutation in a gene discussed in this chapter, be sure to read chapter 13 for the related risk management guidelines. If you are diagnosed with cancer, your mutation status may change your treatment options. You'll

TABLE 7.1 Genes with Inherited Mutations That Are Linked to Hereditary Cancer Risk

CANCER	GENE
blood	*TP53*
bone	*TP53*
brain	*APC, NF1, TP53*
breast	*ATM, BARD1, BRIP1, CDH1, CHEK2* (including male breast cancer), *NF1, PALB2* (including male breast cancer), *PTEN, RAD51C, RAD51D, STK11, TP53*
colorectal	*APC, CHEK2, PTEN, TP53, MUTYH* (*ATM* requires further study)
endometrial (uterine)	*PTEN, STK11*
gastrointestinal	*APC, CDH1, NF1, PTEN, TP53, STK11*
lung	*STK11, TP53*
melanoma	*CDKN2A, CDK4, PTEN* (*PALB2* requires further study)
ovarian	*ATM,* * *BRIP1, PALB2, PTEN, RAD51C, RAD51D*
pancreatic	*APC, ATM, CDKN2A, PALB2, PTEN, TP53, STK11*
prostate	*ATM, CHEK2, HOXB13, NBN* ** (*PALB2* requires further study)
thyroid	*APC, PTEN, TP53, MUTYH* (*CHEK2* requires further study)

*May be slightly increased.

**Increased cancer risk in this gene is only associated with 657del5 mutations.

find more information about tumor testing, postdiagnosis genetic testing, and treatment options in chapters 20–25.

Less Known, Less Studied Genes
APC Gene

A mutation in the *APC* gene produces familial adenomatous polyposis (FAP), a condition that occurs in 1 in 10,000 people and is the source of about 1 percent of colorectal cancers.[1] People who are born with this disorder may have hundreds to thousands of precancerous polyps in the colon and rectum, typically beginning during their teenage years or earlier. A somewhat milder version of this syndrome called attenuated FAP typically causes fewer than 100 colon polyps, which appear at a later age. Left untreated, nearly everyone with FAP develops colorectal cancer by age 40—much earlier than the average age of onset for sporadic colorectal cancer and the age when colorectal cancer screening usually begins. Most people with an *APC* mutation undergo risk-reducing surgery to remove their colon and rectum (see chapter 18). Benign or cancerous growths can grow in the thyroid, stomach, pancreas, small intestine, liver, and brain, although this happens less frequently. Desmoid tumors may begin in the tissue covering the intestines. These fibrous tumors are noncancerous, but they grow aggressively and often recur after they're removed.

About 6 percent of individuals who are of Ashkenazi Jewish ancestry have a specific *APC* gene variant called I1307K. Whether this variant increases cancer risk is unclear. Some studies have shown a mildly increased lifetime risk of colorectal cancer (about 1.5–2 times that of the general population) while other studies have shown no increase in colorectal cancer risk.[2] Unlike other *APC* mutations, I1307K doesn't cause the very high cancer risks that are associated with FAP. Still, increased screening is recommended for individuals with this variant (see chapter 14).

ATM Gene

Inheriting a mutation in one of your *ATM* genes increases the risk of breast cancer and may also increase the risk for ovarian, pancreatic, and prostate cancer. Many experts cite a lifetime breast cancer risk of 15–40 percent for women with an *ATM* mutation; studies in 2021 suggested that the average lifetime risk may be around 25 percent.[3] If you have an *ATM* mutation and have been diagnosed with cancer, your treatment options may be different than the options for someone without a mutation.

Ataxia-telangiectasia (AT) is a very rare disorder that can occur when people inherit two *ATM* mutations (one from each parent). Also called Louis-Bar syndrome, AT is a degenerative disorder that primarily affects the nervous, neurological, and immune systems. It affects 1 in 100,000 births.

BARD1 Gene

The *BARD1* gene works in tandem with *BRCA1* to repair DNA damage, so it's not surprising that mutations in this gene raise the probability for breast cancer, including triple-negative breast cancer. This mutation may also increase ovarian cancer risk.

— *My Story* —
The Information about My Mutation Is Vague

I had trouble finding any information on my inherited *BARD1* mutation. All I know is that it gives me an "elevated risk" for breast cancer. I already knew I had an elevated risk because of my family history, and I don't see why knowing I have this gene is helpful. Sometimes I feel like I'd rather not know I have it. It causes me stress, and there don't seem to be many recommended preventive measures. Many of my family members agree and aren't interested in getting tested.

—*Hayley*

BRIP1, *RAD51C*, and *RAD51D* Genes

Mutations in the *BRIP1*, *RAD51C*, and *RAD51D* genes cause a high risk of breast and ovarian cancers. Mutations in these genes are believed to be more involved in the susceptibility for triple-negative breast cancer, which can be difficult to treat.

CDH1 Gene

Hereditary diffuse gastric cancer (HDGC) syndrome results from a mutation in the *CDH1* gene. It predisposes families to cancer in the lining of the stomach, often before age 40—about 20 years earlier than most gastric cancers in the

Fanconi Anemia

Inheriting two abnormal copies (one from each parent) in the *BRIP1*, *PALB2*, or *RAD51C* genes can cause Fanconi anemia, a disorder characterized by physical abnormalities, bone marrow failure, childhood leukemia, and other cancers.

general population. Less than 1 percent of the US population has any type of stomach cancer; even fewer people have HDGC-related cancer. Little is known about this syndrome or how it affects a person's cancer risk. The estimated lifetime risk for HDGC is estimated to be about 70 percent in men and between 56 and 83 percent in women. Women with HDGC also have a 39–52 percent lifetime risk of developing lobular breast cancer.

CDKN2A and *CDK4* Genes

Although rare, mutations in the *CDKN2A* and *CDK4* genes hold the highest susceptibility for melanoma, the most serious type of skin cancer. Data from *CDKN2A* families in Europe, Australia, and North America show that geographic location influences familial risk, possibly due to different levels of ultraviolet exposure from sunlight.[4] Additionally, people with *CDKN2A* mutations have a high lifetime risk for pancreatic cancer and may be susceptible to lung cancers as well.

CHEK2 Gene

Women with a mutation in the *CHEK2* gene have a 15–40 percent lifetime risk for breast cancer. Breast cancer survivors who have this mutation have a greater risk for a second primary breast cancer. Men with a *CHEK2* mutation are more likely to develop breast and prostate cancer. The chance of developing colorectal cancer is also increased, and the risk for other cancers may be greater as well.

— *My Story* —
Not *BRCA2*, but *CHEK2*

I was diagnosed with breast cancer in 1996. That was before *BRCA* testing was routine, but I've always assumed that I had a *BRCA2* mutation because I'm Ashkenazi Jewish, my mother had pancreatic cancer, and I was diagnosed with breast cancer at a young age. More recently, I had an elevated PSA [prostate-specific antigen], and I knew that *BRCA* status can affect treatment options, so I had multigene panel testing. It turns out that I don't have a *BRCA2* mutation, but I do have a *CHEK2* mutation.

—*Bob*

HOXB13 Gene

Mutations in this tumor suppressor gene, which is critical for the development of the prostate gland, run in some families and increase the risk for early-onset prostate cancer. Men with a *HOXB13* mutation have a lifetime prostate cancer risk of 30–60 percent.

MUTYH Gene

About 1–2 percent of the US population inherits a mutation in one of their *MUTYH* genes, which slightly increases their risk for colorectal cancer. Inheriting mutations in both copies of the *MUTYH* gene results in MUTYH-associated polyposis (MAP). This uncommon condition significantly raises the risk for colorectal and thyroid cancers; more research is needed to identify the specific levels of risk. As is typical of polyposis syndromes, individuals with MAP usually develop numerous polyps, often by the time they're 40. Some have up to 100 polyps, while others may have as many as 1,000.

NBN Gene

One variant in the *NBN* gene, known as 657del5, has been studied for a possible link to cancers. Research results have been conflicting, and more study is needed to determine if this variant raises breast cancer risk. This variant has also been linked to an increased risk for prostate cancer, ovarian cancer, melanoma, and leukemia, although the exact risks are unknown. Current risk management guidelines are based on a person's family history of cancer.

Having a mutation in both of your *NBN* genes (one from each parent) results in Nijmegen breakage syndrome, a disorder that causes small stature and head size, a compromised immune system, and numerous other health issues. Brain and muscle tumors are also likely. Roughly half of people who have this syndrome develop non-Hodgkin lymphoma, usually before age 15.

NF1 Gene

A mutation in *NF1* is linked to a disease known as neurofibromatosis type 1, which causes benign tumors called neurofibromas on or below the skin or in the nerves. People with this disorder often have brain tumors and changes in skin pigmentation. Affected children may develop a rare type of leukemia before age 2. Women with an *NF1* mutation are more prone to have breast cancer before age 50.

PALB2 Gene

The *PALB2* gene works with the *BRCA2* and *RAD51* genes to repair DNA damage. A mutation in *PALB2* increases the lifetime risk for female breast cancer to as much as 40–60 percent and also elevates the likelihood of ovarian cancer. The risk for male breast cancer and prostate cancer with this mutation hasn't been defined, but it's believed to be increased as well. People with *PALB2* mutations are more likely to develop pancreatic cancer. You can read about specific guidelines for managing *PALB2*-associated cancer risks in chapter 13. If you have a *PALB2* mutation and you've been diagnosed with cancer, your treatment options may be different than the options for someone who doesn't have a mutation.

PTEN Gene

One in 200,000 people has Cowden syndrome, a disorder that results from an inherited mutation in a *PTEN* tumor-suppressor gene. Even less frequently, mutations in the *KLLN*, *SDHB*, or *SDHD* genes also cause Cowden syndrome. Families with this syndrome tend to have several types of benign and malignant tumors in the breast, uterus, thyroid, and gastrointestinal tract—the result of the damaged gene's inability to control cellular growth. Ovarian and pancreatic cancer may also show up in family members, although less often. Cancers typically appear between ages 30 and 40 (table 7.2).

STK11 Gene

Peutz-Jeghers syndrome develops from a mutation in the *STK11* gene. It elevates the risk for gastrointestinal cancers, as well as cancers of the cervix, breast, uterus, lung, and pancreas (table 7.3). Children with Peutz-Jeghers often show symptoms by age 10. These might include small dark freckles on the hands or feet, inside the mouth, and around the anus; these usually fade as children become teenagers. Thousands of hamartomas (benign tumors) in the stomach and intestines often occur with Peutz-Jeghers. About half of people with Peutz-Jeghers need surgery by age 18 to resolve complications from polyps. The lifetime risk for cancer, which usually appears by age 50, is about 93 percent.[5]

TABLE 7.2 Estimated Lifetime Risk of Cowden Syndrome Cancers (%)

breast cancer (women)	40–60
thyroid cancer	≤35
kidney cancer	≤33
uterine cancer	≤28
colon cancer	≤9
melanoma	≤6

Source: Tan MH, Mester J, Ngeow J, et al. "Lifetime cancer risks in individuals with germline PTEN mutations," Clinical Cancer Research 18, no. 2, 2012:400–407.

TABLE 7.3 Estimated Lifetime Risk of
Peutz-Jeghers Syndrome Cancers (%)

breast cancer (women)	41–60
colon cancer	≤40
pancreatic cancer	≤35
stomach cancer	≤30
lung cancer	≤20
small intestine cancer	≤15
cervical cancer	≤10
uterine cancer	≤10

Source: McGarrity TJ, Amos CI, Baker MJ. "Peutz-Jeghers syndrome." National Center for Biotechnology Information Bookshelf. https://www.ncbi.nlm.nih.gov/books/NBK1266.

TP53 Gene

An inherited *TP53* gene mutation may result in Li-Fraumeni syndrome, which carries a 50 percent chance of cancer by age 40 and up to a 90 percent chance by age 60.[6] The risk for female breast cancer is very high with this syndrome. Children and young adults who develop cancer most often have cancers of the bone, soft tissue, breast, brain, and blood. Less frequently, they have cancers of the gastrointestinal system, lungs, thyroid, kidneys, skin, and sex organs.

Breast Cancer Basics

Many different factors influence your chance of being diagnosed with breast cancer. While you can control some, others are unavoidable.

Breast cancer receives a great deal of attention—and with good reason. Among women in the United States, it's the second most common cancer (after skin cancer), and it causes more deaths than any other cancer except lung cancer. The emotional attachment that many women have to their breasts can make the threat of breast cancer and the reality of a diagnosis even more daunting. Breast cancer affects men as well, although less frequently; less than 1 percent of breast cancers occur in men.

Many different types of cancer can develop in the breast. Most breast cancers begin in the ducts (the tubes that carry milk to the nipples) or the lobules (the glands that produce milk) (figure 8.1). Cancer develops when damaged cells accumulate in a duct or lobule and eventually form a tumor. On average, it takes 6–8 years before a breast tumor grows large enough to be detected by a mammogram—one reason that having routine screenings with mammograms and magnetic resonance imaging (MRI) is so important. It can take about 10 years before a lump can be felt.

Signs and Symptoms

Breast cancer often develops without pain or other noticeable symptoms until it shows up as a suspicious or questionable area during a self-exam, an

FIGURE 8.1 Inside the female breast

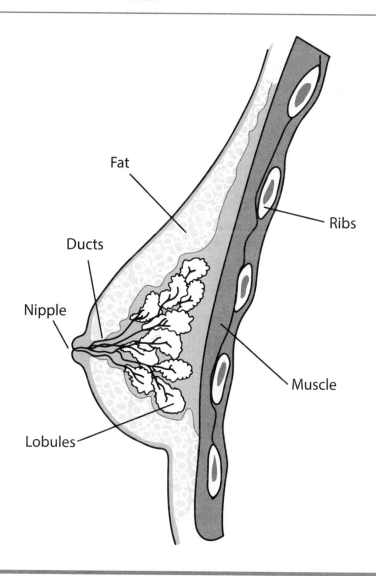

examination by a doctor, or a mammogram or breast MRI. A tumor may show itself as a lump or area of thickness, pain, a skin irritation that refuses to heal, or an unusual discharge from the nipple. While these changes often signal benign conditions, they can be early indicators of cancer. That's why it is important to regularly check your breasts and keep up with recommended screening, which often identifies breast cancers before symptoms appear. Even women who have regular breast screening mammograms or MRIs—high-risk individuals usually have both—may find their own breast abnormalities.

Becoming familiar with the look and feel of your healthy breasts will make it easier to notice any unusual changes, so that you can see a health care provider about them as soon as possible. Most women know to report a lump in their breast, which can be a sign of breast cancer. However, other symptoms may appear with or without a lump. Although the following symptoms don't always signal breast cancer, a doctor should determine the underlying reason for any unusual change in the breast.

- a change in breast size, shape, or appearance
- a painless or painful lump or thickness
- swelling in some or all of the breast
- breast skin that is dimpled like an orange peel (called peau d'orange)
- breast skin that is tender, red, dry, flaky, or thickened
- a nipple that turns inward (if this is a new development)
- nipple discharge that is bloody, dark, or yellow, especially in only one breast
- enlarged lymph nodes in the armpit or above the collarbone

Breast Changes That Don't Affect Risk

While most breast changes aren't cancerous, some changes affect the density of the tissue or the texture of the skin, while others cause thickening or lumps. Some changes mimic breast cancer and may require a biopsy to determine their true nature. Any out-of-the-ordinary changes should be evaluated by your doctor to determine whether the area needs careful monitoring or should be further analyzed.

Facts about Breast Lumps

Finding a lump in your breast that wasn't there before can be scary, but most breast lumps aren't cancer. Here are some facts about breast lumps.

- Normal breast tissue is often lumpy.

- 80 percent of breast lumps are benign.

- Soft cysts and firm fibroadenomas that move easily on the breast aren't usually problematic.

- Scar tissue or natural changes that form in the breast as we age can create benign lumps.

- Abnormal lumps don't usually appear in both breasts at the same time.

- A new lump or mass is the most common symptom of breast cancer.

- A doctor should examine any new lump that feels different than the rest of the breast.

- A biopsy is the only way to be certain that a lump is cancerous.

Breast Cancer in Men

Most men, even those who have an inherited gene mutation, don't develop breast cancer. Abnormalities in the breast or chest may be more noticeable because men have very little breast tissue. The risk of breast cancer is greater for men who are obese or who have gynecomastia, Klinefelter syndrome, or an inherited mutation in a gene that predisposes them to breast cancer. Men who develop breast cancer, particularly before age 50, are more likely to also develop a malignancy in the opposite breast.

- Mammography frequently detects calcifications in breast tissue, especially in postmenopausal women. These tiny mineral deposits result from cysts, infections, excess calcium in blood vessels, and many other factors. Calcifications are generally harmless, but some may indicate precancerous changes in the breast or the presence of ductal carcinoma in situ (DCIS) or invasive ductal carcinoma.
- Many women develop noncancerous fibrocystic changes in the breasts from hormones that are produced during ovulation. Symptoms include swelling, a rope-like texture in the breast, harmless lumps, and pain or tenderness that decreases or disappears after a menstrual period. Excessive caffeine may also worsen fibrocystic changes. Benign, fluid-filled breast cysts are a type of fibrocystic change. They're lumps that move easily, feel firm or soft, and can be painful, especially just before a menstrual cycle. Large or painful cysts can be drained; otherwise, no treatment is needed.
- Fibroadenomas are the most common type of breast mass in women under age 25. These solid lumps of fibrous tissue move easily

beneath the skin when touched. Fibroadenomas may need to be biopsied to confirm they're benign or removed if they become painful or enlarged.

- Inflammation called mastitis can develop in breast tissue. Most often, it's caused by a blocked milk duct or a bacterial infection that develops in women who breastfeed. The breast may become red or tender and feel lumpy or warm to the touch. If antibiotics don't clear the infection, the duct may need to be drained.

- Necrosis (tissue death) occurs as a result of breast surgery, radiation, or blunt trauma to the breast, which damages breast cells, which then die and form a round, hard mass.

- Reddened, tender, or inverted nipples can result from duct ectasia, a condition that develops when breast ducts become blocked with fluid. If the duct becomes infected, a lump may form beneath the nipple or a greenish discharge can develop. Antibiotics, pain medication, or applying moist heat can relieve symptoms. Often no further treatment is required.

What Affects Breast Cancer Risk?

Many different factors influence your chance of being diagnosed with breast cancer. While you can control some, others are unavoidable.

Unavoidable Factors That Increase Risk
- being female
- growing older, although hereditary breast cancer often develops earlier in life than sporadic (nonhereditary) breast cancer
- inheriting a gene mutation associated with higher breast cancer risk (table 8.1)
- a family history of breast cancer
- being diagnosed with breast cancer, which raises the likelihood of another cancer in the same or the opposite breast
- receiving radiation to your chest or breast as a teen or young adult
- starting menstruation before age 12 or beginning menopause after age 55 (both of which heighten lifetime exposure to hormones)
- previous biopsies, especially if an overgrowth of atypical breast cells was found

- never giving birth or having your first child after age 30
- dense breasts
- certain benign breast conditions
- being taller (perhaps due to hormonal, genetic, or nutritional factors)
- exposure to the anti-miscarriage drug diethylstilbestrol (discontinued in 1971), either directly or in utero
- race and ethnicity (see "Racial Disparities" sidebar)

TABLE 8.1 Estimated Lifetime Risk of Breast Cancer (%)

women in the general population	13
ATM mutation	15–40
BARD1 mutation	15–40
BRCA1 mutation	> 60
BRCA2 mutation	> 60
BRIP1 mutation	increased*
CDH1 mutation	41–60
CHEK2 mutation	15–40
NF1 mutation	15–40
PALB2 mutation	41–60
PTEN mutation	41–60
RAD51C, RAD51D mutation	increased*
STK11 mutation	41–60
TP53 mutation	> 60

Source: National Comprehensive Cancer Network. "Guidelines: Genetic/familial high-risk assessment: Breast, ovarian, and pancreatic." Version 1.2022, August 2021.

Note: The NCCN panel provides these estimates in categories of 15%–40%, 41%–60%, and > 60%.

*More research is needed to determine the level of risk for people with mutations in this gene.

Racial Disparities

White women develop breast cancer somewhat more than Black, Hispanic, and Asian women do. Black women, however, are more likely to be diagnosed before age 45 with particularly aggressive cancers that are more difficult to treat. Black women's breast cancer mortality rate at any age is higher than that of any other racial group in the United States. Breast cancer incidence in Asian women is lower, but it's increasing at a fast rate. Disparities in access and quality of health care account for some of these inequities. Other factors related to race or ethnicity may also be involved.

Modifiable Factors That Affect Risk

The chance of developing breast cancer can't be eliminated; however, it can be reduced. The factors listed here decrease breast cancer risk to some degree. Lifestyle risk factors that affect overall cancer risk are discussed in chapter 19.

- Age at first birth and number of births affect breast cancer risk. The risk for breast cancer goes up slightly after giving birth, but declines over time. A first pregnancy while young lowers risk—the younger you are, the more beneficial the effect. If you're a previvor, your risk may be influenced by how many times you've been pregnant and which of your genes carries a mutation.
- Breastfeeding slightly reduces the risk for sporadic breast cancer: the longer you breastfeed, the lower your risk. It may have a similar protective effect for women with *BRCA1* mutations.[1] Whether it affects women with *BRCA2* mutations in the same way is unclear.

- Breast cancer risk may be somewhat reduced after breast reduction surgery.
- Several studies suggest that women who work night shifts may have more risk for breast cancer than those who don't. More research is needed to understand whether this is the case.
- Oral contraceptives slightly elevate breast cancer risk. When you stop using birth control pills, your increase in risk diminishes over time, reverting to the average after 10 years.[2]
- Women of average risk who take combined estrogen and progesterone hormone replacement after natural menopause have a higher risk for breast cancer.
- Risk-reducing medications lower the risk of breast cancer in healthy high-risk individuals (see chapter 15).
- Risk-reducing surgery to remove both healthy breasts reduces hereditary breast cancer risk by as much as 90 percent.[3] Removing the ovaries as well—which greatly reduces the amount of circulating estrogen in the body—may also lower risk (see chapter 17).[4]

Breast Changes That Affect Risk

Adenosis slightly increases breast cancer risk. It develops when breast lobules become enlarged, and it's often found during a biopsy of breast cysts or fibrosis. Sclerosing adenosis occurs when enlarged lobules become distorted by scar-like tissue and form a lump or cause pain. Small, wart-like growths called papillomas can develop in the lining of the milk ducts close to the nipple; they sometimes feel like a small lump and can cause a clear or bloody discharge. Papillomas that become too painful can be surgically removed. Although a single papilloma doesn't affect breast cancer risk, multiple papillomas may slightly raise it.

Radial scars, also called complex sclerosing lesions, aren't true scars. Rather, they're growths that appear as cancer on a mammogram or biopsy and look like scars under a microscope. Radial scars don't often cause symptoms, though they can distort breast tissue if they grow too large. Some physicians recommend careful monitoring; others advise surgical removal. Radial scars slightly increase breast cancer risk.

Gynecomastia is a condition of enlarged breasts in men. Occurring at birth or during puberty, it primarily develops from excessive production of estrogen, but it can also develop from obesity or certain medications. Breast reduction surgery that eliminates excess tissue is usually recommended only for individuals who experience severe pain or emotional discomfort. Gynecomastia can increase a man's risk of breast cancer.

Hyperplasia develops when the normal process of cellular replication is accelerated and an overgrowth of cells appears in the ducts or the lobules. Usual hyperplasia displays these cells in a normal pattern and doesn't affect cancer risk. Moderate hyperplasia inflates cancer risk up to twice as much compared to someone who doesn't have hyperplasia. Atypical hyperplasia is precancerous, and it more significantly affects risk (figure 8.2). Atypical hyperplasia cells that continue to divide and develop more abnormalities can eventually turn into breast cancer. Women with this condition have about four times the breast cancer risk in either breast than women who don't have the condition. Having a strong family history of breast cancer further raises a person's risk. Although treatment isn't usually required, risk-reducing medications (see chapter 15) and frequent screenings (chapter 14) are recommended.

Despite its name, lobular carcinoma in situ (LCIS) isn't breast cancer. Usually diagnosed in premenopausal women, LCIS doesn't require treatment because it doesn't form a tumor or spread beyond the lobules. It does, however, elevate the risk for invasive breast cancer in either or both breasts by 7–12 times.[5] Rarely found by mammography, LCIS is usually discovered during a breast biopsy to explore a lump or other abnormality.

Preventive medication can lower the risk of noninvasive and invasive breast cancers. This can be particularly helpful if you have a strong family history of breast cancer or an inherited mutation that's associated with breast cancer. The affected breast and the healthy breast should be monitored closely so that any cancer that develops can be treated as soon as possible. Some doctors recommend removing the area of LCIS.

Types of Breast Cancer

Ductal Carcinoma in Situ

DCIS is the earliest stage of cancer in the breast. "In situ" means that cancer cells remain in their place of origin; DCIS is confined to the lining of the milk ducts. Too small to be felt, DCIS is usually found by routine screening mammography. Though DCIS isn't life-threatening, early detection is important. Left untreated, some DCIS can become invasive and may metastasize. There's no way to predict with certainty which DCIS will evolve into breast cancer

FIGURE 8.2 How healthy cells evolve beyond hyperplasia

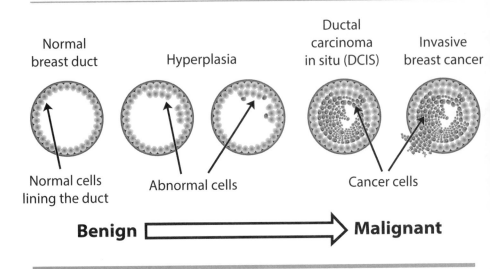

and which won't. If you have DCIS, your risk for a new breast cancer or recurrence is higher than the risk for someone who doesn't have DCIS.

— *My Story* —
I Had DCIS before I Knew That I Have a Mutation

In February 2015, a mammogram that was three years overdue found a suspicious lump. Afterward, one day before my forty-fifth birthday, a breast biopsy confirmed a diagnosis of DCIS. I was treated with lumpectomy and 32 sessions of radiation. I was also tested for an inherited gene mutation because of my young age at diagnosis and because my mom had breast cancer while she was in her 50s. By the end of my treatments, I thought I was done. Then I received my testing results and found that I am *BRCA2*-positive! My mom was tested too, but she was negative. I inherited my mutation from my dad's side of the family.

Dad was an only child, and his son, who is my half brother, hasn't been tested. Therefore, I'm the only one in my family on this journey. I joined a local FORCE group. They gave me helpful information on options to prevent a future reoccurrence of breast cancer. One year later,

Myths about What Causes Breast Cancer

Rumors and myths abound online and elsewhere about the alleged sources of breast cancer. To set the record straight, none of the following factors are at fault:

- breast implants
- large breasts
- an injury to the breast
- deodorant
- abortion
- underwire bras
- coffee
- keeping a cell phone in your bra

I opted for a bilateral mastectomy with reconstruction and a hysterectomy. I'm now five years cancer-free! I continue to help FORCE as a peer navigator to help others with hereditary cancer.

—*Wendy*

Invasive Breast Cancers

Invasive breast cancers are more serious than DCIS because they've penetrated the walls of the ducts or lobules and have entered nearby tissues. If these cancers invade the chest wall or enter the lymph system or blood vessels, they can metastasize to the lungs, bones, liver, or elsewhere in the body. Treatment is then more involved, and remission or cure is less likely.

Invasive Ductal and Lobular Carcinoma

About 80 percent of breast cancers are invasive ductal carcinoma (IDC), cancer that has broken through the walls of the ducts and into the surrounding breast tissue. People of any age can develop IDC, but in the general population, it's more often found after age 55. Only 10 percent of invasive breast cancers are invasive lobular carcinoma (ILC), which begins when abnormal cells accumulate in the lobules. ILC in the general population is more often diagnosed in women who are age 60 and older, and there is a greater risk for another breast tumor and a recurrence after treatment. IDC and ILC that are related to inherited mutations tend to develop at a younger age than the sporadic versions of the same cancers.

Inflammatory Breast Cancer

Less than 5 percent of all breast cancers are inflammatory breast cancer (IBC). IBC often begins with swelling or reddening of the breast, a sign that cancer cells are blocking the lymphatic vessels in the breast skin and preventing the normal flow of lymph fluid. IBC can grow quickly. Most inflammatory breast cancers are invasive ductal carcinomas that develop in the milk ducts of the breast and then spread into the surrounding breast tissue. Symptoms, which include itching, swelling, a feeling of warmth, or breast skin that appears dark or pitted, may advance in a single day, so recognition of the signs and seeking prompt treatment are essential. IBC tends to develop at younger ages than most other breast cancers.

Paget's Disease of the Breast

Paget's disease of the breast is rare. It affects the nipple and/or the areola (the pigmented skin around the nipple), where it is typically characterized by a patch of dry, scaly, itchy, or red skin. These same symptoms occur with a benign skin condition known as topical dermatitis, which sometimes leads to misdiagnosis. Women with Paget's disease often have DCIS or invasive breast cancer at the same time, underscoring the importance of an early diagnosis.

Other Invasive Breast Cancers

Other invasive breast cancer subtypes develop less frequently. Slow-growing mucinous carcinoma begins in the milk ducts and spreads to surrounding tissue. Medullary carcinoma of the breast forms in the breast ducts and divides aggressively, though it usually responds to treatment more than other ductal breast cancers. Medullary carcinoma of the breast is rare, and it may be more prevalent among people with *BRCA1* mutations.

Phyllodes Tumors: Benign, Borderline, Malignant

Phyllodes tumors are an unusual type of breast tumor that develops in the ligaments and fatty tissue of the breast rather than in the ducts or lobules. These tumors are mostly benign, but some are malignant. Removal is recommended in either case, because they can grow quickly and become large enough to stretch the skin of the breast. Although they often return, benign phyllodes tumors don't affect breast cancer risk. When malignant, these tumors can metastasize beyond the breast. Individuals with these tumors should be checked for Li-Fraumeni syndrome, which is linked to this type of tumor.

Diagnosing Breast Cancer

Different diagnostic tools help to determine whether a suspicious area or lump is breast cancer. A lump or unusual area may initially be found during a self-exam, a breast exam by a health care professional, or a routine screening mammogram or breast MRI. Your doctor may then order additional diagnostic tests or imaging to obtain more information about a suspicious area or determine whether a breast lump is a harmless, fluid-filled cyst or a solid mass, which is more likely to be malignant. Depending on the initial screening method, these additional tests might include a diagnostic mammogram, a breast MRI, or an ultrasound. If these results are inconclusive, other imaging or tests may then be used for more clarity. A surgical or needle biopsy that removes a sample of breast tissue or fluid, which is then examined for the presence of cancer cells, is the only sure way to determine the presence of breast cancer.

Chapter 9

Gynecologic Cancers

Vaginal bleeding outside of a normal menstrual period is the most common sign of uterine and endometrial cancers. It's an indication that shouldn't be ignored because it can be the earliest warning of endometrial cancer.

The female reproductive system is a network of organs that prepare and support the body for pregnancy and childbirth. During puberty, the ovaries—two small, almond-shaped glands on either side of the uterus—begin producing hormones. Each month during the reproductive years, the ovaries release an egg into one of the fallopian tubes. Eggs that are fertilized by sperm cells travel through the tube and implant into the endometrium (the lining of the uterus), where they grow into embryos. Eggs that aren't fertilized are shed along with the endometrium during menstruation.

Between puberty and menopause, the ovaries produce estrogen and progesterone, hormones that keep bones strong, stimulate sex drive, regulate the menstrual cycle, and affect other critical body functions. As menopause approaches, the ovaries gradually produce less hormones. The menstrual cycle slows until it stops altogether as a woman reaches menopause. The ovaries, fallopian tubes, and uterus work in tandem but can individually develop cancer, although cancer in these organs is uncommon (figure 9.1). Even less frequently, cancer begins outside the ovaries in the peritoneum, the protective membrane that covers most abdominal organs. Cancers in the cervix and the vagina, which are also part of the female reproductive system, aren't hereditary and aren't covered here.

FIGURE 9.1 The female reproductive system

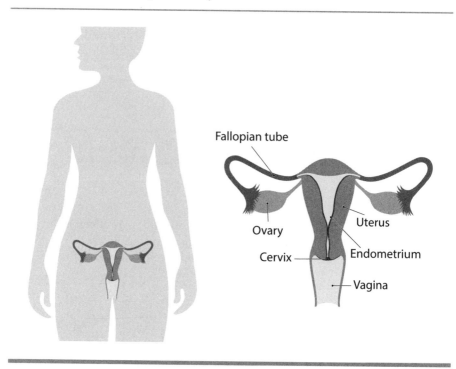

Ovarian, Fallopian Tube, and Primary Peritoneal Cancers

The term "ovarian cancer" includes fallopian tube cancer and primary perito-neal cancer because the three are closely related and are generally treated simi-larly. Pinpointing which organ is the source of a cancer can be challenging.

Ovarian and Fallopian Tube Cancers

Increasingly, experts believe that many ovarian cancers begin in the fallopian tubes and spread to the ovaries. This distinction has opened up new avenues of research into ovarian cancer prevention and early detection. Found early, the cure rate for ovarian cancer is high: five-year survival for individuals diagnosed in the earliest stages is more than 90 percent—nearly double what it was 20 years ago. Almost 60 percent of cases, however, are diagnosed only after metastasis has occurred and when treatment is limited; the five-year survival probability is then 30 percent. Compared to women with nonhereditary ovarian cancers, women with *BRCA* mutations who develop the same types of tumor tend to fare better and are less likely to die from the disease, even when they're diagnosed at later stages.[1] Whether this is due to different tumor traits or simply a better response to treatment is uncertain. Even less is known about differences in prognosis for women with other inherited mutations linked to ovarian cancer.

Signs and Symptoms

Unlike the Pap test for cervical cancer or mammograms that look for breast cancer, no effective screening test has been developed for ovarian cancer. Tucked deep in the abdominal cavity, only 15–20 percent of ovarian tumors are discovered early, when treatment is most successful. Fallopian tube cancer often begins near the opening where eggs enter to be fertilized but usually involves the ovaries as well, making it difficult to determine the exact origin. Many previously diagnosed "ovarian cancers" may have started in the fallopian tubes and then spread to the ovaries. By the time most women are diagnosed, cancer cells have already spread throughout the abdomen and to the lymph nodes and, in some cases, metastasized to other organs. Increasingly, early-stage tumors are unexpectedly found during preventive surgery to remove the ovaries and fallopian tubes of high-risk women.

With no reliable way to screen for these cancers, it's important to be aware of symptoms that may be subtle, easily disregarded, or mistaken for bladder or digestive conditions. Any symptoms that are new, severe, or persist for 12 or more days in a 30-day period should be reported to your doctor. If you're then treated for something other than ovarian cancer and your symptoms linger or become worse, quickly get a second opinion from a gynecologic expert. Symptoms generally aren't painful or noticeable until ovarian cancer has advanced. The pelvic cavity is large, so a mass can continue to grow before it becomes big enough to cause noticeable symptoms.

Common symptoms, which can also be caused by a variety of noncancerous conditions, include

- abdominal bloating
- pelvic or abdominal pain
- feeling full quickly after eating
- needing to urinate urgently or frequently
- vaginal bleeding between menstruation cycles or after menopause

Less common symptoms may include

- fatigue
- upset stomach or heartburn
- back pain
- pain during sex
- heavier-than-normal or irregular menstrual bleeding
- changes in bowel habits, including diarrhea or constipation

Understanding Ovarian Cancer Risk

Your risk of ovarian cancer increases as you grow older. Ovarian tumors usually develop after menopause and rarely before age 40. The risk is higher if you have a predisposing inherited mutation. Mutations in *BRCA1* and *BRCA2* account for almost 40 percent of ovarian cancer cases in women with a family history of the disease. Less is known about the risk for women with mutations in other genes. Inherited mutations in the *BRIP1*, *RAD51C*, *RAD51D*, *EPCAM*, *MLH1*, *MSH2*, and *MSH6* genes are linked to ovarian cancer. Additionally, mutations in the *ATM*, *PALB2*, *PMS2*, and other genes may also increase ovarian cancer risk. Although women with *STK11* mutations are at increased risk for ovarian growths, most of these are benign. If you have a higher-than-average chance for ovarian cancer, it's important to recognize and manage your risk (table 9.1). Genetic testing is recommended if you have a strong family history of breast or ovarian cancer and you haven't already been tested for an inherited mutation. Ideally, if someone in your family has already been diagnosed with ovarian cancer, they should be the first to be tested.

Factors That Increase Risk

Most people who develop ovarian cancer don't have an inherited gene mutation. Other factors that increase ovarian cancer risk include

- growing older
- a personal history of breast, endometrial, or colon cancer
- a family history of breast, ovarian, or colon cancer
- never giving birth or having your first full-term pregnancy after age 35
- obesity (a body mass index of 30 or higher), which raises the risk for some less aggressive ovarian cancers and negatively affects survival

TABLE 9.1 Estimated Lifetime Risk of Ovarian Cancer (%)

women in the general population	1
ATM mutation	may be slightly increased
BRCA1 mutation	≤40
BRCA2 mutation	15–30
BRIP1, RAD51C, RAD51D mutation	≥10*
EPCAM, MLH1, MSH2 mutation	≥10
MSH6 mutation	≤13
PALB2 mutation	5–10
PMS2 mutation	unclear**

Sources: National Comprehensive Cancer Network. "Guidelines: Genetic/familial high-risk assessment: Breast, ovarian, and pancreatic." Version 1.2022, August 2021; National Comprehensive Cancer Network. "Guidelines: Genetic/familial high-risk assessment: Colorectal." Version 1.2021, May 2021.

*Experts agree that mutations in these genes increase risk, but more research is needed to better define risk levels.

**Experts don't agree that the risk is increased.

- endometriosis, a condition in which the uterine lining grows on the outside instead of the inside of the uterus

Factors That Reduce Risk

- Solid evidence shows that oral contraceptives reduce the chance of developing ovarian cancer for women of average or high risk. Taking birth control pills for five or more years lowers risk by about half, and the effect lasts for years after you stop taking them. At the same time, your chance of having breast and cervical cancer slightly increases while you take oral contraceptives.
- Giving birth once or more lowers ovarian cancer risk, especially if you have your first child before age 35.
- Breastfeeding further decreases your risk. The more you breastfeed, the lower your risk, possibly because it delays ovulation. An analysis of 13 studies concluded that women who breastfed for less than three months had an 18 percent reduced risk of ovarian cancer compared

to those who didn't breastfeed; breastfeeding for 12 months or more reduced risk by 34 percent. This lower risk persisted more than 30 years after pregnancy.[2]
- Tubal ligation—blocking or "tying" your fallopian tubes to prevent pregnancy—may lower your chance of ovarian cancer, although not as much as oral contraceptives do. This procedure isn't usually performed solely to reduce ovarian cancer risk. Researchers are investigating whether removing the fallopian tubes (salpingectomy) lowers risk (see chapter 17).
- Premenopausal women with mutations in *BRCA* or other genes that are linked to ovarian cancer who have their healthy ovaries and fallopian tubes removed may reduce their risk by 80 percent or more.[3] A small risk remains for primary peritoneal cancer. (Chapter 17 has more on preventive gynecologic surgeries.)

— *My Story* —
A Second Opinion Led to the Discovery of My Ovarian Cancer

My ovarian cancer diagnosis was delayed despite my family history of cancer; symptoms that included spotting, pain, bloating and urine leakage; and a 5-centimeter cyst (about the size of a lime) on my ovary that was found with ultrasound. My gynecologist never even did an exam and was going to have me come back for a repeat ultrasound in three months. Luckily, I decided to get a second opinion with a gynecologist who did a repeat ultrasound and immediately referred me to a gynecologic oncologist. When the tumor was removed a month later, it was 10 centimeters.

—*Cindy*

Types of Ovarian Cancer
More than 30 different types of ovarian cancer have been identified. Most of them are named for the cells in which they originate.

- About 90 percent of sporadic and hereditary ovarian cancers begin in the epithelial cells that cover the ovaries and fallopian tubes.

These serous epithelial ovarian cancers are the most common type found in individuals with an inherited gene mutation. Epithelial ovarian cancers are usually high-grade serous tumors that begin in the fallopian tubes. Low-grade serous carcinomas in the ovaries occur less often. Other types include endometrioid carcinoma, clear cell carcinoma, carcinosarcoma, and mucinous carcinoma.

- Ovarian germ cell tumors in the cells that produce eggs are rare. Teenage girls and young women are more susceptible to this type of tumor.
- Stromal cell tumors develop in the connective tissue cells that hold the ovaries together and generate estrogen and progesterone. Most of these tumors are benign, but rare cases are cancerous and are seen primarily in adolescents and adults.

Primary Peritoneal Cancer

Primary peritoneal cancer can develop anywhere in the abdominal cavity, affect any of the organs within, and quickly spread to other tissues. The peritoneum is made up of epithelial cells, which are similar to cells that line the ovaries and fallopian tubes, which explains why peritoneal cancer looks and behaves like ovarian cancer, has similar symptoms, and is treated as advanced ovarian cancer. One of the body's four types of tissue—along with muscle, nerve tissue, and connective tissue—epithelial cells cover the outer surfaces of organs and blood vessels.

High-risk women are more likely to develop peritoneal cancer, although it occurs rarely. Importantly, primary peritoneal cancer can develop even after the ovaries and fallopian tubes have been removed. This is why surgery to remove the ovaries and fallopian tubes reduces risk but doesn't eliminate it.

Endometrial Cancers

The uterus is the womb where a baby grows before childbirth. Endometrial cancer, a type of uterine cancer that arises from the lining of the uterus, is diagnosed more than any other gynecologic cancer. The majority of endometrial cancers develop after menopause and are almost always curable. Unlike ovarian cancer, endometrial cancer is often diagnosed at an early stage. Vaginal bleeding outside of a normal menstrual period is the most common sign of uterine and endometrial cancers. It's an indication that shouldn't be

Cysts in the System

Most cysts on the ovaries, fallopian tubes, or peritoneum aren't cancerous and don't affect ovarian cancer risk. Ovarian cysts often come and go with or without symptoms during a menstrual cycle or in early pregnancy. Normal cyclic ovulation often produces detectable ovarian cysts, which are frequently referred to as "functional" cysts, since they are part of normal physiology. Ovarian cysts that grow large enough to cause pain or problems are usually removed. Fallopian tube cysts are usually removed as a precaution because they can become large enough to damage the ovary or fallopian tube, which may then need to be removed. Inclusion cysts in the peritoneum can form when the organ's normal ability to absorb ovarian fluid is damaged. They're usually diagnosed in premenopausal women who've had abdominal or pelvic surgery, trauma to the area, endometriosis, or pelvic inflammatory disease. Inclusion cysts can create pelvic pain or feel like a lump in the pelvis. In some people, they grow large enough to fill the entire abdominal cavity.

Racial Differences in Ovarian Cancer Risk and Mortality

White women are diagnosed with epithelial ovarian cancer somewhat more than women of other races. Yet ovarian cancer disproportionately affects some populations, especially Black women, who are more likely to be diagnosed before age 45 with particularly aggressive cancers. The mortality rate among Black women of any age is higher than that of women of other racial groups in the United States, regardless of the stage of their cancers when they were diagnosed. Between 1975 and 2016, the five-year survival rate for non-Hispanic white women rose from 33 percent to 48 percent, yet it declined during the same period from 44 percent to 41 percent in Black women.[1]

Researchers are studying the causes for these disparities and ways to address them, which is an urgent and unmet need. Black women may ovulate more than white women, raising their lifetime exposure to estrogen.[2] Hispanic women with ovarian cancer are diagnosed earlier and live longer after diagnosis compared to non-Hispanic women. Women of Asian/Pacific Islander ancestry have the highest incidence of endometrioid and clear cell carcinomas, whether they were born in the United States or abroad.

NOTES:
1. American Cancer Society. "Ovarian cancer studies aim to reduce racial disparities, improve outcomes." https://www.cancer.gov/news-events/cancer-currents-blog/2020/ovarian-cancer-racial-disparitiesstudies#:~:text=Three%20recently%20launched%20NCI%2Dsupported,White%20patients%20with%20the%20disease.
2. Peres L, Moorman P, Alberg A, et al. "Lifetime number of ovulatory cycles and epithelial ovarian cancer risk in African American women," Cancer Causes and Control 28, no. 5, 2017:405–14.

ignored because it can be the earliest warning of endometrial cancer. Check with your doctor if you have any of the following symptoms:

- pelvic pain
- pain during sex
- difficult or painful urination
- vaginal bleeding or discharge after menopause or not related to menstrual periods

Risk factors for endometrial cancer include

- having Lynch syndrome or an inherited *PTEN* or *STK11* gene mutation
- taking estrogen-only hormone replacement therapy after menopause (estrogen combined with progesterone doesn't inflate endometrial cancer risk)
- taking tamoxifen to prevent or treat breast cancer
- excessive long-term exposure to natural estrogen, which can be caused by beginning menstrual periods at an early age, never giving birth, and/or starting menopause at a later age
- obesity
- metabolic syndrome, a combination of obesity, high cholesterol, elevated blood pressure, and high blood sugar that heightens the likelihood of cardiovascular disease, diabetes, stroke, and other diseases
- polycystic ovary syndrome, a hormonal disorder that is common during the reproductive years
- endometrial hyperplasia
- type 2 diabetes

Types of Endometrial Cancer

Endometrial cancers are classified as one of two types. Type 1 are low-grade adenocarcinomas, the most common endometrial cancers that develop in the cells of the uterine lining. They're ordinarily found early and have an excellent prognosis. Type 2 endometrial cancers tend to behave more aggressively, are more likely to spread beyond the uterus, and have a worse prognosis. This type includes clear cell carcinomas, high-grade serous carcinomas, and uterine carcinosarcomas. Some research has found a small increase in risk for high-grade serous carcinomas in women with *BRCA1* mutations (and possibly those with *BRCA2* mutations), but other studies have not found such a link. More research is needed to confirm these findings. Women with Lynch syndrome may develop any type of endometrial cancer.

Endometrial Cancer Disproportionately Affects Black Women

In the United States, Black women are more likely to be diagnosed with aggressive, type 2 endometrial cancer and metastatic cancer compared to white, Hispanic, and Asian women. Additionally, Black women with type 2 endometrial cancer have a higher risk of dying of the disease compared to white women.[4] In part this is because Black women are less likely than white women to receive evidence-based care because of the broad effects of systemic racism on health care.[5] Researchers are looking at ways to address these disparities.

Diagnosing Gynecologic Cancers

When an exam or symptoms suggest a possible malignancy, a gynecologic oncologist who is specially trained in diagnosing and treating cancers of the female reproductive system should be consulted. The next step is usually additional imaging and blood tests to try to detect a mass in the ovaries, pelvis, or fallopian tubes. If you have fluid buildup in your abdomen, an ultrasound-guided paracentesis (inserting a needle to remove fluid buildup in the abdomen) may also be used. In some cases, a biopsy may be done with paracentesis or laparoscopy (in which a thin, lighted tube is inserted through a very small abdominal incision). Surgery or biopsy is the only conclusive way to determine whether a pelvic mass is cancerous. For most endometrial cancers, an endometrial biopsy, pelvic exam, and often a pelvic ultrasound are sufficient preoperative testing. If there is concern that the cancer may have spread, imaging such as a computed tomography (CT) scan or pelvic MRI may be used to estimate the extent of the tumors.

Chapter 10

Gastrointestinal Cancers

Almost all colorectal cancers begin as symptomless polyps in the colon or rectum. These are generally harmless in their early stages, but some polyps can become malignant over time.

Everything we eat and drink passes through the gastrointestinal (GI) tract, also called the digestive tract, the body's system that converts foods into energy. The upper GI tract includes the area from the mouth to the stomach and a section of the small intestine known as the duodenum. The remainder of the small intestine and the large intestines comprise the lower GI tract. Aided by nerves, muscles, and intestinal bacteria, the foods and liquids we swallow move down the throat and into the esophagus (figure 10.1). From there, they travel into the stomach and on to the small intestine, where digestive juices from the liver and pancreas help break down the food so that the vitamins, minerals, and other nutrients are absorbed into the bloodstream. Undigested leftovers move through the colon (the large intestine) and into the rectum before being expelled as feces through the anus.

With the exception of colorectal cancer, most malignancies in the gastrointestinal tract are uncommon. Certain inherited gene mutations and syndromes raise the risk for colorectal, gastric, pancreatic, small bowel, and anal cancers (table 10.1). If any of these cancers run in your family, it's important to consult with a genetics specialist, who can determine your risk and management options. Cancers of the liver, esophagus, and gallbladder are rarely seen or associated with inherited mutations and aren't covered here.

FIGURE 10.1 The gastrointestinal tract

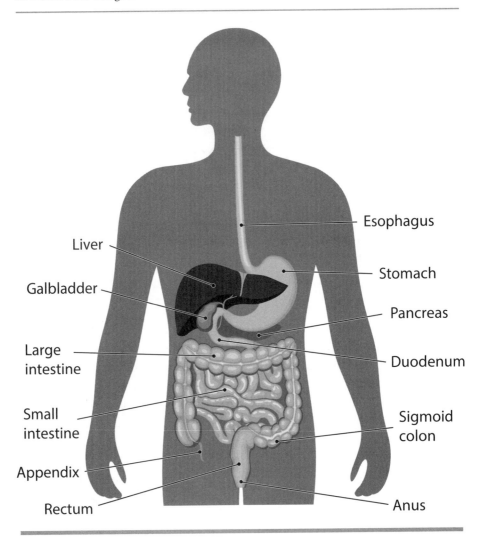

Most gastrointestinal cancers share risk factors and some symptoms (table 10.2). (Other less common symptoms and risk factors are listed throughout the chapter.) Many signs of gastrointestinal cancers, which generally occur over time and progressively become worse, may also be seen with other health conditions. Having one or two symptoms doesn't necessarily mean that you have cancer, but it's important to discuss any persistent symptoms promptly with a doctor so that the root cause can be quickly identified.

TABLE 10.1 Genes with Inherited Mutations That Raise the Risk of Gastrointestinal Cancer

CANCER	GENES
anal	*APC*
colorectal	*APC, CHEK2, EPCAM, MLH1, MSH2, MSH6, MUTYH, PMS2, PTEN, STK11, TP53*
	Other rare mutations: *AXIN2, BMPR1A, GREM1, MSH3, NTHL1, POLD1, POLE, SMAD4* (juvenile polyposis syndrome)
gastric (stomach)	*APC, CDH1, CTNNA1, EPCAM, MLH1, MSH2, MSH6, PMS2, STK11, TP53*
	Other rare mutations: *BMPR1A, SMAD4* (juvenile polyposis syndrome)
pancreatic	*ATM, BRCA1, BRCA2, CDK4, CDKN2A, EPCAM, MLH1, MSH2, MSH6, NF1, PALB2, PMS2, PRSS1* (familial pancreatitis), *STK11*
	Other rare mutations: *MEN1* (multiple endocrine neoplasia type 1), *VHL* (Von Hippel–Lindau syndrome)

Sources: National Comprehensive Cancer Network. "Guidelines: Genetic/familial high-risk assessment: Breast, ovarian, and pancreatic." Version 1.2022, August 2021; National Comprehensive Cancer Network. "Guidelines: Genetic/familial high-risk assessment: Colorectal." Version 1.2021, May 2021; Blair VR, et al. "Hereditary diffuse gastric cancer: Updated clinical practice guidelines." Lancet Oncology 21, no. 8, 2020:e386–97. doi:https://doi.org/10.1016/S1470-2045(20)30219-9.

Colorectal Cancer

Colorectal cancer is the most frequently diagnosed gastrointestinal malignancy. It's sometimes called colon cancer (when it's in the large intestine) or rectal cancer, depending on where it begins. In the United States, colorectal cancer is the third most common cancer. Historically, it's been a disease of the over-50 population. Diagnoses in this group have steadily declined, however, since guidelines for colonoscopy screening were established in the 1990s. Now, younger adults who haven't reached the age for routine colonoscopies are increasingly affected, possibly due to a poor diet, obesity, and an inactive lifestyle—behaviors that can be modified to decrease risk.

The average lifetime risk for colorectal cancer is about 6 percent, but it's higher with certain inherited gene mutations. A personal or family history of colorectal polyps or colorectal cancer, and a low-fiber, high-fat diet

TABLE 10.2 Common Gastrointestinal Cancer Symptoms and Risk Factors

SYMPTOM	COLORECTAL	PANCREATIC	STOMACH	ANAL
dark or bloody stool	x		x	
change in bowel habits	x			
abdominal cramping or pain	x	x	x	
unexplained weight loss	x	x	x	
weakness or fatigue	x	x		
rectal bleeding, itching, pain				x
RISK FACTOR	COLORECTAL	PANCREATIC	STOMACH	ANAL
aging	x	x	x	x
race/ancestry	x	x	x	x
family history	x	x	x	x
inherited mutation/ syndrome	x	x	x	
sedentary lifestyle	x	unclear		
men more than women		x	x	
overweight/obese	x	x	x	
diet	x	unclear	x	
alcohol use	x	x		
tobacco use	x		x	x

that also includes the frequent consumption of red or processed meats and a minimum of fruits and vegetables can heighten colon cancer risk.

Almost all colorectal cancers begin as symptomless polyps in the colon or rectum. These are generally harmless in their early stages, but some polyps can become malignant over time. A change in bowel habits—diarrhea, constipation, stools that appear thinner than usual, or a feeling that the bowels don't empty enough—are common signs of early-stage colorectal cancer. Bloating, cramping, or general discomfort in the abdomen also often occur. Other signs may appear as the cancer advances: jaundice (yellowing of the skin and/or eyes), unexplained weight loss, blood in the stool, and iron-deficiency anemia (low red blood cell count).

Prevention and Early Diagnosis

Routine colonoscopy is the most effective way of preventing colorectal cancer for most average and high-risk people. It's also the most effective way to screen for early-stage cancer in the colon, which is highly treatable. The five-year survival rate for early-stage colorectal cancer is 90 percent. Most colorectal cancers stay within the confines of the colon or rectum for months or years before advancing into the deeper layers of the colon or rectum. Colorectal cancers that reach the lymph nodes can affect the liver, lungs, peritoneum, and other organs. The average five-year survival for late-stage diagnoses is 15 percent.

Types of Colorectal Cancer

Nine of 10 colorectal cancers are adenocarcinomas, which arise from cells that line the inside of the colon and rectum. They can become cancerous if they're not removed. Signet ring cell adenocarcinoma (named for the way it looks under a microscope) is an uncommon subset. Although signet ring cell adenocarcinomas are often more aggressive than other colon adenocarcinomas, they're also more likely to have a biomarker known as microsatellite instability–high (MSI-H, discussed in chapter 20), a characteristic that signals a more favorable prognosis. Less common colorectal tumors include neuroendocrine tumors, which can develop from cells related to hormone production; and sarcomas, which begin in the muscle, blood vessels, or other connective tissues and thus may be found throughout the body, including in the wall of the colon and rectum, although they are very rare.

— My Story —
My Nephew's Diagnosis Was a Wake-Up Call

I have a strong family history of cancer. I thought that maintaining a healthy diet and lifestyle would help me avoid the cancer that plagued both sides of my family. My nephew's diagnosis of colorectal cancer at age 36 was a wake-up call for me and my family. One year later, I was

How Colon and Rectal Cancers Differ

Colorectal cancer includes malignancies of the colon and the rectum, which share several symptoms and are identified similarly. Yet these two cancers can be very different. Colon cancer can grow anywhere along the five-foot length of the colon within the large area between the bottom of the rib cage and the pelvis. Rectal cancer starts in the last five inches of the colon. Because the rectum doesn't have the same protective outer layer that the colon has, cancer that develops there is more likely to spread and to return after treatment. Rectal cancers can be especially threatening because they develop in close proximity to the bowel, bladder, prostate, and vagina, making surgery more difficult. If a tumor affects these organs, a loss of functionality may occur, and additional treatment may be necessary.

also diagnosed with colorectal cancer. Having had breast cancer twice before, I was no stranger to cancer. After my second breast cancer, I was tested for a *BRCA* mutation, which showed that I have a variant of unknown significance in one of my *BRCA2* genes. At the time, I wasn't aware that there were different types of genetic tests, and I was tested only for a *BRCA* mutation. My colorectal cancer was my third primary cancer diagnosis in less than 10 years before I turned 60. Because of all the cancer in my family, including young-onset colorectal cancer, my surgeons recommended that I have expanded genetic testing for a mutation other than *BRCA*. Sure enough, genetic testing proved that I have a Lynch syndrome mutation.

—*Alice*

Racial Differences in Colorectal Cancer Risk and Mortality in the United States

Colorectal cancer diagnoses and deaths have decreased significantly in non-Hispanic white people since colonoscopy screening was introduced, but the same cannot be said for other racial groups.[1] Incidence and mortality are higher in Black people, who are more often diagnosed before age 50. Black people are less likely to be recommended the right care for the type and stage of their cancer. As a result, they are less likely to receive surgical treatments, radiation, and chemotherapy, which may greatly affect their health and survival.[2]

Colorectal cancer is the second most common cancer in Hispanic populations. They're less likely than non-Hispanic white people and Black people to be screened and are more likely to be diagnosed with advanced colorectal cancer. As overall colorectal incidence declines, it's increasing among younger members of all racial and ethnic groups, especially young Hispanics.

Colorectal cancer rates are lowest among Asian Americans and Pacific Islanders. Among Native Americans and Alaskan Natives, colorectal cancer is a leading cause of illness and death.[3]

NOTES:
1. Jackson C, Oman M, Patel A, et al. "Health disparities in colorectal cancer among racial and ethnic minorities in the United States," Journal of Gastrointestinal Oncology 7, Suppl. 1, 2016:S32–43.
2. American Association for Cancer Research. "AACR cancer disparities progress report, 2020." https://cancerprogressreport.aacr.org/disparities.
3. Siegel RL, Miller KD, Sauer AG, et al. "Colorectal cancer statistics, 2020," CA: A Cancer Journal for Clinicians 70, no. 3, 2020:145–64.

Small Bowel Cancer

Cancer is uncommon in the small bowel, which connects the stomach to the colon. This is where most of the digestive process occurs and where nutrients from foods are absorbed into the bloodstream. The small bowel consists of multiple types of cells, so different cancers can start here. Slow-growing gastrointestinal carcinoid tumors (also called neuroendocrine tumors) form in nerve cells that regulate hormone production and cause half of all cancers in the small bowel. Adenocarcinomas, lymphomas, and sarcomas are less common. Tumors can slow the movement of digested food through the intestine, creating abdominal cramping or pain that may worsen after eating. Some tumors can grow large enough to completely block the intestine, causing intense nausea and vomiting. Other symptoms include jaundice (yellowing of the skin and/or eyes) and anemia.

People with chronic intestinal conditions are more prone to small bowel cancer. This includes individuals with celiac disease, a gluten intolerance. Cystic fibrosis also creates a susceptibility to cancer in the small bowel because it prevents the production of enzymes that break down foods.

Diagnosis

If an abnormality is found during an endoscopy, doctors may be able to remove a sample of abnormal tissue to check for cancer cells. When an abnormality can't be reached by a regular endoscope, computed tomography (CT) imaging or a video capsule may be used to pinpoint its location, which is then followed by a biopsy to remove a tissue sample (usually performed with a longer endoscope). In some situations, surgery may be needed to remove the sample.

Pancreatic Cancer

The pancreas aids digestion, secretes insulin, and regulates blood sugar levels in the body. Pancreatic cancer accounts for about 3 percent of all cancers in the United States, but it causes almost 8 percent of all cancer deaths.[1] Situated deep in the abdomen behind the stomach, the pancreas can't be physically examined, and it eludes standard screening, making it difficult to detect early-stage abnormalities. Often called a "silent disease," early-stage pancreatic cancer rarely shows any noticeable symptoms, and symptoms that do appear are often mistaken for less threatening conditions. This cancer spreads quickly and can be very difficult to treat, and possible signs shouldn't be ignored. Signs of pancreatic cancer may include

- jaundice
- urine that is darker than usual
- pancreatitis (swelling of the pancreas)
- dull intermittent pain in the abdomen or the middle or upper back
- painful swelling in an arm or leg
- a burning feeling, bloating, or other discomfort in the stomach
- itchy skin
- nausea
- chills or fever
- recently diagnosed diabetes
- unintentional weight loss

Pancreatic tumors are almost always found after they've already metastasized to the stomach, liver, bowel, lungs, or other organs. Any of the following signs may indicate advancing pancreatic cancer and should be quickly reported to your doctor:

- pain in the abdomen or back that worsens, especially when lying down or after eating
- fluid in the abdomen
- extreme fatigue or weakness
- blood clots
- depression

Risk Factors

Pancreatic cancer is uncommon. The average person has just 1 percent chance of developing this cancer during their lifetime. It does run in some families, although most pancreatic cancer patients don't have a family history of the disease. Inherited mutations are linked to about 10 percent of pancreatic cancers (table 10.1). If you have a strong family history of pancreatic cancer and a gene mutation associated with greater pancreatic cancer risk, your doctor can explain the pros and cons of annual screening and whether you're eligible for pancreatic cancer screening studies. Risk factors for pancreatic cancer include

- being male (slightly higher risk)
- being African American or Ashkenazi Jewish
- a family history of pancreatic cancer
- having chronic pancreatitis
- recently diagnosed diabetes, especially type 2
- a diet that is high in fats and red or processed meats

Tumor Types

Pancreatic tumors are categorized as either exocrine or neuroendocrine based on the type of cell where they begin. These tumors act differently, and they're treated differently. About 93 percent of pancreatic cancers are adenocarcinomas that start in the exocrine cells of the pancreas, which create digestive enzymes. Experts recommend genetic testing for all pancreatic adenocarcinoma patients to better inform their treatment decisions. Other exocrine pancreatic tumors include infrequent acinar cell carcinomas, which overproduce enzymes to help digest fats. Intraductal papillary-mucinous neoplasms in the main pancreatic duct can be benign or cancerous, but even the benign form may increase cancer risk. Women are more likely than men to have an unusual invasive cyst known as mucinous cystic neoplasm with an invasive adenocarcinoma. Less than 10 percent of pancreatic cancers are neuroendocrine tumors that arise from the pancreatic cells that control blood sugar. These grow more slowly than exocrine tumors and have a better prognosis.

Diagnosis

If a pancreatic abnormality is found on an endoscopic ultrasound, in some cases this abnormal tissue can be sampled during the same procedure and then checked for cancer. If an abnormality is found via magnetic resonance cholangiopancreatography (imaging to view the pancreas), your doctor may follow up with an endoscopic ultrasound and biopsy.

Stomach Cancer

Stomach (gastric) cancer is the second most common cause of cancer-related deaths worldwide, although it rarely affects populations in the United States. It is seen more in Asia and Latin America, and diet is suspected to play a significant role. Stomach cancer begins when carcinogenic substances in partially digested foods come into contact with the lining of the stomach or when inflammation persists in the stomach lining. Men are affected more than women. Most stomach cancers are adenocarcinomas that start in the inner lining of the stomach. Gastric adenocarcinomas are either intestinal—chronic inflammation in the lower part of the stomach that's related to *Helicobacter pylori* (see sidebar)—or diffuse, a more aggressive cancer that enlarges quickly in the upper part of the stomach or in the entire stomach.

Like pancreatic cancer, symptoms of stomach cancer don't typically appear until it has advanced. These signs mimic what people experience with an ulcer or a stomach virus. An upper endoscopy is the best way to view the stomach lining to confirm or rule out a diagnosis of cancer. Stomach cancer symptoms may include

- poor appetite
- abdominal pain or swelling
- a sense of fullness after eating
- nausea or vomiting
- anemia
- unintentional weight loss

Risk factors for stomach cancer include

- Hispanic American, African American, Native American, or Asian/Pacific Islander ancestry
- *Helicobacter pylori* infection
- long-term stomach inflammation
- chronic gastritis (a condition that prompts the immune system to attack stomach cells)
- a personal history of mucosa-associated lymphoid tissue lymphoma
- Epstein-Barr virus (an infection that causes herpes and mononucleosis)
- a diet high in salted, smoked, or processed foods and low in fresh fruits and vegetables
- pernicious anemia (reduced red blood cell count from a lack of vitamin B_{12})
- exposure to certain chemicals in the coal, metal, or rubber industries

Helicobacter pylori

Two-thirds of the world's population is estimated to have *Helicobacter pylori*, a common bacterial infection in the mucus of the stomach lining, which causes inflammation and creates precancerous changes. Infection rates are much higher in developing countries than in more industrial nations. The International Agency for Research on Cancer classifies *H. pylori* as a carcinogen in humans. *H. pylori* attacks the protective lining of the stomach, which prevents digestive acids from leaking through and causing ulcers. In fact, it's responsible for many stomach ulcers, including those that were previously thought to be caused by spicy foods and stress. *H. pylori* can even interfere with the immune response in the stomach unless it's treated effectively. Most people who are infected by this bacteria don't have symptoms, although it sometimes causes gastritis (inflammation of the stomach lining). Treatment ordinarily involves two different antibiotics and an acid-suppressing drug to heal the stomach lining.

Anal Cancer

Anal cancer is rare, yet it's one of the fastest-growing cancers in the United States. More people have anal cancer and are dying from it primarily due to a rising trend of human papillomavirus (HPV), a sexually transmitted infection that causes about 90 percent of anal cancers. Nearly all adults will contract HPV at some point during their lives, usually from kissing, intercourse, oral sex, or skin-to-skin contact. The immune systems of most people clear HPV from the body, but this doesn't always happen, especially in those with compromised or suppressed immune systems. Anal cancer is often found early because it can be easily seen and felt during a physical examination or can be identified by colonoscopy. Symptoms of anal cancer may include

- warts in and around the genitals or the anus
- bleeding from the anus or rectum
- pain in the anal area
- a mass or growth in the anal opening
- anal itching that doesn't go away
- change in bowel habits
- discharge or pus from the anus
- swollen lymph glands in the anal or groin areas

Risk factors for anal cancer include

- anal sex
- sexually transmitted diseases
- multiple sex partners
- human immunodeficiency virus/acquired immunodeficiency syndrome (HIV/AIDS)
- a history of HPV-related cancer
- a weakened immune system
- a fistula or another chronic inflammation in or around the anus
- prior pelvic radiation therapy

The Gardasil vaccine protects against the most common cancer-causing strains of HPV. It's recommended for all people ages 9–26. It isn't routinely recommended if you're older than 26. Even those who are already infected may avoid other strains of HPV by being vaccinated. Your doctor can explain whether the vaccine would be of benefit and, if you have a high risk for anal cancer, whether you should have anal cancer screening.

Chapter 11

Genitourinary Cancers

Early-stage prostate cancer often doesn't cause symptoms. Many men don't know that they have it until it's found during a routine medical exam or blood test.

The genitourinary system refers to the organs that produce and excrete urine (the kidneys), transport urine from the body (the ureters, bladder, and urethra), and the reproductive system (figure 11.1). The male reproductive system includes the prostate, testicles, and penis. (The female reproductive system is addressed in chapter 9.) The organs of these two systems are close together. Cancer can begin anywhere in the genitourinary system. It's common in the prostate, but it can also occur in the bladder, ureters, and other organs. If cancer in any part of the genitourinary tract runs in your family or if you have an inherited gene mutation or syndrome that increases the risk for these cancers, it's important to consult with a genetics specialist, who can determine your risk and explain the options for managing it. The focus of this chapter is prostate cancer and other genitourinary cancers that are most closely linked to Lynch syndrome.

Prostate Cancer

Positioned just below the bladder, the prostate produces fluid that combines with sperm cells and other fluids to make semen. A young man's prostate is about the size of a walnut and gets bigger as the person ages. An enlarged prostate doesn't always cause problems, but some men develop benign

FIGURE 11.1 The female (*left*) and male (*right*) genitourinary systems

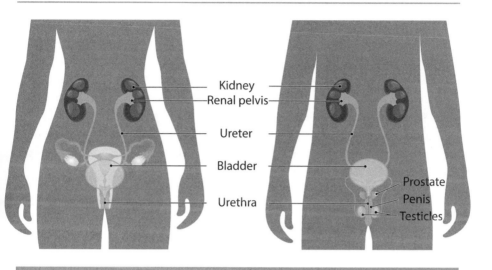

prostatic hyperplasia, a condition that causes an enlarged prostate to squeeze the urethra, causing different types of urinary problems. An enlarged prostate doesn't heighten the likelihood of prostate cancer.

Prostate cancer is the second most common cancer in men in the United States (after skin cancer). About 13 of 100 will develop prostate cancer during their lifetimes—similar to the rate of breast cancer in women. Prostate cancer is more common in older men; about 80 percent of those who reach the age of 80 have cancer cells in their prostate. Most of them, however, aren't diagnosed or negatively impacted by prostate cancer during their lifetime. For many of these individuals, prostate cancer grows slowly and may not cause health issues or require treatment. However, because prostate cancer is the second leading cause of cancer-related death in men, they need to be informed so that they can share decision-making with their doctor for appropriate screening and treatments.

Depending on your specific gene mutation and family history, your lifetime risk may be particularly high for diagnosis at a younger age with a more aggressive cancer that has a poorer prognosis. Cancer that is identified while it's still confined to the prostate is usually curable. Cancers that involve local lymph nodes are treatable but are more difficult to cure. The prognosis declines when cancer cells spread beyond the pelvis or metastasis occurs before diagnosis. Almost all prostate cancers are adenocarcinomas that develop in the cells that make prostate fluid. Small cell carcinomas, neuroendocrine tumors, transitional cell carcinomas, and sarcomas are rare.

Signs and Symptoms

Early-stage prostate cancer often doesn't cause symptoms. Many people don't know that they have it until it's found during a routine medical exam or blood test. While some men notice that they have difficulty urinating—which isn't unusual in older men with enlarged prostates—symptoms rarely show until prostate cancer has advanced. Prostate cancer may cause any of the following conditions:

- difficulty urinating
- painful or burning urination
- a weak or interrupted flow of urine
- urinating more often than usual, especially during the night
- sudden difficulty getting an erection
- blood in semen

Although these same symptoms may be caused by an enlarged prostate, an infection, or conditions other than cancer, they warrant evaluation by a health care provider. Prostate cancer that metastasizes to other areas may cause other symptoms, including

- unexplained weight loss
- swelling in the feet or legs
- pain, especially in the lower back, hip, or pelvis

Understanding Prostate Cancer Risk

Age is the strongest risk factor for developing prostate cancer. The older an individual becomes, the greater the chance of getting prostate cancer; however, 10 percent are diagnosed at age 55 or younger.[1] Men who carry an inherited high-risk gene mutation have a greater risk for prostate cancer, which increases with age (table 11.1). The risk for those with BRCA2 mutations is particularly high.

The following factors increase the risk of prostate cancer. Many individuals with one or more of these risk factors never develop prostate cancer, while some with prostate cancer don't have any of them.

TABLE 11.1 Estimated Lifetime Risk for Prostate Cancer (%)

general population	12
ATM mutation	*
BRCA1 mutation	20–30**
BRCA2 mutation	30–60**
CHEK2 mutation	*
HOXB13 mutation***	30–60
MLH1, MSH6 mutation	≤ 15
MSH2, EPCAM mutation	≤ 25
NBN mutation	*
PALB2 mutation	*

Sources: National Comprehensive Cancer Network. "Guidelines: Genetic/familial high-risk assessment: Breast, ovarian, and pancreatic." Version 1.2022, August 2021; Silvestri V, Leslie G, Barnes D, et al. "Characterization of the cancer spectrum in men with germline BRCA1 and BRCA2 pathogenic variants: Results from the Consortium of Investigators of Modifiers of BRCA1/2 (CIMBA)," Journal of the American Medical Association Oncology 6, no. 8, 2020:1218–30; Shang Z, Zhu S, Zhang H, et al. "Germline homeobox B13 (HOXB13) G84E mutation and prostate cancer risk in European descendants: A meta-analysis of 24,213 cases and 73,631 controls, 2013," European Urology 64, no. 1, 2013:173–76; National Comprehensive Cancer Network. "Guidelines: Genetic/familial high-risk assessment: Colorectal." Version 1.2021, May 2021.

*More research is needed to determine the level of risk for people with mutations in these genes.

**Lifetime to age 85.

***One mutation in this gene, known as G84E, can cause prostate cancer to run in some families and increases the risk for early-onset prostate cancer.

- Being older than 50 is the primary risk factor for prostate cancer. More than half of prostate cancers occur in men who are 65 or older.
- If other individuals in your family have had prostate cancer, you're more likely to have it too, especially if a first-degree relative has been diagnosed, which doubles your risk.
- An inherited mutation in certain genes elevates risk.

- Black men develop prostate cancer more than males of other races. They're more often diagnosed at younger ages with aggressive tumors that grow beyond the prostate. They also die from the disease twice as often as others with prostate cancer.
- Individuals who are obese tend to be diagnosed with more advanced prostate cancer, which is more difficult to treat.

Screening and Diagnosis

Deciding to be screened for prostate cancer should involve a discussion with your health care provider and should be tailored for your individual risk and health factors. Screening is generally not recommended for people who are over the age of 75 or those with other major medical conditions that may shorten their life. When screening is indicated, the prostate-specific antigen (PSA) test is the standard tool for diagnosing prostate cancer. (Current screening guidelines are listed in chapter 14.) A higher PSA result may be caused by one of several conditions, including an infection, an enlarged prostate, or cancer. A biopsy is usually needed to determine whether prostate cancer is the cause. An MRI or transrectal ultrasound can ensure that the biopsy incision is made precisely in the correct spot; it can also be used to determine the stage of the cancer. Biopsy with transrectal ultrasound involves putting a finger-size probe into the rectum, which uses high-energy sound waves to create a computer image of the prostate for an accurate biopsy.

— *My Story* —

My Father Refused Genetic Testing after His Prostate Cancer Diagnosis

I was diagnosed with breast cancer at a young age and tested positive for a *BRCA2* mutation at age 35. I encouraged my father to have genetic testing, but he wouldn't go. When his PSA test rose sharply, I told him he should get it checked and that prostate cancer could be related to a *BRCA2* mutation. Neither my father nor his doctors listened. By the time my father was diagnosed with prostate cancer, it was already advanced. Eventually, treatment stopped working, and he died from metastatic prostate cancer. My father never had genetic testing, but I assume that I inherited my *BRCA2* mutation from him. Sadly, neither of my two brothers have been tested either, although I frequently remind them about the importance of knowing their risk.

—Samantha

Bladder, Ureter, and Renal Pelvis Cancers

The bean-shaped kidneys below the rib cage on both sides of the spine filter liquid waste and extra water from the blood, which is then expelled as urine. Urine collects in the center of each kidney in an area called the renal pelvis. From there, it's funneled into the ureters, the tubes that connect the kidneys to the bladder. The bladder expands as urine collects. When it's full, muscles in the bladder wall contract to force urine through the urethra and out of the body. Because the bladder, ureters, and renal pelvis share common cells, cancers found in these organs often act alike, have similar symptoms, and are diagnosed and treated in the same way.

Bladder and Ureter Cancers

The bladder consists of several tissue layers of different types of cells. Cancer typically starts in the innermost lining of the bladder and can grow into or through other layers of the bladder wall. Over time, cancer cells may grow beyond the bladder and into nearby tissues, spreading to lymph nodes or other organs, such as lungs, liver, or bones. Blood in the urine with or without other urinary symptoms is the most common symptom of bladder cancer, but blood can also be caused by infection or bladder stones (like kidney stones but in the bladder). Blood may be visible in the urine or show up in a routine urine test. Any blood in the urine, even if it disappears, should be reported promptly to a doctor.

Many of the same symptoms that are caused by an enlarged prostate or a common urinary tract infection can also indicate the presence of bladder cancer. These should never be ignored or dismissed. Symptoms of bladder or ureter cancer may include

- blood or blood clots in the urine
- painful or frequent urination
- feeling an urgent need to urinate, even when the bladder isn't full
- difficulty urinating or urinating weakly

Other symptoms may occur as the cancer grows or advances, including

- being unable to urinate
- lower or upper back pain on one side
- loss of appetite
- unexplained weight loss
- fatigue
- swollen feet
- bone pain

Understanding Risk

Smoking is the most common cause of bladder cancer. Having an inherited mutation in a Lynch syndrome gene also increases the chance for bladder or ureter cancer, so it's very important to recognize and manage your risk (table 11.2). Genetic counseling is recommended if you have a strong family history of these cancers and you haven't already been tested for an inherited mutation. Ideally, testing would begin with the person in your family who was diagnosed with either of these cancers.

Risk factors for bladder and ureter cancers:

- Smoking.
- Being older. The average age at diagnosis is 73 years.

TABLE 11.2 Estimated Lifetime Risk for Bladder, Renal Pelvis, and Ureter Cancers (%)

	BLADDER	RENAL PELVIS AND URETER
general population	2.4	1
EPCAM mutation	≤15	2–30
MLH1 mutation	≤10	≤5.0
MSH2 mutation	≤15	2–30
MSH6 mutation	≤10	≤5.0
PMS2 mutation	unclear	unclear

Source: National Comprehensive Cancer Network. "Guidelines: Genetic/familial high-risk assessment: Colorectal." Version 1.2021, May 2021.

- Sex. Men are diagnosed with bladder cancer four times more often than women; they also have ureter cancer more often.
- Family history. A personal or family history of any type of urinary tract cancer.
- Lynch syndrome or an inherited mutation in a *PTEN* gene.
- Race/ethnicity. Non-Hispanic white Americans are diagnosed twice as often as Black or Hispanic Americans. Rates among Asian and Native American people are slightly lower.
- Chronic bladder infections or kidney stones.
- Previous radiation to the pelvis.
- Long-term use of catheters.
- Occupational exposure to industrial chemicals used to make plastics, paints, textiles, leather, and rubber.
- Being a hairdresser or barber who dyes others' hair (a small risk increase). The same risk hasn't been consistently observed in people whose hair is colored.[2]
- Previous treatment with the chemotherapy drug Cytoxan (cyclophosphamide) or the diabetes medication Actos (pioglitazone).
- Drinking chlorine-treated water or water that contains a high level of arsenic.

Types of Bladder and Ureter Cancers

Non–muscle invasive bladder cancer originates and remains in the inside lining of the bladder and is the most common type of cancer there. Muscle-invasive bladder cancers are less common and grow deep into the bladder wall. These can be the most dangerous because they more frequently metastasize, and treatment is more challenging.

Almost all bladder cancers and most ureter cancers are urothelial carcinomas, which start in the cellular lining of the urinary tract. The same type of urothelial cells line segments of the kidneys, the ureters, and the urethra, so when urothelial bladder cancer is identified, the entire urinary tract should be checked for malignancies.

Other types of bladder cancer are less common. Adenocarcinomas, squamous cell carcinomas, sarcomas, or small cell carcinomas develop less often than urothelial carcinomas and may be treated differently.

Diagnosis

No standard screening tests are available for bladder or ureter cancer, although this is an ongoing area of research. People who have already been treated for bladder cancer may be screened with cystoscopy and urine cytology (described below). Diagnosis begins with a thorough physical examination and a review of symptoms. If symptoms are consistent with genitourinary cancer, referral to a urologist is recommended. Tests to identify bladder or ureter cancer may include

- A urinalysis to check for blood in the urine.
- A urine cytology test to look for precancerous or cancer cells in the urine. A negative cytology result doesn't necessarily rule out the possibility of cancer.
- A cystoscopy (an outpatient procedure). A tiny, flexible tube with a lighted lens is passed through the urethra to view the bladder or ureters. This short procedure can identify a suspicious area or growth and help determine whether a biopsy or surgery is required. Blue light cystoscopy is even more accurate. It uses a special injected chemical that is absorbed by tumor cells and makes them more obvious.
- A ureteroscopy (an outpatient procedure), which threads a tube into a ureter. When ureter cancer is suspected, this test can be used to biopsy the questionable tissue. This is the same procedure used to diagnose stones in the kidneys, bladder, and ureters.
- A retrograde pyelography (x-ray imaging that is sometimes used along with cystoscopy to view the urinary tract in better detail). It's also helpful to identify the source of blood in the urine. Performed in an operating room under anesthesia, this test uses a small catheter that's inserted through the urethra and bladder and into a ureter. Contrast dye is then injected into the ureter. If a tumor is confirmed, a biopsy can be done at the same time.
- A transurethral bladder tumor resection—a surgical biopsy procedure—to take a sample of the tumor if cystoscopy finds abnormal tissue.
- A CT scan, MRI, PET scan, or ultrasound to determine whether cancer has spread.

Renal Pelvis Cancers

If you have an inherited mutation in a Lynch syndrome gene, you have a higher-than-average chance of developing urothelial carcinoma that begins in the renal pelvis or a ureter. Symptoms are similar to those of bladder cancers: blood in the urine, persistent back pain, frequent or painful urination, fatigue, and/or unexplained weight loss.

Bladder, ureter, and renal pelvis cancers share some of the same risk factors, including increasing age, smoking, and being male. Other risk factors for renal pelvis cancer include the following:

- obesity
- chronic high blood pressure
- chronic kidney disease
- long-term dialysis
- long-term use of certain pain medications, including aspirin, acetaminophen, or ibuprofen
- Lynch syndrome, Von Hippel-Lindau disease, and certain other inherited syndromes
- family history of kidney cancer

Chapter 12

Melanoma

While the risk factors for many cancers remain a mystery, the primary cause of melanoma is well known. Knowing about sun safety provides opportunities to protect yourself and reduce your likelihood of melanoma and other skin cancers.

Melanoma is the most aggressive and dangerous type of skin cancer. Globally, diagnoses of melanoma are growing rapidly. This may be caused by several factors, including increased screening that leads to earlier detection, excessive unprotected sun exposure, climate change, and use of tanning beds. Melanoma typically develops after age 50. However, it's one of the most common cancers in young adults, especially women, before age 30.[1] Melanoma that runs in families can occur at a younger age.

Skin is the human body's largest organ; the average adult has about eight pounds of it. Except for the eyes, the entire external surface of the body is covered with skin, but there's much more to it than what is readily visible. The epidermis is the outermost layer of skin. It is thinnest in the eyelids and genitalia and thickest in the palms of the hands and soles of the feet. The epidermis is the body's first line of defense against the elements, and it helps to regulate body temperature. It also includes melanocytes, the cells that produce melanin, the natural pigment in hair, skin, and the iris of the eye. A thin layer of cells known as the basement membrane separates the epidermis from the dermis. The next layer of skin is the thicker dermis, which holds blood vessels and the nerve endings that facilitate sensation. It's where hairs on the skin take root and where oil glands lubricate and waterproof the skin. Subcutaneous fat below the epidermis and dermis forms a protective pad for muscles and bones.

Melanoma of the Skin

Melanoma is diagnosed less often than basal cell and squamous cell carcinomas, but it's more dangerous and can be life-threatening. It accounts for about 1 percent of all skin cancers, yet it causes most skin cancer fatalities. Melanoma begins when melanocytes become damaged and evolve into cancer cells (figure 12.1). Although it can start anywhere in the body—in mucous membranes, in the gastrointestinal tract, in reproductive organs, in the eyes, and under the nails—melanoma is primarily found in the skin. Women often develop melanoma on their legs; men tend to have it on their torsos.

Melanoma that grows from the epidermis to the deeper layer of the dermis can enter the blood or lymph vessels and then metastasize to other parts of the body. The five-year survival rate when melanoma reaches the lymph nodes is 65 percent; it is 25 percent when melanoma reaches distant organs. Fortunately, most melanomas are found and treated before that happens. Almost all early-stage melanoma is treated successfully, with a five-year survival rate of 99 percent.[2]

FIGURE 12.1 Types of skin cancer

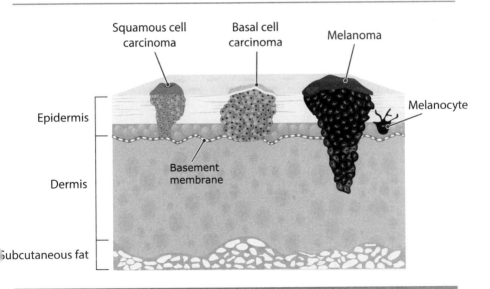

FIGURE 12.2 Melanomas may have traits that differentiate them from ordinary moles

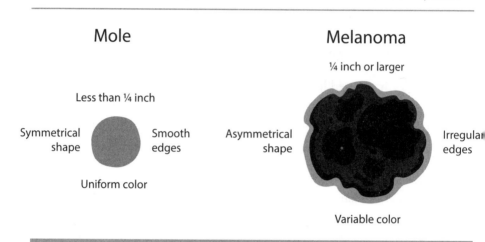

The Mole-Melanoma Connection

Like freckles, moles are common, especially in people who repeatedly expose their skin to sunlight. Unlike freckles, which are created by an overproduction of melanin, moles develop when melanocytes grow in clusters instead of spreading throughout the skin. Melanomas can begin in existing moles, but most moles aren't harmful. Benign atypical moles (dysplastic nevi), however, may indicate a greater risk for melanoma, especially if they're large, irregularly shaped, or change over time (figure 12.2). Atypical moles can run in families. Having one or more moles, or one or more that is one-quarter inch or larger in diameter significantly raises melanoma risk. Although more moles can mean more risk, having fewer moles doesn't necessarily equate to less risk.

— *My Story* —

My Unusual Mole Turned into Melanoma

I was 17 years old when I first heard of melanoma. My mother's doctor noticed a white spot on my back and said that I should see a dermatologist. I waited, and as it quickly grew, a mole formed in the middle with a white ring around it. I got worried and decided to get it checked out.

Ultimately, a 1.5-inch area on my back was removed to get it all. It was a difficult recovery. I've been seen by a dermatologist every year since for the past 28 years. I've had many spots removed, but none have been cancerous. It wasn't until my journey into *BRCA* testing that I found out melanoma is hereditary. This was surprising to me as no one in my family has had melanoma.

—Michelle

Symptoms

The ABCDE rules are an easy way to tell the difference between a normal mole and one that should be assessed by a dermatologist (table 12.1). These characteristics generally apply to melanomas, although some melanomas don't follow these rules.

TABLE 12.1 The ABCDE Rules: Common Differences between Moles and Melanomas

CHARACTERISTIC	MELANOMAS	COMMON MOLES
Asymmetry	half of the area, including the edges, doesn't match the other half	symmetrically round or oval
Border	irregular or jagged	smooth and even
Color	variable shades of tan, brown, or black, with patches of red, white, or blue*	consistent shade of tan, brown, or black
Diameter	usually ¼ inch (about the size of a pencil eraser) or larger**	usually less than ¼ inch**
Evolving	changes size, shape, color, or texture, or becomes itchy, is painful, or bleeds	remains the same

*Not all melanomas are different colors. Some can be the same color as the rest of the skin.

**Most moles and melanomas follow this rule, but some melanomas can be smaller than ¼ inch, and some harmless moles can be larger than ¼ inch in diameter.

The Ugly Duckling Rule

Generally, a person's benign moles look alike and are of similar size. Melanomas, however, can look different and stand out. These "ugly ducklings" may meet one or more of the ABCDE rules for melanoma. They may be lighter or darker or shaped differently than other moles, and they should be assessed by a dermatologist.

Types of Melanoma

Melanomas of the skin are classified into four major types:

- Superficial spreading melanoma, the most common type, develops as a flat or somewhat raised spot in the skin and may have a variety of colors ranging from pink or white to black or brown. This type of melanoma may take months or years to grow across the epidermis before it reaches deeper into the skin. While superficial spreading melanoma can be found nearly anywhere on the body, it's most likely to appear in areas that have been exposed to high levels of ultraviolet (UV) light: the torso, legs, and upper back.
- Nodular melanoma forms as a firm, rounded bump on the skin that may tend to bleed. Unlike other melanomas, this kind has often grown deep into the dermis by the time it's identified, and it has a poorer prognosis.
- Acral lentiginous melanoma is the most common melanoma among people with dark skin. It ordinarily appears as a brown or black area—like a bruise that doesn't heal—under the nails, on the soles of the feet, or on the palms. These cancers tend to have poorer prognoses.

- Lentigo maligna melanoma is usually found in older people. It's a slow-growing, invasive cancer that is caused by chronic sun exposure on the face, ears, or arms. It may be flat or somewhat raised on the skin with uneven edges. This type of melanoma most often appears bluish-black, although it can be light brown, dark brown, red, white, or gray.

Other less common types, such as mucosal melanoma, don't fit into any of these categories. Ocular melanoma, although it has a similar name, is a disease that behaves differently in terms of natural history, genetic altera-tions, and response to treatment (see below).

Melanoma Risk

About 1 in 50 people in the United States develop melanoma in their lifetime (table 12.2). Ultraviolet light is a known carcinogen and the primary (and pre-ventable) cause of melanoma. Exposure to UV, whether the source is the sun, sun lamps, or tanning beds, damages skin. Tanning beds result in more mela-noma and other skin cancers than the number of lung cancers caused by smok-ing.[3] People with a rare condition known as xeroderma pigmentosum have

TABLE 12.2 Estimated Lifetime Risk for Melanoma (%)

general population	0.1–2.8*
BAP1 mutation	undetermined increase**
BRCA2 mutation	***
CDK4 mutation	≤80.0
CDKN2A mutation	28.0–67.0
PTEN mutation	***

Sources: National Comprehensive Cancer Network. "Guidelines: Genetic/familial high-risk assessment: Breast, ovarian, and pancreatic." Version 1.2022, August 2021; Pilarski R. "The role of BRCA testing in hereditary pancreatic and prostate cancer families," American Society of Clinical Oncology Educational Book 39, 2019:79–86; Puntervoll H, Yang X, Vetti H, et al. "Melanoma prone families with CDK4 germline mutation: Phenotypic profile and associations with MC1R variants," Journal of Medical Genetics 50, no. 4, 2013:264–70.

*Risk varies by race, ethnicity, gender, and melanoma subtype.

**Ocular melanomas are one of the main cancers associated with this mutation.

***The risk for melanoma is believed to be increased, but the exact risk is unclear.

inherited mutations in one of at least nine different genes that ordinarily repair DNA damage from ultraviolet radiation. These people can be severely burned after just a few minutes in the sun. Individuals with xeroderma pigmentosum have a 10,000-fold increased risk for skin cancer, including melanoma, compared to the average person.[4] Most people with this condition develop skin cancer during childhood.

While the risk factors for many cancers remain a mystery, the primary cause of melanoma is well known. Knowing about sun safety provides opportunities to protect yourself and reduce your likelihood of melanoma and other skin cancers. Risk factors for melanoma include the following:

- frequent exposure to intense ultraviolet rays from the sun, tanning beds, or sun lamps
- increasing age (most melanoma occurs after age 60)
- dysplastic nevus syndrome (atypical mole syndrome), a condition that can cause 100 or more moles on the body, especially with a family history of melanoma
- Caucasian ancestry
- 10 or more atypical moles
- multiple moles larger than the tip of a pencil eraser
- a personal history of melanoma
- a family history of melanoma
- a weakened or suppressed immune system
- light skin that freckles or burns easily
- blue or green eyes
- red or blond hair
- a history of blistering sunburns, especially during childhood, and/or multiple sunburns between ages 15 and 20[5]
- Parkinson's disease (having melanoma also raises the risk of Parkinson's)[6]
- certain high-risk genetic mutations (see table 12.2)

Familial Melanoma

Compared to sporadic melanoma, which usually occurs after age 50, familial melanoma may develop much earlier. Most sporadic melanomas occur in people with no apparent family history or known family mutation, and most familial melanomas develop from shared environmental factors rather than predisposing gene mutations. Family members who have an inherited *CDKN2A* gene mutation can develop multiple atypical moles (familial atypical multiple mole melanoma syndrome). More frequently, this same syndrome occurs in people who don't have a *CDKN2A* mutation. Inherited mutations in other genes, including *BRCA2*, *CDK4*, and *PTEN*, may also amplify melanoma risk. Inherited mutations in the *BAP1* gene raise the likelihood of melanoma in the skin and the eye. Genetic counseling and consideration of testing are recommended for individuals with one or more of the following:

- three or more melanomas, especially before age 45
- three or more blood relatives on the same side of the family with melanoma or pancreatic cancer
- one or more Spitz nevus moles that affect children and adolescents, a close blood relative with melanoma in the eye, mesothelioma (cancer that is related to asbestos exposure), or meningioma or astrocytoma (types of brain tumor)

— EXPERT VIEW —
Melanoma and Family History

BY JOANNE JETER, MD

When we think about melanomas and family history, we can put families into one of three categories. The first category, which is the most common, is sporadic melanoma. Individuals in this category have a personal history of melanoma, but they don't have a family history of melanoma or associated cancers, such as pancreatic cancer. The second category is familial melanoma, which means that multiple individuals in the family have melanoma, but no inherited gene mutation cause can be identified. This can be due to shared physical characteristics, such as skin, hair, or eye color; number of moles; shared behaviors; or environmental factors. The third category, which is by far the least common, is hereditary melanoma or melanoma due to an increased risk from an inherited genetic alteration.

Ancestry Affects Melanoma Risk

Anyone can develop melanoma, regardless of their skin color. Even though everybody has the same number of melanocytes, the amount of melanin produced determines the degree of lightness or darkness of a person's skin. White people are significantly more prone to melanoma than are individuals of color, who have more skin pigment. Compared to white people, the incidence in Native Americans and Native Alaskans is 80 percent lower and in Hispanics about 84 percent lower.[1] Black people and Asian/Pacific Islanders rarely have melanoma; when they do, it tends to develop on the palms, soles of the feet, under the nails, and in mucous membranes.

Despite the lower incidence among Black people, they tend to develop the more aggressive subtypes of melanoma, and they more often die from the disease. The five-year melanoma survival rate is 70 percent for Black people compared to 94 percent among white people. The prognoses for acral lentiginous and mucosal melanoma, the most common subtype found in African Americans, are worse for all races.

NOTE:

1. Centers for Disease Control and Prevention. "Rate of new cancers: Melanomas of the skin, United States, 2017." https://gis.cdc.gov/Cancer/USCS /DataViz.html.

Screening and Diagnosis

The best cure for melanoma is early detection. Identifying melanoma isn't always easy, however, because the shape, size, color, and texture can vary widely. Sometimes, none of the ordinary warning signs appear. It's crucial to thoroughly inspect your skin, including areas that don't ordinarily see the sun. Using the ABCDE rules as a guide, look carefully each month, even during the winter, for any changes: a new freckle or mole; an existing mole that grows, itches, or becomes swollen; a sore spot that doesn't heal; or any irregular skin change. (Use a handheld mirror or ask a partner to examine your back and other hard-to-see areas.) Any skin abnormality that doesn't heal or is unexpectedly dark, regardless of size, should be examined by a dermatologist, who can determine whether a biopsy is appropriate. A head-to-toe skin check by a doctor should be part of your annual physical exam. You may need more frequent professional screening if you have higher-than-average risk for melanoma or another skin cancer.

Ocular Melanoma

Melanoma doesn't often affect the eyes. When it does, it starts from DNA damage that prompts pigment cells in an eye to multiply out of control. The mutated cells collect in or on the eye and form ocular melanoma, a condition that can cause vision loss if it develops in critical parts of the eye.

The eye has three layers: the outer sclera, the middle uvea (which includes the pigmented part of the eye), and the inner retina. Ocular melanoma almost always starts in the uvea. In rare cases, it affects the conjunctiva, the lubricating protective cover inside the eyelids and over the sclera. Melanoma can also form in the cells that produce eye color.

Having light-colored eyes or an inherited mutation in the *BAP1* gene raises the risk for ocular melanoma. Some data suggest that an inherited mutation in *BRCA2* may also slightly increase the risk for ocular melanoma.

Symptoms

Early-stage ocular melanoma can be difficult to detect on your own because it doesn't always show symptoms. In most cases, it begins in a part of the eye that can't be seen in a mirror, underscoring the importance of routine eye exams by an ophthalmologist (a doctor who specializes in eye and vision care).

Eight Steps to Lower Melanoma Risk

1. Limit sun exposure. If possible, stay in the shade or avoid exposure between 10:00 am and 4:00 p.m., when the sun is strongest.

2. Wear protective, UV-sensitive clothing when outside.

3. Wear a hat with a brim that shades your face, neck, and ears.

4. Use a broad-spectrum sunscreen with an SPF of 30 or higher every day, even on cloudy days. Apply generously to all exposed parts of the body 15–30 minutes before going outside. Reapply every couple of hours or hourly if you swim or sweat. Use a lip balm or lipstick that has an SPF of at least 30.

5. Wear sunglasses that block out 100 percent of UVA and UVB rays.

6. Avoid sun lamps and tanning beds.

7. Be extra cautious if you take medication that increases sensitivity to the sun.

8. Protect children from the sun. Sunburns early in life affect melanoma risk later.

Melanomas inside the eye may be orange, may be thicker than expected, and may leak fluid. Symptoms of ocular melanoma may include

- a dark spot on the iris or the conjunctiva
- flashing lights or shadows in the eyes
- pain in an eye
- floaters (small spots that move around in your field of vision)
- a change in the shape of the pupil
- blurred or distorted vision in one eye
- a blind spot in your side vision

Risk factors for ocular melanoma include

- white ancestry and over age 50
- blue or green eyes
- certain inherited mutations in the *BAP1* or *BRCA2* genes
- xeroderma pigmentosum
- extended exposure to natural or artificial sunlight (may cause conjunctival melanoma)
- abnormal skin pigmentation of the conjunctival lining of the eyelids or increased pigmentation on the uvea
- a mole or freckle in or on the surface of the eye

Screening and Diagnosis
In many cases, ocular melanoma is identified during a routine eye exam. When symptoms appear, an ophthalmologist will first dilate the eye and then examine it. Additional tests may be needed to either rule out melanoma or make a diagnosis:

- Ultrasound or MRI provides initial images of the eye.
- Angiography involves a dye that is injected into the arm and travels to your eye, which highlights abnormalities on the inside of the eye.
- Autofluorescence uses a special camera that reveals abnormalities, which show up as small points of light in a photograph.
- Optical coherence tomography provides very detailed images of the inside of the eye.
- A biopsy may be required when conjunctival melanoma is suspected.

Part III
Strategies for Risk Reduction and Early Detection

The chapters in this part focus on strategies and recommendations regarding screening for cancers and lowering the likelihood of developing them. Screening tests and exams are important tools that often find cancer before it causes symptoms like a lump that can be felt or unexplained fatigue. Cancers discovered in their earliest stages are more likely to be smaller and still confined to the area where they began. That means that other parts of the body aren't affected, which broadens treatment options and may make treatment more likely to succeed. Some screening, such as removing precancerous polyps or precancerous moles, can detect changes early enough to prevent cancer.

Screening methodologies aren't perfect, however. Some produce false-positive results, which can cause anxiety and unnecessary additional procedures. Some screening may not find cancer that has already developed, producing a false-negative result that can lead to a false sense of security. Even so, screening for certain cancers is an important part of overall health care, especially if you're at high risk.

While you can't control every facet of life that increases cancer risk, you can take steps to minimize many risk factors. Of course, some risk management actions are more easily accomplished than others. You can't avoid growing older, or fix the mutated gene that you inherited, or erase the cancer history in your family. But there may be factors that you can modify to lower your risk. Poor nutrition, excess weight, lack of physical activity, insufficient sleep, stress and anxiety, smoking, and drinking alcohol may inflate your risk for numerous cancers. Ignore these influences, and your likelihood of developing multiple cancers grows. Manage them, however, and you reduce the odds while improving your overall health.

Taking risk-reducing medications or having surgical procedures are more aggressive ways to decrease cancer risk. These actions can cause both short-term and long-term side effects, but they also reduce risk more dramatically. Preventive actions don't guarantee that you'll never develop cancer, but they may be your most effective option to lower your high cancer risk. Carefully consider the benefits and limitations of each alternative before you decide to pursue it.

Chapter 13

Risk Management Guidelines

Screening recommendations and risk management guidelines for Lynch syndrome vary by mutation and family cancer history. . . . It's important to speak with your genetic counselor and doctor to determine which options are best for you.

There is no foolproof method to eliminate cancer risk, but following expert-endorsed risk management guidelines can lower your chance of a cancer diagnosis or increase your chance of finding cancer at its earliest and most treatable stage. The cancer screening and risk management guidelines in this chapter are based on the most current research. They're recommended by the National Comprehensive Cancer Network (NCCN) or other expert organizations for people who are predisposed to cancer because of their family history or an inherited high-risk gene mutation. Most of these guidelines are updated annually, so if you have a high risk for cancer due to your family history or an inherited gene mutation, it's a good idea to regularly check with your doctor or genetic counselor for any changes. Each recommendation has benefits and risks, which you should discuss with your doctor and carefully consider before you make decisions about treatment. Some of the gene mutations covered here are rare, and risk management for some is complex.

Whenever possible, you should seek out health care professionals who have specific expertise in managing people who have the same mutation that you have. In addition to the guidelines in this chapter, which are listed by gene to help you easily find information that is most meaningful to you, chapters 14–18 provide detailed information about strategies. NCCN guidelines also state the following:

- Genetic counseling and genetic testing should be considered for at-risk relatives.
- Individuals of reproductive age should be advised about their options for prenatal diagnosis and assisted reproduction, including pre-implantation genetic testing (see chapter 27).

Guidelines for *BRCA1* or *BRCA2* Gene Mutations

Mutations in the *BRCA1* and *BRCA2* genes raise the risk for breast, ovarian, pancreatic, and prostate cancers and may raise the risk for melanoma (table 13.1).

Guidelines for Lynch Syndrome Gene Mutations (*MLH1, MSH2, MSH6, PMS2, EPCAM*)

Lynch syndrome mutations raise the risk for colorectal, endometrial, and other cancers. Screening recommendations and risk management guidelines for Lynch syndrome vary by mutation and family cancer history (table 13.2). It's important to speak with your genetic counselor and doctor to determine which options are best for you.

Guidelines for Mutations in Other Genes

Inherited mutations in other genes can also increase the likelihood of a cancer diagnosis. National guidelines address screening and risk management for people with these mutations (tables 13.3–13.12).

APC and FAP

Specific risk management guidelines apply to people with *APC* mutations who have familial adenomatous polyposis (FAP) or attenuated FAP (AFAP) (table 13.3). Because of the very high risk for multiple cancers and the complexities of risk management, the NCCN recommends that people with these mutations receive care at a facility with expertise in managing those with FAP.

TABLE 13.1 Summary of Guidelines for *BRCA1* and *BRCA2* Gene Mutations

BEGINNING AGE	RECOMMENDATIONS
For women	
18	learn to be aware of breast changes; may include monthly breast self-exams
25	clinical breast exam every 6–12 months
25*	annual breast MRI with contrast until age 75
30	annual mammogram; consider 3D mammography, if available, until age 75
no specified age	consider risk-reducing mastectomy; consider medication to reduce breast cancer risk
30–35	consider annual transvaginal ultrasound and CA-125 blood test (at doctor's discretion)
35–40 (*BRCA1*)**	remove ovaries / fallopian tubes; discuss risks and benefits of removing the uterus at the same time
40–45 (*BRCA2*)**	remove ovaries / fallopian tubes
75	consider whether to continue breast screening
For men	
35	breast self-exam education/training; annual clinical breast exam
40 (*BRCA1*)	consider annual prostate cancer screening with PSA testing and digital rectal exam (after discussion with your doctor about limitations and benefits of screening)
40 (*BRCA2*)	recommend annual prostate cancer screening with PSA testing and digital rectal exam (after discussion with your doctor about limitations and benefits of screening)
50 (for men with gynecomastia)***	consider annual mammogram
For men and women	
no specified age	learn about signs and symptoms of *BRCA*-related cancers; consider annual full-body skin examination

TABLE 13.1 (*continued*)

BEGINNING AGE	RECOMMENDATIONS
50 with family history of pancreatic cancer****	consider magnetic resonance cholangiopancreatography (MRCP) and / or endoscopic ultrasound (EUS); consider participating in a pancreatic cancer screening study

Sources: National Comprehensive Cancer Network. "Guidelines: Genetic/familial high-risk assessment: Breast, ovarian, and pancreatic." Version 1.2022, August 2021.

*Or earlier, based on family history of breast cancer.

**Upon completion of childbearing.

***Or earlier, based on family history of male breast cancer.

****Or 10 years before the earliest pancreatic cancer diagnosis in the family. Screening should be performed by a facility that is experienced with screening for pancreatic cancer.

TABLE 13.2 Summary of Guidelines for Lynch Syndrome Gene Mutations

BEGINNING AGE	RECOMMENDATIONS
For women	
30	be aware of endometrial and ovarian cancer symptoms
30–35	consider endometrial biopsy every 1–2 years
no specified age	consider taking an oral contraceptive (after discussion with your doctor about limitations and benefits)
	consider annual transvaginal ultrasound* and CA-125 blood test (at doctor's discretion)
after childbearing	consider risk-reducing hysterectomy; discuss risk-reducing removal of your ovaries and fallopian tubes with your doctor (*EPCAM, MLH1, MSH2, MSH6*)
For men	
40	consider annual prostate cancer screening with PSA testing and digital rectal exam (after discussion with your doctor about limitations and benefits of screening)

TABLE 13.2 (*continued*)

BEGINNING AGE	RECOMMENDATIONS
For men and women	
adulthood (and after childbearing)	consider daily aspirin use (discuss risks, benefits, and dose with your doctor)
20–25**	high-quality colonoscopy every 1–2 years (*EPCAM*, *MLH1*, *MSH2*)
30–35**	high-quality colonoscopy every 1–2 years (*MSH6*, *PMS2*)
30–35	consider annual urinalysis, especially if you have a family history of urothelial cancer or you have an *MSH2* mutation (especially men)
40	consider baseline esophagogastroduodenoscopy with random stomach biopsy; consider continued surveillance every 3–5 years if you're in a high-risk category for gastric cancer;*** consider *H. pylori* testing, and treatment if detected
50 with family history of pancreatic cancer****	consider annual magnetic resonance cholangiopancreatography (MRCP) and/or endoscopic ultrasound (EUS) (*EPCAM*, *MLH1*, *MSH2*, *MSH6*); consider participating in a pancreatic cancer screening study
no specified age	consider annual physical and neurological exam; know the signs and symptoms of neurologic cancer and the importance of prompt reporting of abnormal symptoms to your doctor; consider a clinical skin exam every 1–2 years

Source: National Comprehensive Cancer Network. "Guidelines: Genetic/familial high-risk assessment: Colorectal." Version 1.2021, May 2021.

*The NCCN does not recommend using transvaginal ultrasound for endometrial cancer screening before menopause.

**Or earlier, based on a family history of colon cancer.

***Includes men, older people, and individuals who are of Asian ethnicity; have an *MLH1* or *MSH2* mutation or a first-degree relative with gastric cancer; and those who live in or are from countries with high rates of gastric cancer, chronic autoimmune gastritis, gastric intestinal metaplasia, or gastric adenomas.

****Or 10 years before the earliest pancreatic diagnosis in the family. Screening should be performed by a facility that is experienced with screening for pancreatic cancer.

TABLE 13.3 Summary of Guidelines for *APC* Gene Mutations*

BEGINNING AGE	RECOMMENDATIONS
infants	physical exam to screen for liver tumors; abdominal ultrasound and AFP (alpha-fetoprotein) blood levels every 3–6 months until age 5
10–15**	annual high-quality colonoscopy or flexible sigmoidoscopy
late teenage years	thyroid ultrasound every 2–5 years, with referral to thyroid expert if findings are abnormal***
no specified age (depends on personal history of polyps and individual preferences)	risk-reducing colectomy; speak with health care experts about benefits and risks of each colectomy surgical option
after colectomy	sigmoidoscopy (frequency depends on type of surgery and amount of tissue remaining)
20–25****	upper endoscopy (frequency depends on number, size, and type of polyps found)
no specified age	consider small intestine screening with capsule endoscopy; learn signs and symptoms of other FAP-related tumors, including central nervous system cancers and desmoid tumors; consider imaging with abdominal MRI with and without contrast or CT with contrast at least annually, if personal history includes desmoid tumors

Source: National Comprehensive Cancer Network. "Guidelines: Genetic/familial high-risk assessment: Colorectal." Version 1.2021, May 2021.

*Guidelines for people with *APC* variant I1307K are shown in table 13.12.

**People with AFAP may start screening at age 18.

***Or more frequently, based on family history of thyroid cancer.

****Or earlier, based on family history.

People who have a specific *APC* gene variant called I1307K have only a slightly increased risk for colon cancer, and they do not develop FAP (table 13.12).

ATM

Inheriting a mutation in an *ATM* gene increases the risk of breast cancer, and it may also raise the risk for ovarian, pancreatic, and prostate cancers (table 13.4).

TABLE 13.4 Summary of Guidelines for *ATM* Gene Mutations

BEGINNING AGE	RECOMMENDATIONS
For women	
40*	annual mammogram; consider 3D mammography, if available; consider annual breast MRI with contrast
no specified age	not enough evidence to recommend risk-reducing mastectomy to all women; manage based on family history
For men	
40	consider annual prostate cancer screening with PSA testing and digital rectal exam (after discussion with your doctor about limitations and benefits of screening)
For men and women	
50 with family history of pancreatic cancer**	consider magnetic resonance cholangiopancreatography (MRCP) and/or endoscopic ultrasound (EUS); consider pancreatic cancer screening trial

Sources: National Comprehensive Cancer Network. "Guidelines: Genetic/familial high-risk assessment: Breast, ovarian, and pancreatic." Version 1.2022, August 2021; National Comprehensive Cancer Network. "Guidelines: Prostate cancer early detection." Version 2.2021, July 2021; Giri VN, Knudsen KE, Kelly WK, et al. "Implementation of germline testing for prostate cancer: Philadelphia prostate cancer consensus conference 2019," Journal of Clinical Oncology 38, no. 24, 2020:2798–2811.

*Or earlier, based on family history of breast cancer.

**Or 10 years before the earliest pancreatic cancer diagnosis in the family. Screening should be performed by a facility that is experienced with screening for pancreatic cancer.

CDH1
Inheriting a *CDH1* mutation increases the risk for stomach and breast cancers (table 13.5).

CHEK2
The NCCN provides guidelines for managing the increased risk of breast, colorectal, and prostate cancers due to an inherited *CHEK2* mutation (table 13.6).

TABLE 13.5 Summary of Guidelines for *CDH1* Gene Mutations

BEGINNING AGE	RECOMMENDATIONS
For women	
30*	annual mammogram; consider 3D mammography, if available; consider annual breast MRI with contrast
no specified age	discussion of risk-reducing mastectomy with health care provider based on family history of breast cancer
For men and women	
18 (for those with a stomach)	upper endoscopy and multiple random biopsies every 6–12 months
18–40	total gastrectomy to remove stomach

Sources: National Comprehensive Cancer Network. "Guidelines: Genetic/familial high-risk assessment: Breast, ovarian, and pancreatic." Version 1.2022, August 2021; National Comprehensive Cancer Network. "Guidelines: Gastric cancer." Version 5.2021, October 2021.

*Or earlier, based on family history of breast cancer.

TABLE 13.6 Summary of Guidelines for *CHEK2* Gene Mutations

BEGINNING AGE	RECOMMENDATIONS
For women	
40*	annual mammogram; consider 3D mammography, if available; consider annual breast MRI with contrast
no specified age	not enough evidence to recommend risk-reducing mastectomy to all women; manage based on family history
For men	
	no specific guidelines for managing the risk for prostate cancer and male breast cancer; discuss the benefits and risks of increased screening with a genetic counselor and doctor; consider enrolling in a prostate cancer screening study
For men and women	
40**	high-quality colonoscopy every 5 years

Sources: National Comprehensive Cancer Network. "Guidelines: Genetic/familial high-risk assessment: Breast, ovarian, and pancreatic." Version 1.2022, August 2021; National Comprehensive Cancer Network. "Guidelines: Genetic/familial high-risk assessment: Colorectal." Version 1.2021, May 2021.

*Or earlier, based on family history of breast cancer.

**Or earlier, based on family history of colon cancer.

MUTYH and MAP

People who inherit mutations in both of their *MUTYH* genes develop *MUTYH*-associated polyposis (MAP). This condition significantly raises the risk for colorectal and thyroid cancers. The NCCN has guidelines for people with MAP (table 13.7). People who inherit a mutation in one copy of their *MUTYH* gene have a slightly increased risk for colon cancer, but they do not develop MAP. NCCN screening guidelines address individuals who have a single *MUTYH* mutation and at least one first-degree relative with colon cancer (table 13.12).

TABLE 13.7 Summary of Guidelines for People with Two *MUTYH* Gene Mutations*

BEGINNING AGE	RECOMMENDATIONS
25–30**	high-quality colonoscopy every 1–2 years, depending on findings
25–30	risk-reducing colectomy (when polyps cannot be controlled with colonoscopy and removal); discuss benefits and risks of colectomy options with health care experts
after colectomy	sigmoidoscopy (frequency depends on type of surgery and amount of tissue remaining)
25–30	annual physical exam; thyroid ultrasound
30–35	baseline upper endoscopy (frequency of follow-up depends on number, size, and type of polyps found)

Sources: National Comprehensive Cancer Network. "Guidelines: Genetic/familial high-risk assessment: Colorectal." Version 1.2021, May 2021; Cancer.net. "MUTYH (or MYH)-associated polyposis." https://www.cancer.net/cancer-types/mutyh-or-myh-associated-polyposis.

*Table 13.12 includes guidelines for people with a mutation in one *MUTYH* gene.

**Or earlier, based on a family history of colon cancer.

PALB2

Inheriting a *PALB2* mutation raises the chance of developing breast, ovarian, and pancreatic cancers (table 13.8).

TABLE 13.8 Summary of Guidelines for *PALB2* Gene Mutations

BEGINNING AGE	RECOMMENDATIONS
For women	
30*	annual mammogram; consider 3D mammography, if available; annual breast MRI with contrast
no specified age	consider risk-reducing mastectomy
50**	consider risk-reducing salpingo-oophorectomy
For men	
	no specific guidelines for managing the risk for male breast cancer; discuss the benefits and risks of increased screening with a genetic counselor and doctor
For men and women	
50 with family history of pancreatic cancer***	consider magnetic resonance cholangiopancreatography (MRCP) and/or endoscopic ultrasound (EUS); consider pancreatic cancer screening trial

Sources: National Comprehensive Cancer Network. "Guidelines: Genetic/familial high-risk assessment: Breast, ovarian, and pancreatic." Version 1.2022, August 2021; Tischkowitz M, Balmaña J, Foulkes WD, et al. "Management of individuals with germline variants in PALB2: A clinical practice resource of the American College of Medical Genetics and Genomics (ACMG)," Genetics in Medicine 23, no. 8, 2021:1416–23. doi:10.1038/s41436-021-01151-8.

*Or earlier, based on family history of breast cancer.

**Or earlier, based on family history of ovarian cancer.

***Or 10 years before the earliest pancreatic cancer diagnosis in the family. Screening should be performed by a facility that is experienced with screening for pancreatic cancer.

PTEN

PTEN mutations (Cowden syndrome) increase the risk for breast, uterine, thyroid, colon and kidney cancers and for melanoma (table 13.9).

STK11

STK11 mutations (Peutz-Jeghers syndrome) increase the risk for breast, colon, pancreatic, cervical, uterine, stomach, lung, and small intestine cancers (table 13.10).

TP53

TP53 mutations (Li-Fraumeni syndrome) raise the risk for childhood cancers; breast, colon, liver, bone, adrenal, pancreatic, and connective tissue cancers; brain tumors; and leukemia (table 13.11).

Mutations in various other genes increase the probability of developing one or more cancers. Where sufficient study data are available, we have included expert risk management recommendations for these mutations (table 13.12).

Gene Mutations without NCCN Guidelines

More research is needed before the NCCN can establish risk management recommendations for rare or less studied mutations in other genes. If you have an inherited mutation in a gene that is not included in this chapter, it's important to consult with a genetics expert to determine the best risk management plan based on your personal and family medical history and other circumstances.

TABLE 13.9 Summary of Guidelines for *PTEN* Gene Mutations

BEGINNING AGE	RECOMMENDATIONS
For children	
at age of diagnosis of a mutation	consider neurologic assessment followed by brain MRI if symptoms are found
7	annual thyroid ultrasound (continue into adulthood)
For women	
18	learn to be aware of breast changes
25*	clinical breast exam every 6–12 months
30–35*	annual mammogram; consider 3D mammography, if available, until age 75; annual breast MRI with contrast until age 75
no specified age (based on family history)	discuss risk-reducing mastectomy
35	learn about endometrial cancer symptoms; consider having an endometrial biopsy every 1–2 years
after childbearing	consider hysterectomy
after menopause	consider transvaginal ultrasound (at doctor's discretion)
75	consider whether to continue breast screening
For men and women	
no specified age	learn cancer signs and symptoms; annual dermatology exam
18*	annual physical exam
35*	high-quality colonoscopy every 5 years
40	consider kidney ultrasound every 1–2 years

Source: National Comprehensive Cancer Network. "Guidelines: Genetic/familial high-risk assessment: Breast, ovarian, and pancreatic." Version 1.2022, August 2021.

*Or earlier, based on family history.

TABLE 13.10 Summary of Guidelines for *STK11* Gene Mutations

BEGINNING AGE	RECOMMENDATIONS
For children	
8 (girls)	annual physical exam for observation of precocious puberty*
10 (boys)	annual testicular exam and observation for feminizing changes or precocious puberty*
8–10 (all children)	high-quality colonoscopy and upper endoscopy every 2–3 years; small bowel CT, magnetic resonance enterography, or video capsule endoscopy (follow-up by age 18)**
For women	
18–20	annual pelvic exam and Pap smear
30	clinical breast exam every 6 months; annual mammogram; consider 3D mammography, if available; annual breast MRI with contrast
For men and women	
no specified age	smoking cessation
18	small bowel CT, magnetic resonance enterography, or video capsule endoscopy every 2–3 years; high-quality colonoscopy every 2–3 years;** upper endoscopy every 2–3 years**
30–35***	consider magnetic resonance cholangiopancreatography (MRCP) with contrast and/or endoscopic ultrasound (EUS) every 1–2 years; consider participating in a pancreatic cancer screening study

Source: National Comprehensive Cancer Network. "Guidelines: Genetic/familial high-risk assessment: Colorectal." Version 1.2021, May 2021.

*A child with precocious puberty prematurely develops some physical characteristics of an adult. Girls may have their first menstrual period and begin developing breasts before the age of 8. Boys may develop facial hair, a deepening voice, and an enlarged penis and testicles before age 9.

**Frequency of follow-up screening may depend on presence and size of polyps.

***Or 10 years before the earliest pancreatic cancer diagnosis in the family. Screening should be performed by a facility that is experienced with screening for pancreatic cancer.

TABLE 13.11 Summary of Guidelines for *TP53* Gene Mutations

BEGINNING AGE	RECOMMENDATIONS
For women	
18	learn to be aware of breast changes
no specified age	discuss risk-reducing mastectomy with your doctor
20	clinical breast exam every 6–12 months
20*	annual breast MRI with contrast until age 75
30	annual mammogram; consider 3D mammography, if available, until age 75
75	consider whether to continue breast screening
For men and women	
no specified age	learn the signs and symptoms of cancer; physical exam, including neurologic exam, every 6–12 months
18	annual skin cancer screening
no specified age (based on personal and family history)	annual whole-body MRI; annual brain MRI
25**	colonoscopy and upper endoscopy every 2–5 years
50 with family history of pancreatic cancer***	consider magnetic resonance cholangiopancreatography (MRCP) and/or endoscopic ultrasound (EUS); consider participating in a pancreatic screening clinical trial
no specified age	consider additional screening based on family cancer history; address psychosocial, social, and quality-of-life aspects related to the complex management of Li-Fraumeni syndrome; alert pediatricians to the mutation in the family and the associated risk of childhood cancers

Sources: National Comprehensive Cancer Network. "Guidelines: Genetic/familial high-risk assessment: Breast, ovarian, and pancreatic." Version 1.2022, August 2021.

*Or the age of the earliest breast cancer diagnosis in the family, if there is a history of breast cancer before age 20.

**Or earlier, based on family history of colon cancer.

***Or 10 years before the earliest pancreatic cancer diagnosis in the family. Screening should be performed by a facility that is experienced with screening for pancreatic cancer.

TABLE 13.12 Summary of Guidelines for Mutations in Other Genes

GENE	BEGINNING AGE	RECOMMENDATIONS
APC variant I1307K, *MUTYH* single mutation*	40**	high-quality colonoscopy every 5 years
BARD1	40**	annual screening mammogram; consider 3D mammography, if available; consider annual breast MRI with contrast
BARD1, NF1	no specified age	not enough evidence to recommend risk-reducing mastectomy to all women; manage based on family history
BRIP1, RAD51C, RAD51D	no specified age	manage breast cancer risk based on family history of cancer
	45–50	consider risk-reducing salpingo-oophorectomy
CDKN2A	40***	consider magnetic resonance cholangio-pancreatography (MRCP) and/or endoscopic ultrasound (EUS); consider pancreatic cancer screening study
CDKN2A, CDK4	10	skin exam by dermatologist every 3–12 months (frequency based on number, location, and type of skin changes and other risk factors); consider monitoring using digital dermoscopy and clinical photography; be aware of melanoma symptoms; perform monthly self-examinations for skin changes
HOXB13	40**	consider annual prostate cancer screening with PSA testing and digital rectal exam (after discussion with your doctor about limitations and benefits of screening)

(*continued*)

TABLE 13.12 (*continued*)

GENE	BEGINNING AGE	RECOMMENDATIONS
*NF1*****	30**	annual screening mammogram; consider 3D mammography, if available; consider breast MRI with contrast annually until age 50

Sources: Giri VN, Knudsen KE, Kelly WK, et al. "Implementation of germline testing for prostate cancer: Philadelphia prostate cancer consensus conference 2019," Journal of Clinical Oncology 38, no. 24, 2020:2798–2811; National Comprehensive Cancer Network. "Guidelines: Prostate cancer early detection." Version 2.2021, July 2021; National Comprehensive Cancer Network. "Guidelines: Genetic/familial high-risk assessment: Breast, ovarian, and pancreatic." Version 1.2022, August 2021; National Comprehensive Cancer Network. "Guidelines: Genetic/familial high-risk assessment: Colorectal." Version 1.2021, May 2021; Leachman SA, Lucero OM, Sampson JE, et al. "Identification, genetic testing, and management of hereditary melanoma," Cancer and Metastasis Review 36, no. 1, 2017:77–90; Rossi M, Pellegrini C, Cardelli L, et al. "Familial melanoma: Diagnostic and management implications," Dermatology Practical and Conceptual 9, no. 1, 2019:10–16.

*Only if a first-degree relative has or had colon cancer.

**Or earlier, based on family history of cancer.

***Or 10 years before the earliest pancreatic cancer diagnosis in the family. Screening should be performed by a facility that is experienced with screening for pancreatic cancer.

****Only applies to people who have been diagnosed with neurofibromatosis.

Chapter 14

Early Detection Strategies for High-Risk People

The ideal test for cancer is sensitive and specific: someone who tests positive has the disease, while someone who tests negative doesn't. But it's difficult, if not impossible, to create the perfect test, and most screening methods compromise one quality or the other.

The next best thing to preventing cancer is catching it early before cancer cells can multiply and grow. That's why surveillance is so important. Screening tests can be lifesaving because they often find cancer before it spreads. With the exception of colonoscopy, routine screenings don't prevent cancer or reduce risk, but if cancer develops, surveillance creates an opportunity to find it when treatment has a better chance of succeeding. A biopsy may be needed to verify whether an abnormal change in an organ or tissue is benign or malignant.

Recommended cancer screenings for the general population aren't always adequate for high-risk individuals, who have a higher lifetime cancer risk and tend to develop tumors at younger ages, sometimes before routine screenings in the general population begin. Talk to your doctor about the benefits and risks of the tests and procedures covered in this chapter. In addition to those guidelines, the NCCN also recommends the following for high-risk people:

- Learn to recognize the signs and symptoms of each of the cancers for which you have heightened risk.

- Have annual physical exams by a doctor or nurse practitioner.
- Consider participating in a screening clinical study for the cancers for which you have heightened risk.

The Vocabulary of Screening

Scientists use certain criteria to describe the utility of screening tests. "Sensitivity" is the probability of a true positive test among those who have the disease. If 2 people in a group of 100 have cancer, a highly sensitive test would correctly identify both of them. A highly sensitive test doesn't miss many cancers, though it's more likely to identify normal tissue as suspicious (a false positive), leading to unnecessary biopsies.

"Specificity" is the probability of a true negative test among those who don't have the disease. A highly specific test correctly identifies healthy tissue. If only 2 people in the group of 100 have cancer, yet 10 falsely test positive, the test isn't very specific. A highly specific test is less likely to produce a false-positive result, but it may also miss more cancers (false negatives).

The ideal test for cancer is sensitive and specific: someone who tests positive has the disease, while someone who tests negative doesn't. But it's difficult, if not impossible, to create the perfect test, and most screening methods compromise one quality or the other.

Surveillance for Breast Cancer

Breast Exams

If you're at high risk for breast cancer, you should become familiar with how your breasts look and feel so you'll recognize areas that change. For people with inherited mutations, this breast awareness may include breast self-exam (BSE), a technique for carefully examining your breasts for any changes or abnormalities. For premenopausal women, this should be done at the same time each month a few days after your period. Individuals who do not menstruate (including high-risk men, postmenopausal women, and transgender men) should practice BSE around the same day each month.

Routine breast self-exams aren't recommended for everyone, as they may cause false positives. People who practice regular BSE have more biopsies for benign lumps than people who don't. Yet many individuals, particularly those at high risk, discover their early-stage breast tumors during BSE or

Cancer Screenings for Transgender People

Regardless of your gender identity, it's important to have all of the recommended screenings for your biological organs, including those you retain after gender-affirming surgery. This is especially important if you have a high risk for developing any cancer. For example, if you're a trans man and still have your cervix, you should have routine Pap smears. Likewise, if you're a trans woman, you still need regular PSA tests for prostate cancer.

Cancer screening guidelines for transgender people are an evolving area of medicine with respect to the type of screening, recommended starting age, and frequency. The National LGBT Cancer Network has a database of LGBT-friendly cancer screening centers on its website (https://cancer-network.org).

while they're dressing, showering, or bathing. A lump, discharge, or other suspicious symptom shouldn't be ignored, even if you believe you're too young to have breast cancer. Notify your doctor right away. If you have a gene mutation linked to breast cancer or a family history of cancer, choose doctors with expertise in managing high-risk people, and let them know of your genetic status.

A clinical breast exam (CBE) is usually performed as part of your annual physical by your primary doctor, a gynecologist, or other health care professional. You might wonder why you should bother with monthly BSE if a doctor is going to examine your breasts anyway. A CBE is an important part of your screening regimen—it's an opportunity for an expert to detect any suspicious breast changes—but it only occurs once or twice a year. You, on the other hand, have 12 opportunities during that year to find anything unusual. Although CBE is a somewhat ineffective method of detecting breast cancer, the combination of self-exams, mammography, and breast magnetic resonance imaging (MRI) improves the odds of finding tumors early.

Breast Magnetic Resonance Imaging with Contrast

NCCN guidelines recommend breast MRI beginning at age 25 for many high-risk women, who are more likely to develop breast cancer at a younger age than other women. (A person's starting age may vary, based on their mutation and family history of breast cancer.) Breast MRI uses magnetic fields to produce hundreds of detailed images of the breast from several angles. MRI with contrast uses a dye that is injected into a vein to highlight areas in breast tissue that have increased blood flow, as cancers do. MRI machines that are specifically designed for the breast produce the best images, but not all facilities have them.

During a 30- to 60-minute breast MRI, you'll be positioned face down with your breasts hanging through openings on a sliding table. Once you're appropriately positioned, the table slides into the narrow tube of the MRI machine. You'll need to stay still and in position during the scan. You'll feel nothing unusual, but it is quite noisy—you'll hear what sounds like loud hammering. If you're claustrophobic, keeping your eyes closed or covered can help you remain relaxed and calm. If you anticipate being anxious, you can ask your doctor to prescribe a mild sedative for you to take before the procedure.

Breast MRI is sensitive. It's particularly good at finding abnormalities, including those that prove to be benign, which means it's less specific than other breast cancer tests. It may also find cancers that are missed by mammograms, especially in premenopausal women. Before making an appointment, ask how many breast-screening MRIs a facility has performed, what their biopsy recommendation rate is, and whether they can perform MRI-guided biopsies if the screening finds an abnormality that can't be seen by mammography or ultrasound.

Even when biopsies turn out to be unnecessary, experts believe the benefit of MRI outweighs the risk for high-risk women. It's also important to let the technician know if you have an artificial joint, heart valve, pacemaker, bone

Is MRI with Contrast Safe?

The contrast dye used with MRI includes the metal gadolinium, which is excreted by the kidneys within 24 hours. However, there is some concern that small traces may accumulate in the brain, bones, and kidneys over several years and adversely affect health. Even though the FDA considers the dye to be safe for most people, it doesn't recommend gadolinium for individuals with kidney issues. Let your doctor know if you're allergic to imaging dyes, pregnant, have kidney problems, or have previously had scans with gadolinium. Request a copy of the patient information for the dye, and read it carefully. If you're concerned about safety, ask which type of gadolinium will be used. The macrocyclic type, which is more often used for breast imaging, doesn't appear to have the same risk as the linear type.

screw, or other metal or electronic implants. MRI isn't generally recommended during pregnancy, especially during the first 12 weeks.

— *My Story* —
The Ups and Downs of High-Risk Screening

Screening gives me an opportunity that previous generations of high-risk women didn't have. I'm grateful to have this knowledge about my mutation, and I'm privileged to be able to be proactive about my health at a young age. Nevertheless, the MRI experience isn't always easy. For my third MRI, I got a low dose of anxiety-relieving medication for the MRI, had a ride set up, and was feeling positive. Unfortunately, the contrast dye wouldn't inject, and I had to reschedule. The act of going through the MRI at age 27 to catch cancer, as well as the anxiety that follows, is a unique experience for young previvors. It's an experience my peers don't understand.

—*Carissa*

Mammogram

Mammography has been the gold standard for detecting early-stage breast cancer since the 1970s. Mammograms use low-dose x-rays to produce images of the internal breast structure. Mammography misses some breast cancers (false negatives), especially in younger women with dense breasts, and it isn't highly sensitive. It frequently identifies suspicious changes that require a biopsy, even though cancer isn't present in the breast (false positives). But expert guidelines still recommend mammograms because they may find cancers missed by MRI.

They also can often find microcalcifications in the breast. These small calcium deposits are generally benign, but they are sometimes the first indication of cancer developing in the breast. Because high-risk women are more likely to develop breast cancer at a younger age, NCCN guidelines recommend that they start having mammograms at age 30, which is 10 years before the age when most expert organizations recommend mammograms for women of average risk. If you're a man with a high risk for breast cancer, talk to your doctor about having a baseline mammogram.

Most mammography in the United States uses digital x-ray technology to create images of the breast. (Check the US Food and Drug Administration's mammography facility database, www.accessdata.fda.gov/scripts/cdrh/cfdocs/cfMQSA/mqsa.cfm, to verify that your mammogram facility is certified by the FDA.) Digital mammography produces instant computerized images that can be enlarged to more easily spot breast abnormalities. It's more sensitive than the older mammography, which produced images on film, so fewer people are called back to repeat the process. Traditional mammograms produce a single image taken from the front and side of the breast. 3D mammography (also known as tomosynthesis) captures multiple images from different angles, which allows radiologists to view breast tissue in layers and more easily see abnormalities. For high-risk individuals, 3D mammography can be used for breast imaging when breast MRI is unavailable. People who have 3D mammograms have lower call-back rates, but the technology is more expensive than other types of mammography, so it's important to check with your health insurer to determine what your plan covers.

The total amount of radiation from digital mammography is small—less than film-based mammography and well below the maximum level set by the FDA. In women with *BRCA* mutations, exposure to diagnostic radiation before age 30 has been associated with an increased risk of breast cancer.[1] (Research hasn't yet determined how radiation from early mammography might affect people with other predisposing mutations.) Experts point out that the benefits of mammography outweigh its limitations and that, in many cases, mammograms save lives. One exception is people with *TP53* gene mutations, who are extremely sensitive to the DNA damage caused by radiation. Experts recommend that these individuals avoid mammograms and have breast screening only with MRI.

Used together, mammograms and breast MRIs are complementary, with each finding some cancers missed by the other. Mammography is better at finding microcalcifications that may be DCIS. MRI does a better job of finding early cancers in premenopausal, high-risk women whose dense breast tissue can obscure mammography images.

Mammogram Screening when You Have Breast Implants

If your natural breasts have been enlarged with implants, your mammograms should be performed by a specially trained technician. Ask your doctor for a referral or inquire about a facility's experience with breast implants when making your appointment. Always let the radiology technician know before your screening that you have implants.

Mammogram Screening after Breast Cancer Treatment

If you've previously been treated for breast cancer with radiation or chemotherapy, your doctor will likely recommend a new baseline mammogram six months after your final treatment and then annually thereafter. Some doctors recommend mammograms at six-month intervals for two or three years after radiation treatments are completed. If you've had one breast removed, you should continue with recommended screenings of your healthy breast to address your elevated risk of developing another breast cancer. Most doctors don't recommend mammograms after a bilateral mastectomy, whether or not your breasts have been reconstructed, since almost all of your breast tissue has been removed.

Surveillance for Gynecologic Cancers

No exam, test, or imaging reliably finds early-stage ovarian or fallopian tube cancers. Because symptoms are often vague, many women are not diagnosed with ovarian cancer until it's advanced. In the hopes of earlier detection, some gynecologic experts use ovarian cancer screening tests for high-risk patients who have not had risk-reducing surgery, although this has not been proven to help women live longer. Endometrial cancer is more likely than ovarian cancer to be detected early due to the presence of symptoms (see chapter 9). The most utilized screening methods are pelvic exam, transvaginal ultrasound, the CA-125 blood test, and endometrial biopsy.

Pelvic Exam

A pelvic exam by a health care professional isn't a sensitive or specific test for ovarian or fallopian tube cancer, but it's recommended because it sometimes detects abnormalities that indicate cancer. High-risk pelvic exams have three components:

- Visually checking the vaginal opening, vulva, and labia, and then using a speculum to widen the vaginal walls so that the vagina, cervix, ovaries, and uterus can be checked for abnormalities. A Pap smear (gently removing a small sample of cells from the cervix to test for precancerous changes or cancer) is sometimes then taken. Contrary to common perception, Pap smears don't screen for ovarian or fallopian tube cancer. All women with a uterus are at risk for cervical cancer, which is caused by the HPV virus, and should undergo screening Pap smears per guidelines. Genetic syndromes that increase the risk of endometrial or ovarian cancer do not increase the risk of cervical cancer.
- Feeling the ovaries by inserting one or two gloved fingers into the vagina while pressing down on the abdomen with the other hand. Even though this procedure isn't sensitive or specific enough to identify cancer with certainty, it might detect a cyst, a growth, or another abnormality that could indicate cancer.
- Rectovaginal examination. This is the best way to feel for abnormalities in the uterus and ovaries. The health care provider inserts a gloved, lubricated finger into the rectum and another finger of the same hand into the vagina. The other hand lightly presses on the abdomen to evaluate the tissue between the uterus and the vagina, the ligaments that hold the uterus in place, and the alignment of the ovaries and fallopian tubes. A rectovaginal exam may be uncomfortable, but it shouldn't be painful.

Transvaginal Ultrasound

Transvaginal ultrasound uses high-frequency sound waves to examine the vagina, uterus, fallopian tubes, ovaries, and bladder. A small probe connected to a computer is inserted into the vagina. Gently moving the probe creates sound waves that bounce off the pelvic organs, causing echoes that are sent to the computer, which then creates a picture of the internal tissues and organs. Even though transvaginal ultrasound isn't highly sensitive or specific and a false-positive result can lead to unnecessary surgical biopsy, some experts perform this screening for high-risk people who still have their ovaries and/or uterus.

CA-125 Blood Test

Cancer antigen 125 (CA-125) is a blood protein that can be elevated when a woman has ovarian cancer. As a method of routine screening, CA-125 produces less than optimal results in most women: about 50 percent of women with early-stage ovarian cancer and 20 percent who have advanced disease don't have elevated CA-125 levels.[2] Liver disease, other cancers, and some benign conditions, including uterine fibroids, can also raise CA-125 levels, especially in premenopausal women, making the test difficult to interpret, producing false positives, and requiring surgery to confirm a diagnosis. Combined with transvaginal ultrasound, CA-125 may find some ovarian cancers before symptoms appear, so some experts order the test for their high-risk patients who still have their ovaries.

Endometrial Biopsy

An endometrial biopsy is usually a short outpatient procedure. Like a pelvic exam, the test involves a doctor using a speculum to open the vaginal canal. A small tube is then passed through the cervix and into the uterus. The tube suctions samples of endometrial tissue as it is moved through different areas of the uterus. A pathologist then studies the tissue under a microscope to look for abnormal cells.

Surveillance for Gastrointestinal Cancers

Colonoscopy

Colonoscopy is the most effective way to screen for early-stage colorectal cancer. Removing colon polyps during colonoscopy can prevent colon cancer from developing. It's an outpatient procedure that usually lasts for 20–30 minutes. The preparation is somewhat inconvenient, but it's necessary to thoroughly clean the colon to make it easier to see abnormalities. Your doctor will prescribe a special diet for a few days before your procedure, and you will be given a liquid laxative to drink the day before and possibly the morning of your test. Once you've been lightly sedated, a gastroenterologist will insert a colonoscope (a flexible tube with a camera on the end) through your rectum and into your colon. You'll be asleep, so you shouldn't feel any discomfort or pain. Carbon dioxide or air will then be used to distend the colon for better viewing. Any polyps or questionable areas will be removed or sampled during the procedure and will be checked by a pathologist (figure 14.1). You'll awaken shortly after the procedure, but you'll need a ride home. Most people are back to normal after the sedation wears off or within 24 hours.

Colonoscopy is a sensitive test. If you have prepared properly, the gastroenterologist can completely examine most areas of the colon for growths and abnormalities. Because colonoscopy involves removing abnormal growths that may turn into cancer if left in place, it's one of the few types of screening that also prevents cancer from developing. Because colonoscopy requires anesthesia and may involve a biopsy, it's not without risk.

Other methods of checking for colorectal cancer, including fecal occult blood tests, which use a stool sample, are less effective and aren't recommended as standard screening for high-risk people.

Esophagogastroduodenoscopy

Esophagogastroduodenoscopy (EGD), also called an upper endoscopy, is an outpatient procedure used to view, find, and biopsy abnormalities of the

FIGURE 14.1 Polyps found during a colonoscopy are removed and examined

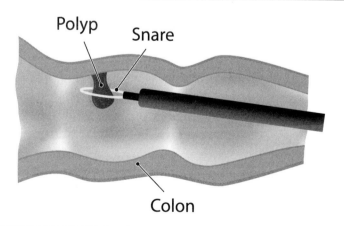

esophagus, stomach, and duodenum. EGD is well tolerated with minimal discomfort and is typically done in less than 15 minutes. Before the procedure begins, your doctor will give you a sedative. Once you're asleep, an endoscope will be placed into your throat, through your esophagus, and into your stomach and duodenum. As the endoscope moves downward, it sends images to a computer, so that your doctor can view different parts of your gastrointestinal tract. If necessary, samples of tissue or digestive fluid can be obtained during the procedure.

Endoscopic Ultrasound

Pancreatic cancer is difficult to detect, and most often it's diagnosed at a late stage. Minimally invasive endoscopic ultrasound (EUS) is a way to examine the pancreas. It involves passing a tiny scope with an ultrasound probe down the esophagus, into the stomach, and through the top of the small intestine. EUS can sometimes provide visual details of the pancreas that can't be seen with CT or other methods of imaging. The small probe emits sound waves that bounce off the surrounding tissue and are converted into detailed computerized images of the pancreas. EUS is a 30- to 45-minute outpatient procedure that's performed under sedation or general anesthesia. If a biopsy is required, a small needle can be fitted into the scope to collect a tissue sample at the same time.

EUS alone has a small risk of bleeding or tearing of the GI tract, but a pancreatic biopsy may cause bleeding, infection, or inflammation of the pancreas. Sometimes, abnormalities found with EUS can be tested for cancer during the procedure, but some require additional testing, which may include general anesthesia and surgery. For this reason, most experts recommend this screening only for people who have the highest risk for pancreatic cancer. Unfortunately, few other options for pancreatic cancer screening are available. Pancreatic cancer screening, either with EUS or magnetic resonance cholangiopancreatography (described below), should be performed at a high-volume cancer center with expertise in screening individuals who are at high risk for pancreatic cancer.

Magnetic Resonance Cholangiopancreatography

MRCP is a special 15- to 40-minute MRI that provides images of the pancreas, liver, gallbladder, and bile duct. MRCP uses a strong but harmless magnetic field to obtain images of the upper abdomen, so it's important to let the technician know if you have an artificial joint, heart valve, pacemaker, bone screw, or any other metal or medical implant. Like other types of MRI, MRCP is noninvasive, not painful, and generally causes no downtime or side effects. Some people, however, have reactions to the contrast dyes that may be used during the scan.

Like endoscopic ultrasound, magnetic resonance cholangiopancreatography is sensitive but not specific. Abnormalities that are found require additional testing, which may include general anesthesia and surgery. For this reason, most experts recommend MRCP only for people with the highest risk for pancreatic cancer.

Magnetic Resonance Enterography

Magnetic resonance enterography creates detailed images of the small intestine. Before the test, you'll need to drink a contrast material, which will highlight your intestine. You'll also be given medication to reduce any movement in the bowel that could interfere with the images. Before the test begins, an additional contrast material will be administered intravenously.

Magnetic resonance enterography is a type of MRI. It uses a harmless but strong magnetic field, which can interfere with some medical devices, so it's important to tell the technician if you have hearing aids, a pacemaker, or any other metal implant in your body. You should also let them know if you are or suspect that you're pregnant. The exam takes about 20 minutes.

Testing for *H. pylori*

Helicobacter pylori is a bacteria that can cause chronic inflammation in the stomach and increase the risk for stomach cancer. *H. pylori* infections are treatable and can be identified by several different tests:

- A blood test looks for *H. pylori* antibodies. The presence of these antibodies in your blood means that you're currently infected with the bacteria or have been in the past.
- A urea breath test checks for *H. pylori* bacteria in the stomach.
- A stool antigen test checks your feces for *H. pylori* molecules, which trigger your immune system to fight the infection.
- A small biopsy of the stomach lining can be performed during an endoscopy.

Video Capsule Endoscopy

A video capsule endoscopy lets your doctor view your small intestine, an area that can't be reached by a traditional upper endoscopy or colonoscopy. You'll need to abstain from eating or drinking anything for at least 12 hours before your test, and you may also need to cleanse your bowels. You'll first swallow a pill-size video camera. As it passes through your small intestine, the tiny camera will send video images to a small recorder worn on your belt for about eight hours. You then return to your doctor's office so that the recorder can be removed and the images uploaded to a computer. This type of endoscopy isn't painful, and under most circumstances, your body will expel the capsule in a few hours or a few days.

Small Bowel Computed Tomography Scan

A CT scan uses x-rays with or without a contrast dye. This procedure reveals the entire thickness of the bowel wall. If your doctor prefers to use contrast with the scan, you'll need to drink up to 1.5 liters of a liquid that contains a contrast material before your procedure. The scan is performed as you lie face up on a table that slides through the CT machine. It takes about an hour to drink all of the liquid and about 45 minutes for the scan.

— *My Story* —

A Daughter's Pancreatic Screening

My mother was a two-time breast cancer survivor, and like her, I carry a *BRCA2* gene [mutation]. I was already being screened for breast cancer twice a year when I received my diagnosis in 2015. I wasn't surprised. I had always expected a diagnosis knowing our family history, and I quickly opted for a double mastectomy.

Six months after my diagnosis, my mother was diagnosed with Stage 4 pancreatic cancer. While this wasn't her first cancer diagnosis (she survived breast cancer twice), her pancreatic cancer came as a surprise. Various chemotherapies and experimental drugs, subsequent tumors in her brain and lungs, and then pulmonary embolisms followed. Almost three years after being diagnosed, my mother died.

Based on the recommendations of her oncologist, I found a pancreatic specialist in my area, who recommended yearly screening. Instead of alternating breast MRIs and mammograms, I now alternate abdominal MRIs and endoscopic ultrasounds, as well as fasting blood sugar tests (elevated blood sugar levels can be an early indicator of pancreatic cancer). The screening is relatively easy, all things considered, though the ultrasound does require anesthesia.

Deciding to have pancreatic screening was easy for me. Early detection of my breast cancer gave me more options and a better chance of survival than I otherwise would have had. I take comfort in knowing that if I develop pancreatic cancer, it will also likely be caught early and will be treatable. Though I may carry a *BRCA2* gene mutation like my mother, I believe that early detection of the disease will give me a chance for survival that she didn't have.

—*Rebecca*

Surveillance for Prostate and Other Genitourinary Cancers

Prostate-Specific Antigen Test

PSA is a protein in semen and blood that can be elevated when a man has prostate cancer. PSA tests aren't specific because numerous benign conditions, including urinary tract infections and inflammation or enlargement of the prostate, can also raise a person's PSA level. A false-negative test result may show that the PSA level is low, even though the individual has prostate cancer. A false-positive test result, which shows an elevated PSA level when cancer doesn't exist, can lead to a biopsy, which can be painful and cause infection.

Due to the risk of unnecessary biopsy and overtreatment of slow-growing cancers, PSA testing is not routinely recommended for all men. However, before deciding whether it's right for them, people with inherited mutations or other risk factors for prostate cancer are advised to speak with their doctors about their level of risk and the benefits and limitations of testing. If your PSA level is elevated, your doctor may recommend repeating the test to confirm or question the original result. If your PSA level remains high, your doctor may suggest that you continue having routine PSA tests along with digital rectal exams to watch for any changes.

Using a small sample of blood, PSA testing can pick up prostate cancers in the earliest stage, especially tumors that might be missed by a digital rectal exam. Testing often identifies individuals who may have otherwise died from their disease, yet the benefits don't always outweigh the potential harm of unnecessary treatment. For people at high risk for aggressive prostate cancer (especially men with a *BRCA2* mutation), the benefits of PSA testing outweigh the risks.

Digital Rectal Exam

A DRE is a physical inspection that may detect prostate growths or other changes in the bladder and rectum. DRE is less effective than the PSA blood test in finding prostate cancer, but it sometimes identifies cancers in people who have normal PSA levels. During a digital rectal exam, you'll bend over a table or lie on your side with your knees bent to your chest. Your doctor will gently insert a gloved, lubricated finger into your rectum to feel your prostate for any irregularities. Applying pressure to your prostate may cause brief discomfort if it's inflamed or swollen, and you might feel that you have to urinate. Tell your doctor before your DRE if you have hemorrhoids or an anal fissure.

Testicular Exam

A testicular exam is a complete physical inspection of the testicles and scrotum (the sac of skin surrounding the testicles). During this exam, a doctor checks each of these organs for lumps, bumps, and other unusual features.

Urinalysis

A urinalysis assesses the color, odor, clarity, and pH level of a person's urine and checks for the presence of bacteria. It can also identify small amounts of blood in the urine, which can be a sign of bladder cancer. Often performed as part of a routine health checkup, urinalysis is neither sensitive nor specific. Additional tests may be required if an abnormality is found.

Ultrasound

Ultrasound provides views of the kidneys and bladder. Your doctor may ask that you come for the test with a full bladder, so that the scan can be performed before and after you urinate. A technician will spread a clear, warm gel on your abdomen over the kidneys to help transmit the sound waves. A small wand called a transducer is then moved slowly over the gel. It emits high-frequency sound waves, which are changed into computer images. The procedure can usually be completed in about 30 minutes. Ultrasounds don't emit radiation or use contrast dye, so they're safe during pregnancy and for people who are allergic to dyes.

Surveillance for Melanoma

Education

It's important to learn the signs and symptoms of melanoma, especially those associated with inherited gene mutations that increase melanoma risk. Become familiar with your skin, examine it monthly, and notify your doctor if you discover any new moles or unusual changes.

Full-Body Skin Examination

During a head-to-toe examination of your skin, you'll be checked for any unusual moles or skin irregularities. Ideally, this exam should be performed by a dermatologist who has expertise in diagnosing skin cancer. The entire exam usually takes about 15–20 minutes, but it may last a bit longer if tissue samples need to be taken from any questionable or suspicious areas.

Eye Cancer Screening

If you're at high risk for ocular melanoma, annual eye exams by an ophthalmologist that include pupil dilation and examination of the retina can help detect melanoma in the eye. Talk with your oncologist, genetic counselor, and eye doctor about when you should begin these screenings and how frequently you should have them.

Screening for Other Hereditary Cancers

Neurological Exam

A neurological exam is a painless, 30- to 60-minute evaluation of your nervous system. A neurologist begins by asking about your symptoms, medical history, and any medical issues. Testing the nervous system generally includes the following:

- Your level of awareness is gauged by talking with you and observing the clarity of your speech.
- Your motor function is tested by having you push and pull against the neurologist's hands with your arms and legs. The neurologist will observe the way you walk as well as your posture, balance, and coordination.
- Your sensory ability and reflexes are checked by observing your reaction to touch with or without instruments on various parts of your body.
- Your vision, smell, hearing, ability to distinguish different tastes, and eye movement are evaluated.
- Your facial movements, including your ability to swallow and stick out your tongue, are checked. Your gag reflex and your ability to feel facial sensations are also evaluated.

Brain Scan

This test provides images of the internal structure of your brain and measures how your brain uses oxygen. A painless outpatient test, a brain scan may include

- A CT scan with or without a contrast dye, which usually takes about 15–30 minutes.
- An MRI brain scan, which uses magnetic radio waves to produce images. MRI brain scans last between 30 and 60 minutes.
- A positron emission tomography (PET) scan, which shows your real-time brain function (unlike CT and MRI scans, which only look at brain structure). Before the PET scan, a small amount of a radioactive tracer is injected through an intravenous line in your hand or arm. You'll need to wait about an hour for the tracer to collect in your tissues and organs before you enter the PET machine. The entire procedure takes up to two hours.

Thyroid Ultrasound

This test produces pictures of the thyroid gland. A technician will spread a clear, warm gel on your neck to transmit the sound waves. A small wand will then be moved slowly over the gel. The wand emits high-frequency sound waves, which are changed into computer images. The procedure is typically completed in about 30 minutes.

Insurance and Payment Issues

Always be sure to check with your health insurer to determine whether the screening you need is a covered benefit. For people of average risk, the Affordable Care Act (ACA) requires most health plans to cover the entire cost of the following cancer screenings with no out-of-pocket costs:

- Screening mammogram every 1–2 years for women ages 40–74.
- Colon cancer screening with colonoscopy or other screening method for people ages 45–75. Colonoscopy is covered every 10 years, while the covered frequency of other screenings depends on the method chosen.
- Pap test for cervical cancer every three years between ages 21 and 65; human papillomavirus (HPV) test combined with a Pap smear every 5 years for people ages 30–65 who don't want to have a Pap smear every 3 years.

Most health insurers cover medically necessary screening for high-risk individuals for whom more frequent, more intensive, or earlier screenings are recommended, but copays or other out-of-pocket costs may apply. These costs vary, depending on the type of health plan, the kind of screening. and the demonstrated medical necessity. Some state laws also require health insurance coverage of additional preventive services, such as PSA tests and digital rectal exams for high-risk men who are age 40 and over. Medicare pays for the following screening tests for eligible individuals, including those with disabilities under age 65:

- Breast cancer. One baseline mammogram for women ages 35–39; annual screening mammograms and 3D mammograms for women age 40 and older. Medicare covers a clinical breast exam as part of the well-woman annual exam.

- Cervical and other gynecologic cancers. One Pap test and pelvic exam every 24 months. Medicare covers these screening tests every 12 months if you're at high risk for cervical or vaginal cancer or if you're of childbearing age and you've had an abnormal Pap test in the past 36 months.

- Prostate cancer. Screening with a digital rectal exam and a PSA blood test once every 12 months for men age 50 and over.

- Colon cancer. Screening colonoscopy once every 2 years for those at high risk of colorectal cancer. If you're not considered to be at high risk for colorectal cancer, colonoscopy is covered once every 10 years or 4 years after a previous flexible sigmoidoscopy. There is no minimum age requirement for these guidelines.

Medicare generally doesn't cover cancer screenings beyond those outlined above, although additional coverage may be available through Medicare Advantage plans or secondary insurance. The Part B deductible applies to other or more frequent cancer screenings that are considered to be diagnostic, for which you will pay 20 percent of the Medicare-approved amount.

Medicaid coverage of cancer screenings varies by state. Medicaid beneficiaries in states that have expanded their programs under the ACA are entitled to the same screening and preventive services as those who are covered by private insurance. Most Medicaid programs cover the cost of basic screening for breast, cervical, prostate, and colorectal cancer. If your health insurer denies coverage of recommended cancer screenings, you may be able to successfully appeal the decision. The FORCE website (www.facingourrisk.org) has templates for appeal letters to contest various denials.

Chapter 15

Medications That Reduce Cancer Risk

It's important to understand and weigh the benefits and risks of any chemopreventive option before deciding if it's right for you. Some studies of these medications haven't specifically focused on high-risk people; fewer have focused on people with *BRCA* mutations, Lynch syndrome, or other inherited risk factors.

Prevention is the most effective approach to controlling cancer, but not all cancer types have reliable preventive options. Chemoprevention, as described in this chapter, and surgery (chapters 16, 17, and 18) are two of the most effective approaches to lower cancer risk. Chemoprevention is the use of drugs, vitamins, or other natural or synthetic substances to reduce risk in healthy individuals. The transition from healthy cell to malignancy sometimes takes years, providing opportunities along the way to inhibit or slow the growth of cancer cells. Chemoprevention isn't the same as chemotherapy, a type of cancer treatment that can cause many side effects. Chemoprevention reduces the chance of developing cancer, usually with fewer side effects than chemotherapy.

Chemoprevention doesn't guarantee that you'll never develop cancer, but it improves your chances of staying cancer-free. The degree of protection may vary, depending on the type of cancer and your existing level of risk. Even if you take a preventive medication, you'll still need recommended screenings to find any early cancers that may develop.

Chemoprevention isn't recommended for the general population, but it may be a reasonable way to lower your high probability of developing certain cancers. The higher your current risk, the greater your benefit will be. It's important to understand and weigh the benefits and risks of any chemopreventive option before deciding if it's right for you. Some studies of these medications haven't specifically focused on high-risk people; fewer have focused on people with *BRCA* mutations, Lynch syndrome, or other inherited risk factors. A health care team with expertise in managing high-risk patients can give you a clear sense of how various chemoprevention interventions might influence your risk.

Researchers continue to explore ways to reduce cancer risk with medication. This chapter includes chemoprevention methods for hereditary breast, gynecologic, and colorectal cancers. Diet, exercise, sleep, and other lifestyle factors that affect overall cancer risk are discussed in chapter 19.

Questions to Ask Your Doctor about Chemoprevention

- What is my risk of developing cancer?
- Is chemoprevention an option for me?
- What method of chemoprevention would benefit me the most?
- How long will I need to stay on the medication?
- How much will chemoprevention lower my cancer risk?
- What side effects may occur?
- Is my insurance likely to pay for it?
- Is a chemoprevention clinical trial an option for me?

Risk-Reducing Medications for Breast Cancer

Some medications that are used to treat breast cancers can also prevent them. If you have a high risk for breast cancer, you might benefit from preventively taking tamoxifen, raloxifene, or an aromatase inhibitor.

Tamoxifen and Raloxifene

As a means of prevention, raloxifene is less effective than tamoxifen, but it has fewer harmful side effects, and for some women, it's a better choice. Low-dose tamoxifen may be better tolerated than standard-dose tamoxifen, but less is known about its long-term effectiveness. Tamoxifen and raloxifene are alike in some ways and different in others.

- Both are selective estrogen receptor modulators (SERMs), which block the effects of estrogen and progesterone on breast tissue.
- Both are FDA-approved to prevent hormone-dependent breast cancer in women. Neither drug reduces the chance of breast cancers that aren't hormone-sensitive.
- Tamoxifen is used to prevent and treat breast cancer. Raloxifene is given only as a preventive medication.
- Tamoxifen is appropriate for premenopausal women who are age 35 or older and postmenopausal women. Raloxifene is prescribed only for postmenopausal women.
- Tamoxifen lowers the likelihood of invasive breast cancers, DCIS, and LCIS in high-risk women by as much as 50 percent. Raloxifene reduces risk slightly less.[1]
- For women who have been diagnosed with DCIS or LCIS, which are precursors for invasive breast cancer, both medications reduce the chance of a future breast cancer.
- For breast cancer survivors, tamoxifen decreases the chance of recurrence by 30–50 percent in premenopausal women and by 40–50 percent in postmenopausal women. It also reduces the risk of a new cancer in the opposite breast by about half.[2]
- The protective benefits of both drugs last for several years after you stop taking them. Compared to tamoxifen, the

benefits of raloxifene decline more quickly when you stop taking it.

- Both drugs are taken as a daily pill for at least five years.

Other Benefits and Side Effects

Reliable and effective, tamoxifen and raloxifene have beneficial aspects as well as mild to serious side effects. Both drugs improve bone density, which helps to prevent osteoporosis (raloxifene is primarily an osteoporosis medication), and both reduce cholesterol. However, hot flashes, vaginal dryness, mood changes, and other menopause-like symptoms can occur with either drug. Tamoxifen and raloxifene can also cause vaginal bleeding or discharge, headaches, nausea, leg cramps, and rashes.

Other side effects can be more serious. Tamoxifen slightly elevates the risk for endometrial cancer. Raloxifene doesn't have the same estrogen-like effect on the uterus, so it's less likely than tamoxifen to increase the chance of developing endometrial cancer. These medications can raise the chance of stroke and blood clots, particularly if you smoke or have clotting disorders. They're not appropriate if you're prone to blood clots or if you're taking estrogen replacement.

— *My Story* —
Surveillance Alone Isn't Enough for Me

When I tested positive for a *BRCA1* mutation at age 27, I wasn't ready for prophylactic surgery, so my oncologist suggested I take tamoxifen for five years. If my body didn't react well to surgical menopause or I had complications from mastectomy, that could affect my life forever. Taking a pill didn't feel that way, and I would be doing something more than just surveillance. After researching carefully, I decided to try tamoxifen for six months. I was comfortable with my decision, and I had an easy out if I didn't want to continue. If I didn't like how I felt or couldn't handle the side effects, I would stop taking it. As it turned out, I tolerated tamoxifen well, maybe because I was young when I started taking it or because I was proactive with my diet and lifestyle. Maybe I was just lucky. I took a risk with tamoxifen. It was the best decision I could have made.

—*Cari*

Aromatase Inhibitors

Postmenopausal women who have hormone receptor–positive breast cancers are treated with aromatase inhibitors (AIs), including Aromasin (exemestane) and Arimidex (anastrozole). AIs don't influence estrogen that is made by the ovaries, which is why they're not effective for premenopausal women. Although neither medication is FDA-approved specifically for chemoprevention, both are often used off-label for that purpose. Even though the ovaries don't produce much estrogen after menopause, the aromatase enzyme in fat converts other hormones into estrogen, which can stimulate receptors on the breast. This may be one reason that carrying extra postmenopausal weight raises the chance for a breast cancer diagnosis. AIs inhibit aromatase and reduce up to 95 percent of postmenopausal estrogen.

Five years of Aromasin or Arimidex reduces breast cancer risk by about half in high-risk, postmenopausal women.[3] The NCCN and the American Society of Clinical Oncology list these drugs as risk-lowering options for this population. The Arimidex, Tamoxifen, Alone, or in Combination (ATAC) trial also reported that in breast cancer survivors, Arimidex reduces the risk of a new cancer in the opposite breast by 58 percent.[4] (The study didn't specifically include women with inherited gene mutations.) Another aromatase inhibitor, Femara (letrozole), may also lower the likelihood of breast cancer in high-risk, postmenopausal women, but more study is needed to determine whether this is the case.

Aromatase inhibitors don't have the bone-protective benefit of tamoxifen and raloxifene; AIs can accelerate postmenopausal bone loss because estrogen is also decreased in bone cells. AIs cause some of the same side effects as those medications, including hot flashes, vaginal dryness, headaches, and muscle or joint pain. AIs don't cause uterine cancers and are less likely than tamoxifen and raloxifene to cause serious blood clots.

— THE FORCE PERSPECTIVE —

Why Don't More People Embrace Chemoprevention?

Despite the effectiveness of tamoxifen and raloxifene, they're not widely used, possibly because individuals don't consider the benefit to be worth the risk of side effects. They may also fear taking a medication that they perceive as a cancer treatment, or they may hear from a family member or friend that cancer treatment with tamoxifen was difficult.

In a FORCE poll of previvors who still had their natural breasts, fewer than 10 percent had ever taken tamoxifen or raloxifene. About 66 percent indicated that their doctors had never recommended tamoxifen to reduce their risk. Forty percent said that they were willing to participate in research to test new methods of chemoprevention—which is significant because more research specific to high-risk individuals is needed. Perhaps doctors would recommend preventive drugs more frequently if they could more accurately predict how well the medicines would work for high-risk people, particularly those who have inherited mutations.

Risk-Reducing Medications for Gynecologic Cancers

Developing risk management options for ovarian cancer is challenging. Learning how to prevent ovarian cancer short of removing the ovaries requires more long-term research with large groups of participants. There is evidence, however, that medications can reduce your risk of some gynecologic cancers.

Oral Contraceptives

More than 60 years after oral contraception (birth control pills) gave women control over their fertility, it is now recognized as a way to protect high-risk women against ovarian cancer. By reducing the frequency of ovulation, oral contraceptives lower a person's overall exposure to estrogen. It's the most effective way to reduce your risk if you want to keep the option to bear children and you aren't ready to have your ovaries and fallopian tubes removed. Women who take birth control pills lower their risk for ovarian cancer by 30–50 percent compared to those who have never used them.[5] This protective effect increases the longer oral contraceptives are used and continues for up to 30 years after you stop using them.[6] Although this same benefit extends to women with BRCA mutations, it's unclear whether oral contraceptives reduce risk to the same degree in other high-risk women.[7]

Oral contraceptives also lower the risk for endometrial cancer. The longer they're used, the greater the protection. Data suggest that oral contraceptives reduce the risk of endometrial cancer in women with and without Lynch syndrome.[8]

Birth control pills aren't without side effects, however, including a slightly greater risk for blood clots. The risk for breast cancer is also slightly elevated, although it declines when you stop taking the pills, and it disappears altogether 10 years after use stops.[9]

Risk-Reducing Medications for Colorectal Cancers

Nonsteroidal anti-inflammatory drugs (NSAIDs), including aspirin, Advil and Motrin (ibuprofen), and Aleve (naproxen), are sold over the counter to reduce fever, inflammation, and pain. Stronger NSAIDs are the most commonly prescribed medications for these same conditions. Observations of

Searching for a Way
to Prevent Prostate Cancer

Numerous studies have explored different medications, vitamins, and supplements that might prevent prostate cancer. A clinical trial of selenium and vitamin E concluded that neither substance lowered prostate cancer risk, and participants who took vitamin E had a higher risk. The Prostate Cancer Prevention and the REDUCE trials studied the potentially protective effects of Propecia (finasteride) and Avodart (dutasteride), medications that are used to treat enlarged prostates. Individuals who took the drugs had about 25 percent reduced risk for low-grade prostate cancer. However, whether these drugs increase the risk for high-grade prostate cancers is debatable. The FDA declined approval for using either medication as chemoprevention, citing the fact that low-grade prostate cancers don't necessarily require treatment or affect a person's health and the concern that the drugs may affect the risk of high-grade cancer.

people who use NSAIDs for therapeutic purposes show that when they're taken regularly for 10 or more years, these drugs lower the frequency of intestinal polyps, which can become colorectal cancer. The clinical trial known as CAPP2 concluded that taking daily aspirin for two years lowered the risk for colorectal cancer in people with Lynch syndrome.[10] It may take several years to determine the effects of aspirin use on risk, but its protection may last up to 20 years. More research is needed to determine the best dose and duration of aspirin usage for people with Lynch syndrome. Long-term use of NSAIDs can cause bleeding; lung, liver, and kidney issues; a greater chance of heart disease; and other side effects. If you have Lynch syndrome, NCCN guidelines recommend that you discuss the benefits and risks of taking aspirin with your doctor.

Chemoprevention in a Bottle

We usually think of chemoprevention in the form of a pill, but it can also come in a bottle. Sunblocks and sunscreens meet all of the desired characteristics of a chemopreventive. They're safe, effective, affordable, easily obtained, and other than allergic reactions in some people, are without side effects. Yet many people don't use them in sufficient quantity, frequency, or at all. Products that are SPF 30 or higher are recommended to prevent melanoma and other skin cancers.

Insurance and Payment Issues

Chemoprevention for Breast Cancer

The Affordable Care Act (ACA) requires most private health plans to pay for tamoxifen, raloxifene, and aromatase inhibitors used as chemoprevention with no out-of-pocket expenses for high-risk women who are 35 and older and who meet other specific guidelines. Health insurers generally cover the medications even for high-risk women who don't meet the guidelines, but deductibles, coinsurance, or copays may apply. All Medicare Part D and Medicare Advantage plans cover tamoxifen, raloxifene, and aromatase inhibitors with a minimal copay or none at all.

Chemoprevention for Gynecologic Cancers

The ACA requires most private health insurers to pay for FDA-approved contraceptives with no out-of-pocket costs. Similarly, federal law requires insurance coverage of contraceptives for federal employees and their dependents. Some health insurance plans, including self-funded, short-term, and exempt "religious employer" plans, aren't required to abide by all of the ACA rules and may have different policies.

If you have Medicare Part D prescription drug coverage, your plan may pay for some types of hormonal contraceptives. Look for the medications on your plan's formulary (list of covered prescription drugs). Pricing may vary based on the drug you choose and whether you use an in-network pharmacy or a mail-order service.

Most Medicaid programs offer free contraceptives, although eligibility requirements and benefits vary by state, and all FDA-approved birth control methods may not be covered. Many states have expanded family planning services and access to hormonal contraceptives for low-income individuals who would not otherwise be eligible for Medicaid.

Resources

Many hospitals and medical practices have nurse navigators, social workers, or financial counselors who can help identify financial assistance and other resources. Most pharmaceutical companies have financial assistance programs for people who are uninsured or underinsured and struggling to afford their medications. Some clinical trials study medications to lower cancer risk, and the cost of the drugs in these studies may be covered for participants. The FORCE website (www.facingourrisk.org) provides links to financial assistance resources and sample appeal letters if your insurer denies coverage.

Chapter 16

Surgeries That Reduce Breast Cancer Risk

Removing healthy breasts to avoid breast cancer isn't an easy decision, and it isn't acceptable to everyone. For some women, removing their breasts to prevent cancer that they may never develop seems extreme. For others, the decision remedies the concern they feel, especially if they've seen loved ones wage war against breast cancer.

Mastectomy is a surgical procedure that removes one or both breasts to treat breast cancer. Risk-reducing mastectomy (RRM) removes a woman's healthy breasts to prevent or greatly reduce her risk of breast cancer. Risk-reducing mastectomy is an aggressive action, but it's also the most effective way to prevent breast cancer from developing. It lowers breast cancer risk by 90–95 percent.[1] If your estimated lifetime risk is now 60 percent, RRM will reduce it to about 3–6 percent, lower than the average risk of women who don't have an inherited mutation. A small risk remains after mastectomy because it's not possible to remove every bit of breast tissue.

Experts consider risk-reducing mastectomy to be a reasonable option for women who have a high risk of developing breast cancer. It isn't recommended for women with average or slightly increased risk or for high-risk men. Your doctor may recommend that you consider RRM in the following situations:

- Genetic testing shows that you've inherited a mutation in a *BRCA1*, *BRCA2*, *PALB2*, *PTEN*, or *TP53* gene. If you have a mutation in a different gene that raises breast cancer risk, the NCCN recommends that you consider RRM based on your personal and family history.

- You have a strong family history of breast cancer.
- You've been diagnosed with breast cancer in one breast, which raises the risk for a diagnosis in your opposite breast.
- You've been diagnosed with lobular carcinoma in situ, which increases the risk of developing invasive breast cancer.

Mastectomy Procedures

RRM is a total mastectomy, which is less severe than the modified radical mastectomy that is performed to treat invasive breast cancer. Both procedures remove the breast tissue. Modified radical mastectomy also removes lymph nodes in the axilla (underarm) to check if cancer cells have spread beyond the breast. Because previvors are presumed to be free of breast cancer, a total mastectomy leaves their lymph nodes intact. In a small percentage of high-risk women, invasive breast cancer is discovered during RRM, and one or two lymph nodes may be removed and checked for cancer cells as a precautionary measure. (This is called a sentinel lymph node biopsy, which is discussed in more detail in chapter 21.) While the goal of mastectomy is always to remove as much breast tissue as possible, the location and length of your mastectomy incisions and the amount of breast skin removed depend on whether you decide to have your breasts reconstructed and when.

Mastectomy without Reconstruction

If you choose to forgo breast reconstruction and "go flat" after mastectomy, your breast surgeon will make a broad elliptical incision across the entire expanse of each breast (figure 16.1). Breast tissue from the collarbone to the underarm and across to the middle of the rib cage will be separated from the underlying chest muscle and the overlying skin, and then the tissue will be removed. Most of the breast skin, including your nipple, areola, and scars from any previous biopsies will also be removed. Just enough skin will be left to close the wound. The edges of the incision are then pulled together and sutured in a straight or diagonal line. You can ask your surgeon to perform an aesthetic flat closure, so that the remaining skin is tight and smooth, making the chest wall appear flat rather than concave. If you decide to have breast

FIGURE 16.1 A total mastectomy removes breast tissue and most of the breast skin, including the nipple and areola (*left*). Mastectomy scars remain on the chest (*right*).

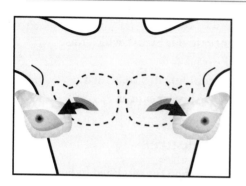 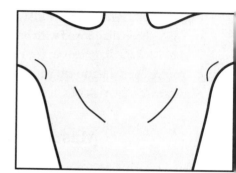

reconstruction sometime in the future—this is called delayed breast reconstruction—it will be performed by reopening your mastectomy scar.

A total mastectomy without breast reconstruction lasts two to three hours and requires at least one night in the hospital. If you want to fill out your clothes once you've healed, you can use breast prostheses. These temporary breast forms are made of cotton, foam, latex, or silicone and stick to your chest or fit into a pocket in your bra, bathing suit, or lingerie. Prostheses come in a variety of shapes, weights, and prices. A qualified fitter in a mastectomy boutique or department store can ensure that your prostheses fit correctly.

— *My Story* —

My Breasts Don't Define Me

I chose no reconstruction because I wanted to be done with surgery. I didn't want to risk infection, reconstructive failure, or additional operations. Part of me will always miss my breasts, but they don't define me, and reconstruction would not have given them back. Coming to terms with my new reality meant accepting that my breasts were gone. I knew if I ever changed my mind, reconstruction would still be an option. Six years later, I haven't changed my mind. I am undeniably different, but I'm still me. I have no regrets about forgoing reconstruction. My choice may not be right for everyone. It was simply the right one for me.

—*Lisa*

Mastectomy with Reconstruction

If you choose to have immediate breast reconstruction, you'll enter the operating room with your natural breasts, which will be removed, and then new breasts (or the beginnings of new breasts) will be created while you're still sedated. Your breast surgeon will perform a bilateral skin-sparing mastectomy through incisions made around your areolas (figure 16.2). Sometimes, an additional vertical or horizontal incision is made. Your breast tissue, nipples, and areolas will then be removed, while most of your breast skin will be preserved to hold your new breast. Once this is completed, your plastic surgeon will step in to perform your reconstruction.

You also have the option for nipple-sparing mastectomy, which will preserve almost all of your visible breasts, including your nipples and areolas. Having your natural nipples on your reconstructed breasts is safe, and you may prefer to retain a small part of your natural breasts. This procedure requires special surgical skill to carefully remove breast tissue from the skin without damaging the delicate blood vessels that support the nipple. If this vital blood supply is compromised, some or all of the nipple may die. To reduce the chance of that happening, nipple-sparing mastectomy incisions are made under the breast, beneath the areola, or just outside of the areola (figure 16.3). Your nipples may be flatter, look different, and/or have less sensation or response than they did before your surgery.

FIGURE 16.2 Skin-sparing mastectomy incisions

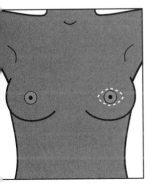 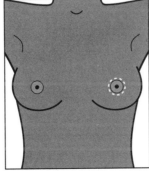 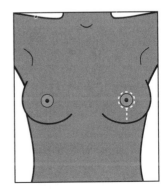

FIGURE 16.3 Nipple-sparing mastectomy incisions

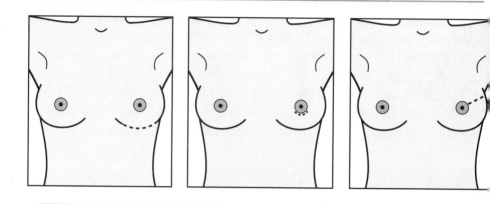

— *My Story* —

Acting on My Test Results

Eight of 10 women in the three generations before me had breast cancer, so I was pretty sure if I had a *BRCA* mutation my odds of developing breast cancer were very high. My father's family has a strong history of breast cancer that includes four of his six sisters, two aunts, and both great-aunts. After I found out about my *BRCA2* mutation on my thirty-fifth birthday, I was on the operating table just six months later, having a bilateral mastectomy.

—*Bethany*

Is Risk-Reducing Mastectomy Right for You?

Removing healthy breasts to avoid breast cancer isn't an easy decision, and it isn't acceptable to everyone. For some women, removing their breasts to prevent cancer that they may never develop seems extreme. For others, the decision remedies the concern they feel, especially if they've seen loved ones wage war against breast cancer. Your circumstances and tolerance for risk will greatly influence your decision.

Mastectomy is irreversible, so it's important to have a clear sense of your own risk and to speak with your health care team about all of your options. Weigh the benefits and limitations of close surveillance and taking tamoxifen

Routine Care after Mastectomy

Very little breast tissue remains after mastectomy, and mammography is no longer required. Most experts recommend an annual clinical breast exam to feel for any abnormalities in the scar or within the reconstructed breast. It's important to regularly perform breast self-exams to discover any lump or irregularity as soon as possible. Examine the area around your breasts up to the collarbone and down below the ribs, looking for hard, pea-size lumps or anything that feels or looks unusual. Report any irregularities to your doctor.

or raloxifene before deciding if RRM is the best way for you to reduce your breast cancer risk. (*The Breast Reconstruction Guidebook* by Kathy Steligo describes mastectomy and reconstructive options and issues in detail.) Women share their postmastectomy photos—with and without reconstruction—on the FORCE website (www.facingourrisk.org/reconstruction).

If the idea of breast reconstruction appeals to you, consult with two or three plastic surgeons about what you can realistically expect in the way of results and recovery. Take the time you need to make a decision you can live with.

— THE FORCE PERSPECTIVE —

Mastectomy Lowers Risk, but Does It Improve Survival?

Some women report that their health care professionals question the choice of risk-reducing mastectomy because it hasn't been shown to improve survival. You might wonder how a procedure that almost eliminates the possibility of cancer doesn't automatically ensure that you'll live longer, but that's what the research reflects. While RRM greatly improves your odds of never developing breast cancer or enduring chemotherapy, radiation, or other treatment, it doesn't necessarily mean improved survival.

The majority of high-risk women who are diagnosed early, particularly those who are screened with breast MRI, survive their breast cancer, so perhaps risk-reducing mastectomy doesn't improve that already strong survival rate. Maybe researchers haven't studied high-risk women after RRM long enough. A survival benefit may emerge as more long-term studies follow women beyond 10 years after mastectomy.

Breast Reconstruction Choices

If you're contemplating risk-reducing mastectomy, you have a lot to think about, including whether you want to have breast reconstruction at the same time to replace the volume and shape of your breasts. While breast reconstruction can't remove mastectomy scars or restore lost sensation, for many women it softens the harshness of mastectomy and restores confidence in their physical appearance. Among the range of reconstructive options, no one method is right for every woman. From an aesthetic perspective, some of the best reconstruction is achieved immediately following RRM.

Reconstruction with Breast Implants

Reconstruction with breast implants accomplishes reconstruction with the shortest surgery and recovery. Most implant reconstruction uses silicone gel implants, which are softer and feel more like natural breast tissue than saline-filled implants. Although more streamlined procedures are available, many surgeons still prefer the traditional three-step process over several months. After the breast tissue has been removed, temporary implants called tissue expanders are placed beneath the chest muscles. Over several weeks, the plastic surgeon gradually fills the expanders with saline to stretch the muscles and the skin. Some women find this process uncomfortable; others sail through it without a second thought.

When the area behind the muscles stretches sufficiently, the expanders are replaced with breast implants. Later, a revision surgery can be performed to correct minor problems and improve the appearance of the new breasts.

Fat grafting—transferring fat liposuctioned from your back, thighs, or abdomen to your new breasts—can improve contour and symmetry, create cleavage, and even increase breast size. If your nipples were removed during your mastectomy, they can be re-created at this stage from a small amount of breast skin and then later tattooed to add color and simulate the areolas. This is an optional step that some women choose to forgo since reconstructed nipples lack the nerves required for sensation or response. An alternative to nipple reconstruction is to have 3D tattooing that realistically simulates nipples and areolas.

If you have a nipple-sparing mastectomy, you're a candidate for direct-to-implant breast reconstruction, a procedure that places full-size implants immediately after mastectomy, thereby avoiding the need for tissue expansion. You leave the operating room much as you entered: with fully formed breasts and your natural nipples. Unless a cosmetic or medical problem arises, you will need no further reconstructive procedures. Direct-to-implant reconstruction uses patches of an acellular dermal matrix (donated human tissue), which are sewn onto the chest muscles. This matrix forms an immediate sling to hold the implants under the muscles, eliminating the need for expanders. Implants can also be placed over the chest muscles and covered with an acellular dermal matrix, which provides a cushioning layer between the implant and the breast skin.

Eventually, almost all implants must be replaced for one reason or another: wrong size or shape, an infection that won't heal, a shift in position, or a leak or rupture. Some women need their implants replaced within a year of reconstruction while others have theirs for 15 years or longer. Capsular contracture—scar tissue that squeezes the implant and thus distorts breast shape and causes discomfort or pain—may require an operation to remove the scar tissue and replace the implant, but there's no guarantee that the same thing won't happen again.

Implants are a good option if you

- haven't had radiation to your chest
- don't mind having additional surgery to eventually replace your implants
- want the least invasive method of breast reconstruction
- want to avoid a longer surgery and recovery
- don't want to scar another area of your body

Are Breast Implants Safe?

Millions of women worldwide have had augmentation or reconstruction with breast implants. Most of them are satisfied and have
few if any problems. However, breast implants aren't lifetime
devices, and they can wrinkle, ripple, rupture, and cause other issues
that may require additional surgery to resolve.

Implants have been linked to breast implant–associated anaplastic large-cell lymphoma (BIA-ALCL), a serious but rare cancer
of the immune system that can develop years after the devices are
placed into the chest. Most BIA-ALCL has been found in the scar
tissue that naturally forms around the implants in women who have
textured expanders or implants that have a roughened surface.
When diagnosed early, BIA-ALCL can be treated successfully by
removing the implant and scar tissue, but some women may require
additional treatment. Left untreated, BIA-ALCL can spread
throughout the body, and it can be fatal.

Some women report experiencing breast implant illness (BII),
with symptoms that may include fatigue, brain fog, reduced memory, and joint pain. Even after years of research, it's still unclear
whether these conditions are directly related to implants or other
causes. Some women have said that their symptoms disappeared
when their implants were removed and not replaced.

The FDA website (www.fda.gov) includes breast implant information and updated safety information about BIA-ALCL and BII.

— *My Story* —
Better than Ever

My mother was diagnosed at age 59 with metastasized inflammatory breast cancer. She died the next year. When my gynecologist suggested I get tested for a *BRCA* mutation, I refused. What would I do if I inherited this risk—worry even more about getting breast cancer? The years passed. Finally, I felt I had to be tested only when I knew what to do if I was positive. Thankfully, I found the FORCE message boards, where I read about women who had prophylactic mastectomy, kept their nipples intact, and had implants placed in a single surgery. For the first time, I felt hope. If I tested positive, I had an option I could live with. Within three months of testing positive for a *BRCA2* mutation, I had nipple-sparing mastectomies with direct-to-implant reconstruction. It wasn't easy. Once I recovered, my body looked better than ever. This procedure gave me the impetus to save my life, and I've never looked back.

—Andrea

Breast Reconstruction with Your Own Tissue

Autologous tissue flap reconstruction is another way to re-create breasts after mastectomy. An area or "flap" of tissue can be removed from your abdomen, hip, thigh, back, or buttocks and transferred to your chest to replace lost breast tissue. Some flap procedures also use muscle, which adds to recovery time and may compromise strength and flexibility at the donor site. Advanced procedures use only fat, which is all that is needed to create a new breast. When there is minimal scarring or fat necrosis, breasts made with your own living tissue are soft and move like your natural breasts. Necrosis is an area of transferred tissue that dies from an inadequate blood supply. A small area of necrosis may harden and feel like a lump. It may resolve on its own or require surgical removal. Rarely, an entire flap fails and must be replaced.

Not all plastic surgeons have the advanced surgical skills to perform flap reconstruction, which can add several hours to mastectomy surgery. The total reconstruction timeline is often shorter than reconstruction with tissue expanders and implants, although recovery from the surgery is longer and more intense. Like most breast implant procedures, flap surgeries usually require a later revision procedure to refine the shape and appearance of the new breast and, if desired, create new nipples (unless you have nipple-sparing mastectomies).

Tissue flaps are a good option if you

- want reconstructed breasts that look and feel the most natural
- are willing to accept additional scarring at the donor site
- have previously had radiation to your chest or breast
- don't want to spend the time needed for tissue expansion
- want reconstructed breasts that aren't likely to require replacement

— *My Story* —

My DIEP Flap Experience

Soon after I found that I carried a *BRCA2* mutation, I decided to have risk-reducing mastectomies and learned that I was a candidate for deep inferior epigastric perforator (DIEP) flap breast reconstruction. I chose to use my abdominal tissue to eliminate the need for foreign objects (breast implants) in my body. My age (45) at the time of surgery, physical well-being, and life stage were all contributing factors, as the recovery and rehabilitation time with DIEP is longer and more intense than reconstruction with implants.

The whole process took about six months. I had three procedures. The initial surgery was the most invasive and lengthy. For the first 24 hours after surgery, I was in the ICU so that the flaps could be continuously monitored. I spent the next five days in the hospital and then went home with six drains, which were removed within two weeks. My entire recovery took about 12 weeks. With two young children, I needed additional help at home for the first few weeks. Eight weeks after my initial surgery, my plastic surgeon created nipples with flaps from my breast skin and improved the contour of my breasts. This was a simple outpatient procedure with minimal recovery time. Several weeks later, my areolas were tattooed, and I was done.

Nineteen months after my mastectomies, my new breasts look natural, and I am comfortable with the results. The sense of empowerment that I have felt throughout this journey has been humbling,

allowing me to nearly eliminate my risk of breast cancer. Importantly, my body has demonstrated a resilience beyond what I knew existed.
—*Heather*

Side Effects, Risks, and Recovery

Initially, you'll be sore at the surgery sites after mastectomy or breast reconstruction. Your surgeon will prescribe pain medication so that you'll be comfortable. You'll feel weak and tired, but your strength, flexibility, and energy will gradually improve. Carefully following your surgeon's instructions for recovery and giving yourself plenty of time to rest will help you heal. You may need three to four weeks to recover from a mastectomy alone or with implant reconstruction and eight weeks or more to get back to your normal activities after mastectomy with tissue flap reconstruction. No matter which procedure you choose, you'll go home from the hospital with surgical drains in your incisions; these need to remain in place for several days to siphon fluids away from the surgery sites and encourage healing. Before you're discharged from the hospital, your nurse will show you how to manage the drains until they're removed. You should also be instructed on how to perform exercises that will restore range of motion in your shoulders and chest. It's important to perform these movements as directed. If needed, your surgeon can refer you to a physical therapist.

Most women recover from mastectomy and reconstruction without serious problems. Like all operations, however, issues can occur, and some may require additional medical intervention. Developing an infection after these surgeries is uncommon, but it sometimes happens; a round of antibiotics usually takes care of the problem. Broader infections can be more difficult and may delay healing. Seromas (buildup of fluid) or hematomas (buildup of blood) that collect deep in the incision site are often absorbed by the body over time. Larger seromas and hematomas can cause swelling, bruising, or pain that requires medical attention. If draining the area with a needle doesn't resolve the problem, surgery may be needed.

Less common problems may include delayed healing, blood clots, and long-term postoperative pain. (Postmastectomy pain syndrome, a chronic condition that many women develop after mastectomy, is described in chapter 29.) Although complications can develop after mastectomy, they are more likely to occur with breast reconstruction, which is more invasive than mastectomy alone. Nerves in the chest are severed when breast tissue is

Choosing Your Surgeon

You should select a general surgeon, breast surgeon, or surgical oncologist who regularly performs mastectomies. If you're considering a nipple-sparing mastectomy, ask how many of these procedures the surgeon has performed and the rate of success. Ask to see postoperative photos of the surgeon's nipple-sparing results, and try to speak with other women who have had the same procedure. If you decide to have breast reconstruction, choosing the right plastic surgeon can make the difference between being satisfied and being disappointed. Not all surgeons perform all procedures, and experience varies widely. Get a second and even a third opinion. Verify the certifications for the surgeons you are considering at the American Board of Medical Specialties website (www.abms.org).

removed, and much of the sensation in the area is permanently lost. Though some feeling may return over time as nerves regenerate, especially if you have flap reconstruction, sensation in your reconstructed breast won't be the same as it was in your natural breast. If you have flap reconstruction, the area around the donor incision will also likely remain permanently numb.

Will Your Health Insurance
Pay for Your Surgeries?

Federal law doesn't require health insurers to cover mastectomy solely to reduce the risk of breast cancer. Several states, however, require this coverage when it's "medically necessary," which insurance companies may define in different ways. Some health insurance providers will pay some or all of the costs with either a letter from your doctor recommending mastectomy to lower your high risk or a second confirming opinion. If your insurance carrier refuses to cover your procedure, ask your doctor to write a supportive appeal letter explaining why mastectomy is necessary to reduce your higher-than-average breast cancer risk. (Find sample appeal letters at www.facingourrisk.org.)

The Women's Health and Cancer Rights Act of 1998 requires health insurance that covers mastectomy to also pay for breast reconstruction, although some plans are exempt, and out-of-pocket costs may apply. This law also requires health plans to pay for costs related to breast prostheses, achieving breast symmetry (including lifting, reducing, or augmenting the opposite breast to match the reconstructed breast), and lymphedema therapy, if needed.

Discuss coverage with your surgeons and your health insurer before you schedule your surgeries. Get clarity on the amount of out-of-pocket costs, including deductibles and copays for which you may be responsible, and whether you're required to use in-network surgeons. If you're underinsured or uninsured, contact your local affiliate of the American Cancer Society or Susan G. Komen about accessing donated surgical services.

Chapter 17

Surgeries That Reduce the Risk of Gynecologic Cancers

If you're premenopausal, RRSO will create a sudden drop in hormone production that will cause early menopause. You may then have the same symptoms you would experience with natural menopause: hot flashes, vaginal dryness, changes in concentration or memory, depression or anxiety, sleep issues, bone loss, and/or other short-term and long-term symptoms.

If you have a high risk for ovarian, fallopian tube, or primary peritoneal cancers, preventive surgery can greatly decrease your chance of a diagnosis. This is especially important since these gynecologic cancers often develop without symptoms, and screening tests are either not available or not sufficiently accurate to detect these cancers in their earliest stages.

Gynecologic surgeries are performed for contraception, to remove cysts or fibroids, to remedy painful intercourse, and to treat numerous other medical conditions, including cancer. Some of the same surgeries also reduce the risk of certain hereditary gynecologic cancers in high-risk women.

- Oophorectomy removes the ovaries.
- Salpingectomy removes the fallopian tubes.
- Salpingo-oophorectomy removes the ovaries and fallopian tubes.
- Partial (supracervical) hysterectomy removes the uterus, leaving the cervix intact.
- Total hysterectomy removes the uterus and cervix.

Salpingo-Oophorectomy to
Reduce the Risk of Ovarian Cancer

The most effective method of counteracting an inherited predisposition to ovarian cancer is risk-reducing salpingo-oophorectomy, the removal of both ovaries and both fallopian tubes. It is the standard of care for most high-risk women. Much of the research on the benefits and risks of RRSO has involved high-risk women with *BRCA1* or *BRCA2* mutations. RRSO benefits high-risk women in the following ways:

- It reduces ovarian, fallopian tube, and primary peritoneal cancer risk by 80 percent or more.[1]
- It lowers the risk of hormone-sensitive breast cancer when surgery is done before menopause.[2]
- It's associated with reduced risk for death from ovarian cancer and all other causes.[3]

If you have an inherited mutation in a *BRCA1* gene, your risk of ovarian cancer rises sharply between ages 40 and 49. You may also have a slightly increased risk for an aggressive type of endometrial cancer. National guidelines recommend that you have RRSO between the ages of 35 and 40 and when you're finished having children and that you speak with your surgeon about the benefits and risks of having a hysterectomy at the same time. You're less likely to develop ovarian cancer before age 50 if you have a *BRCA2* mutation; in that case, RRSO is recommended between ages 40 and 45.

Less is known about the beneficial effects of RRSO in women with other mutations. Experts use the results of available research to try to predict outcomes and create guidelines for women with other gene mutations. You're encouraged to discuss the benefits and risks of RRSO with your doctor after you've completed childbearing if you carry a mutation in a *BRIP1*, *RAD51C*, *RAD51D*, *EPCAM*, *MLH1*, *MSH2*, or *PALB2* gene. Researchers are still studying the risk for ovarian cancer in people with an *ATM*, *MSH6*, or *PMS2* mutation. It may be reasonable to consider risk-reducing salpingo-oophorectomy if you have a mutation in one of these genes, especially if you also have a family history of ovarian cancer. Your genetic counselor can help you understand your risk for ovarian cancer so that you can discuss the benefits and risks with your surgeon.

After RRSO, a small risk for primary peritoneal cancer remains. This is an uncommon cancer with no effective method of screening, so no specific follow-up to RRSO is advised other than the recommended well-woman screenings and being aware of the symptoms of primary peritoneal cancer.

Salpingo-Oophorectomy Procedures

Risk-reducing salpingo-oophorectomy is typically done with minimally invasive laparoscopic surgery. Once you're sedated, a laparoscope—a narrow tube with a video camera at one end—is inserted through a small incision made in your navel. Carbon dioxide is then introduced into the abdomen to create more space between the abdominal wall and the internal organs. The scope lights up the abdomen and sends magnified images to a viewing screen

Removing the Fallopian Tubes to Reduce Ovarian Cancer Risk

The discovery that many ovarian cancers begin in the fallopian tubes has led to research into whether salpingectomy—removal of the fallopian tubes—safely and effectively reduces ovarian cancer risk. Researchers are studying whether it's safe for premenopausal high-risk women to remove only their fallopian tubes and delay removing the ovaries until after menopause. Until these studies are complete, experts can't recommend salpingectomy alone over RRSO for women at high risk for ovarian cancer. Risk-reducing salpingo-oophorectomy is recognized as the most effective method of decreasing that high risk.

so that the surgeon can clearly see your pelvic organs. Guided by the laparoscopic images, the surgeon inspects the abdominal organs and uses laparoscopic tools to remove the ovaries and most of the fallopian tubes through two or three additional small cuts (figure 17.1). The resulting scars are small and eventually may become nearly invisible. Laparoscopic RRSO is usually a short outpatient operation.

Serial sectioning of the ovaries and fallopian tubes after RRSO is critically important. This is a close pathological examination of several thin cross-sections of the fallopian tubes and ovaries to look for any precancerous changes or cancer cells. In some high-risk people, this pathology reveals a small, previously undetected invasive cancer that may require chemotherapy and/or additional treatment. An abdominal wash should also be done: sterile liquid is flushed into the pelvic cavity, the fluid is removed, and then it is sent to a pathologist, who looks for any evidence of cancer.

If cancer is suspected or found, or if you have a history of endometriosis, prior pelvic infection, or prior pelvic surgery, you might benefit from a robotic-assisted RRSO. Surgeon-controlled robotic surgery provides better optics so that the surgeon can proceed with more precision and accuracy while minimizing trauma to surrounding tissues. However, additional incisions are often needed to perform robotic surgery, and not all people need the higher level of technology. In addition, not all facilities have robotic capabilities, and not all surgeons have the required expertise or experience.

It's normal to feel tired after RRSO. You'll be sore around your incisions and abdomen, and you may have temporary discomfort in your back. You'll be prescribed medication to control your pain during the first couple of weeks after surgery. You may experience some vaginal discharge or spotting. Most people recover fully within two weeks.

A laparotomy may be necessary if you have scar tissue from previous surgeries, if your organs appear abnormal, or if cancer is suspected or found. A laparoscopic oophorectomy can end up as a laparotomy if a larger incision is needed to control bleeding or rectify a complication.

During laparotomy, a four- to six-inch abdominal incision is made through the skin, fascia (connective tissue), and peritoneum. It may run horizontally across the lower abdomen or vertically from the navel to the pubic bone (figure 17.1). Although a horizontal incision minimizes the scar that forms, a vertical incision may provide greater visibility into the upper abdomen when cancer is suspected. The surgeon gently separates the abdominal

FIGURE 17.1 Incisions for oophorectomy and hysterectomy: laparoscopic (*top left*), robotic-assisted laparoscopic (*top right*), and two types of laparotomy (*bottom*)

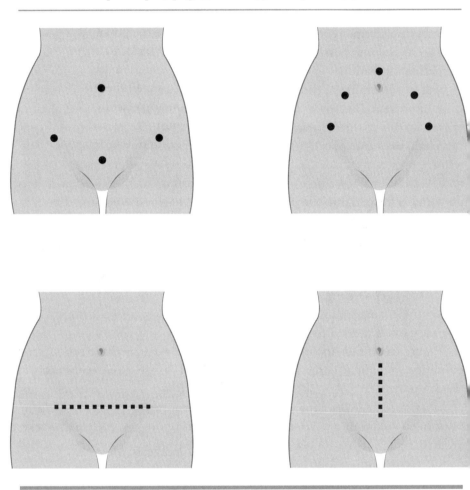

muscles and inspects the ovaries and the fallopian tubes before removing them. The abdominal layers are then stitched back together, and the incision is closed with sutures or surgical staples. Laparotomy takes two to four hours and is performed under local or general anesthesia. Because it's more invasive than laparoscopy, laparotomy can cause more bleeding and has a greater risk for complications. You'll need to stay in the hospital for one or two days. You may need six weeks or more before you fully recover.

Side Effects of Salpingo-Oophorectomy

While the benefits of RRSO are significant, it forever ends menstrual periods, which you may welcome, but it also eliminates the possibility of natural pregnancy.

If you're premenopausal, RRSO will create a sudden drop in hormone production that will cause early menopause. You may then have the same symptoms you would experience with natural menopause: hot flashes, vaginal dryness, changes in concentration or memory, depression or anxiety, sleep issues, bone loss, and/or other short-term and long-term symptoms (see chapter 28). The younger you are when you have this surgery, the more intense these symptoms are likely to be. You're less likely to have symptoms if you're already perimenopausal or postmenopausal when you have RRSO.

In addition to the general side effects of surgery, including possible infection, delayed wound healing, blood loss, and postoperative pain, RRSO may cause blood clots and may damage nerves or internal organs.

— EXPERT VIEW —

Focus on the Fallopian Tubes

BY BARBARA NORQUIST, MD

Oncologists have long assumed that ovarian carcinomas arise in the surface layer (epithelium) of the ovary or the epithelial lining of small ovarian cysts. However, we now understand that many so-called ovarian cancers originate in the fallopian tubes and then spread to the ovaries. Several lines of evidence support this tubal hypothesis. Most early BRCA-associated gynecologic cancers are found not in the ovary, but in the fallopian tubes during prophylactic surgery. (Some sporadic ovarian cancers may also begin in the fallopian tubes.) People whose ovaries are removed without also removing the fallopian tubes are at higher risk of later developing peritoneal cancer than those who have their tubes removed during ovarian surgery.

The current standard of care and the only proven method to prevent ovarian cancer in high-risk women is to have both the ovaries and fallopian tubes removed. However, as awareness of the tubal hypothesis increases, so has interest in the alternative of salpingectomy with delayed oophorectomy: removing the fallopian tubes in one procedure and then removing the ovaries later. This approach may decrease the risk of ovarian cancer while avoiding or delaying the side effects of surgical menopause. The most important downside to this approach is that we do not yet know how safe it is or how effective it is at preventing ovarian cancer. People choosing this strategy need two surgeries instead of one. Removing the fallopian tubes results in sterilization and is therefore not appropriate for individuals who desire future fertility. Multiple clinical trials are currently investigating the safety and side effects of salpingectomy with delayed oophorectomy, with the hope of providing an additional option for those who face an inherited risk of ovarian cancer.

Making Decisions about Risk-Reducing Salpingo-Oophorectomy

Deciding whether RRSO is right for you and when to have it can be challenging. A genetic counselor can clarify how the surgery will affect your cancer risk and identify the best time to have it. The younger you are when you have your ovaries and fallopian tubes removed, the greater your chance of preventing ovarian cancer. Having RRSO closer to age 35 helps you to avoid ovarian cancer, but it also causes early menopause. (Knowing that short-term hormone use for menopausal symptoms doesn't appear to affect breast cancer risk in previvors after RRSO may help your decision.)[4] If you're confident that you don't want a future pregnancy, you may decide that RRSO is the best way to lower your chance of developing ovarian cancer. The decision can be more difficult if you believe that RRSO is in your best interest but you also want to become pregnant now or in the future. A fertility expert can explain your options (see chapter 27), and your doctor can help you understand and manage your risk in the meantime.

Your current menopausal status may also influence what you decide. If you're high risk and postmenopausal, your doctors may recommend oophorectomy as soon as possible, because your risk increases as you age, your ovaries are producing few if any hormones, and milder side effects can be expected after RRSO. Even though some women develop hereditary ovarian cancer before age 50, most diagnoses occur after that age. While postponing salpingo-oophorectomy until you reach natural menopause means more years with your natural hormones, it also raises the chances of being diagnosed with cancer in the interim.

Other considerations that may influence your decision:

- your level of risk
- your tolerance for risk
- the lack of reliable screening for ovarian cancer
- you have relatives who developed ovarian cancer at a young age
- the risk-reducing benefits compared to menopausal symptoms and other side effects of surgery
- you're years away from menopause
- you've had ovarian cysts, menstrual problems, or other gynecologic issues
- the time needed for surgery and recovery

If you have an inherited mutation in a Lynch syndrome gene—*MLH1, MSH2, MSH6,* or *EPCAM*—you have a high risk for ovarian cancer and a high risk for endometrial cancer. (The associated risk with a *PMS2* mutation is less clear.) In this case, you face another decision. Should your uterus be removed in addition to RRSO? (See the section "Salpingo-Oophorectomy, Hysterectomy, or Both?" later in this chapter.)

— *My Story* —

Breaking the Family Curse

For as long as I can remember, the fear of breast cancer cast a shadow over my life. My grandmother died from it before I turned 5. When my mother was diagnosed at age 39, I viewed it as some kind of curse. My family was secretive, and I felt alone with this. When my daughter was born, my joy was tempered by the thought that she would have breasts one day. Five years ago, when my aunt got ovarian cancer, a genetic counselor recommended my mother have testing. She later found that she carried a *BRCA* mutation. I was then tested and learned that I had the same mutation. I knew something was going on with the breast cancer in my family and felt sure I would not escape it, yet having it confirmed was devastating. I immediately had an oophorectomy. Having the mutation was beyond my control, but eventually knowing about it was a kind of blessing.

—Randi

Oophorectomy and Mastectomy: Either, Neither, or Both?

If you have a mutation in a *BRCA1*, *BRCA2*, or *PALB2* gene, you have an elevated risk for breast and ovarian cancer. (Mutations in the *ATM*, *BRIP1*, *RAD51C*, and *RAD51D* genes may also raise the risk for both cancers, but more research is needed to confirm the associations.) Even without surgery, you may never develop either cancer, making the decision to remove healthy organs more difficult. Mastectomy is the most effective means of reducing breast cancer risk. Oophorectomy is the most effective way to lower ovarian cancer risk and may reduce breast cancer risk as well. Having both surgeries provides the greatest overall risk reduction.

Some people opt to have both surgeries at the same time and be done with it. Others have one operation when they learn of their high-risk status and the other surgery later. As a 35-year-old woman who wants to bear children, for example, you might have a prophylactic bilateral mastectomy right away, then have RRSO after your children are born. Another person of the same age might prefer to have both mastectomy and RRSO immediately to reduce the risk as much as possible and as soon as possible. Someone else may opt for more frequent surveillance with or without chemoprevention.

Deciding if and when to have these surgeries is a personal choice and one that should be made only after you've had time to research and thoughtfully consider all the ramifications of each surgery (table 17.1). A genetic counselor and a gynecologic expert can help you sort these issues, clarify the different risk management options, and explain how each affects your risk. Talking to other high-risk people who have faced these same choices can also be helpful. Though they're not medical professionals, peers offer a "been there, done that" sounding board for someone who is struggling with these perplexing decisions. The FORCE message boards are an excellent resource where other previvors share their experiences.

Hysterectomy to Reduce the Risk of Endometrial Cancer

Hysterectomy (removal of the uterus) is the second most common surgery after cesarean delivery among women of reproductive age in the United States. It's often recommended to control vaginal bleeding, remove fibroids, and remedy other problems in the uterus. A partial hysterectomy removes the uterus, while a total hysterectomy removes the uterus and the cervix. Most often, surgeons remove the fallopian tubes and the uterus at the same time. If the ovaries are preserved, the risk of ovarian and primary peritoneal cancer remains.

If you have Lynch syndrome or an inherited *PTEN* mutation, NCCN guidelines recommend that you discuss the benefits and risks of a hysterectomy after you finish having children in order to reduce your risk of endometrial cancer. Women with a *BRCA1* mutation, who have a slightly increased risk for endometrial cancer, should discuss the benefits and risks of hysterectomy at the time of their risk-reducing salpingo-oophorectomy. Unlike ovarian cancer, endometrial cancer often has signs and symptoms that indicate early cancer. For this reason, some high-risk individuals who have no symptoms choose not to have a risk-reducing hysterectomy.

Hysterectomy Procedures

If you decide to have a risk-reducing hysterectomy, your surgeon is likely to perform a procedure known as a laparoscopic-assisted vaginal hysterectomy (LAVH). A laparoscope is inserted through a small incision in the navel, and surgical instruments are used to perform the surgery through separate small incisions (figure 17.1). The uterus, which is separated from the vagina and moved away from the bladder and rectum, is cut into sections and removed through the laparoscope or directly from the vagina. The abdominal cuts and the vaginal incision are then stitched closed. LAVH is often performed as outpatient surgery, although some people stay overnight in the hospital. The risk of infection is reduced, scarring and pain are significantly less, and recovery is shorter than with non-laparoscopic surgery. Small scars remain on the abdomen after the procedure.

Some facilities perform a robotic-assisted laparoscopic hysterectomy. The uterus can also be removed with an abdominal hysterectomy, through a four- to six-inch horizontal or vertical incision in the abdomen, similar to the incision used in oophorectomy (figure 17.1). An abdominal hysterectomy requires a hospital stay of two to three days and six weeks or more of recovery.

Vaginal bleeding and discharge are normal for several weeks after a hysterectomy. Constipation is common, and some individuals also have problems urinating. Other potential complications include infection, excessive bleeding, and/or damage to the urinary tract or bowel. Bladder prolapse, a condition in which the bladder sags down into the vagina, is a risk with hysterectomy, although it doesn't happen often. Reduced sexual satisfaction is sometimes mentioned as a possible side effect after hysterectomy, yet studies of women in the general population don't support this claim. Long-term problems may include a greater risk for urinary problems, heart attack, and stroke. Emotionally, you may feel sad that you can no longer bear children, or you may be relieved that you no longer have to worry about birth control.

Salpingo-Oophorectomy, Hysterectomy, or Both?

Deciding whether to have a hysterectomy, an oophorectomy, or both can be confusing. While both procedures reduce cancer risk to some degree, a total hysterectomy with risk-reducing salpingo-oophorectomy (TAH/RRSO)—removal of the uterus, cervix, ovaries, and fallopian tubes—more broadly decreases the chance of gynecologic cancer. Some people who have a high risk for endometrial cancer may choose to remove their ovaries at the same time that they have their hysterectomy. Some who have a high risk for ovarian cancer may choose to have a hysterectomy along with RRSO.

If you plan to have an RRSO, your doctor can help you decide whether you should also have a hysterectomy (table 17.1). You may be more likely to choose hysterectomy if your circumstances include any of the following:

- You're at high risk for endometrial cancer due to family history, your health or medical circumstances, or other factors.
- You've had previous abnormal Pap smears, heavy bleeding, uterine fibroids, endometriosis, or other abnormalities of the uterus or cervix.
- You're considering hormones after surgery and prefer to take estrogen alone, rather than a combination of estrogen and progesterone (see chapter 28).

If you plan to have a hysterectomy, your doctor can help you decide whether you should also have an RRSO (table 17.1). You may be more likely to choose TAH/RRSO if your circumstances include any of the following:

- You're at high risk for ovarian cancer due to family history, your health or medical situation, or other factors.

- You've had previous issues with your ovaries, such as frequent or painful cysts.
- You're postmenopausal.

The procedures for TAH/RRSO and abdominal hysterectomy are similar, except that during an abdominal hysterectomy, the ovaries, fallopian tubes, uterus, and cervix are removed through an abdominal incision. An RRSO with laparoscopically assisted hysterectomy (RRSO/LAVH) removes the uterus and cervix through a vaginal incision. Each operation lasts two to four hours. You'll

TABLE 17.1 Benefits and Limitations of Risk-Reducing Gynecologic Surgeries

	BENEFITS	LIMITATIONS
risk-reducing salpingo-oophorectomy (RRSO) only	• reduces ovarian and fallopian tube cancer risk • eliminates menstrual period • typically done as a laparoscopic, outpatient procedure	• leads to surgical menopause (if performed before natural menopause) • doesn't lower endometrial cancer risk • complicates the decision regarding hormone replacement • eliminates ability to conceive (in vitro fertilization is possible with previously stored embryos)
hysterectomy only	• eliminates menstrual periods • doesn't cause surgical menopause • you can still conceive, but you'll require a pregnancy surrogate	• doesn't lower ovarian cancer risk
RRSO and hysterectomy combined	• provides maximum risk reduction for ovarian and endometrial cancers • simplifies hormone replacement therapy decision	• eliminates ability to conceive (in vitro fertilization is possible if you have previously stored embryos) • leads to surgical menopause (when performed before natural menopause)

stay in the hospital for a few hours or overnight after RRSO/LAVH and one or two nights after TAH/RRSO. You'll need six weeks or more for a full recovery.

Who Should Perform Your Surgery?

Even though gynecologists are trained to perform oophorectomy and hysterectomy, it can be beneficial to consult with a gynecologic oncologist. If a gynecologist performs your surgery and cancer is found, a second surgery may be needed to stage and determine the extent of the disease. Gynecologic oncologists, however, have advanced training. They're familiar with the specific protocol for high-risk women, which includes exploring the pelvic organs for abnormalities or evidence of cancer, performing a peritoneal wash, and removing the ovaries, fallopian tubes, uterus, and cervix. If cancer is found, a gynecologic oncologist can remove lymph nodes and as much of the tumor as possible, and then continue to manage your treatment. The Foundation for Women's Cancer (https://specialist.foundationforwomenscancer.org) can help you find a gynecologic oncologist in your area.

— THE **FORCE** PERSPECTIVE —

When Prophylactic Surgery Finds Cancer

While the goal of prophylactic surgery is to prevent cancer, sometimes during surgery an unexpected tumor is discovered. If this happens to you, give yourself time to adjust to your diagnosis. Being diagnosed with cancer as you were taking steps to prevent it can be disheartening, even if you're grateful that the cancer was discovered early. Necessary treatment may shift your preventive timeline. Be patient and kind with yourself. Try not to second-guess your decisions. Without a crystal ball, there's no way you could have foreseen a diagnosis that seemed to come out of the blue. Gather your resources, assemble a health care team that you trust, and rally your support system around you. Do your homework and create a plan of action, just as you did when you decided to have genetic testing and when you made your decisions about prophylactic surgery. You'll get through this and move forward.

Questions for Your Gynecologic Surgeon

- Do you recommend a hysterectomy, a salpingo-oophorectomy, or both?

- What are my options for surgery?

- Am I a candidate for minimally invasive surgery?

- What can I expect from these operations?

- How many of these surgeries have you done in high-risk people?

- What complications may occur, and how will you address them?

- How long will I be in the hospital?

- What should I expect during recovery, and how should I prepare for it?

- What long-term follow-up care will I need?

Insurance and Payment Issues

Many health insurance companies will cover some or all of the costs of risk-reducing salpingo-oophorectomy and hysterectomy, although the conditions for coverage may vary. Some insurers may require a second opinion or a letter of medical necessity from your health care provider. If you're considering preventive surgery for endometrial and/or ovarian cancer, review your insurance policy to determine whether a particular risk-reducing method is covered. Discuss insurance coverage issues with your doctor and your insurance company before you have the surgery. Some health insurers consider payment based on individual circumstances, while others view prophylactic surgeries as elective and not medically necessary. If your request is denied, your physician and genetic counselor are your best defense. Ask them to provide letters of medical necessity on your behalf and to assist with any appeals if coverage is denied.

— *My Story* —

My Preventive Surgery Found Cancer

My sister, a nurse practitioner, knew instantly that the mass on my father's chest was breast cancer. Treatment and genetic testing followed, confirming a *BRCA2* mutation in the family. My sister and I both tested positive, and one day before her fortieth birthday, she too was diagnosed with breast cancer. She urged me to have prophylactic surgery. At 37, I had bilateral mastectomy almost joyously, thinking I could relax about cancer.

I desperately wanted a second child, but I couldn't conceive, and after much consideration, I decided to have an oophorectomy. Although my surgeon wasn't worried about my risk because of my young age, I felt my risk was too great. After the procedure, he said everything appeared normal and that 99 percent of the pathology results had come back clear. I rebounded quickly, and I was shopping when I received the call with my final pathology report. I cried and shook as I heard "serous tubal intraepithelial carcinoma, Stage 0 in both fallopian tubes." I had cancer. It was caught before it could become invasive, and I required no further treatment. My diagnosis helped me find peace with my decision not to have that second child. My father had to develop breast cancer to save my life and my sister's, and I know how lucky I am to be alive.

—*Kisaria*

Surgeries That Reduce the Risk of Gastrointestinal Cancers

While it might seem surprising, people can live well without a stomach. Yet eating and drinking in a more controlled way can be difficult. It takes planning, effort, and patience to change your preoperative eating habits and learn what your new system can and can't tolerate.

Risk-reducing surgeries are recommended for some individuals who have inherited mutations that greatly increase their risk of cancer in the gastrointestinal tract. Removing the colon and rectum is advised for some people with very high risk for colorectal cancer, and stomach removal is advised for people who have an inherited *CDH1* mutation and hereditary diffuse gastric cancer syndrome.

Total and Segmental Colectomy to Reduce the Risk of Colon Cancer

Colectomy is a surgical procedure that removes a portion or all of the colon (the large intestine). It's used to treat Crohn's disease, ulcerative colitis, other bowel diseases, and some colon cancers. Risk-reducing colectomy may also be recommended if you have an inherited mutation that increases your risk for colorectal cancer, depending on the type of mutation and your personal situation. For some people, doctors may recommend the surgery before cancer develops. For others, doctors may recommend it to prevent a new diagnosis in people who already have colorectal cancer.

If you've already been diagnosed with cancer, depending on its extent and location you'll have either an open colectomy (laparotomy) with a single long incision in the abdominal wall or a laparoscopic colectomy with several small incisions near your navel. Both methods are performed under general anesthesia and are completed in one to four hours, depending on the procedure. Once you're sedated, your colon is separated from nearby organs and removed. Some colectomies temporarily or permanently reroute the way stool leaves the body. In some cases, waste will be collected in a surgically created internal pouch until it's eliminated. In other cases, waste may be routed via a stoma, a permanent opening made on the abdomen, to a colostomy bag worn on the outside of your body. If you have a colostomy bag, you'll be shown how to manage it before you're discharged from the hospital. The type of colectomy you have depends on your medical history and your preference. You may not be a candidate for all surgical options.

- Segmental colectomy removes the portion of the colon that is affected by cancer, a large polyp, or multiple polyps. Segmental colectomy is used as treatment but not for prevention.
- Total abdominal colectomy with ileorectal anastomosis removes the entire colon but retains the rectum so that you remain continent after surgery. This surgery may be used preventively, but it's less ideal if you have a very high risk for rectal cancer due to rectal polyps.
- Total proctocolectomy with ileal pouch and anal anastomosis removes the colon and rectum and leaves the anal sphincter (the muscle that controls the release of stool) in place. A portion of the small intestine is used to create an internal pouch, which may allow you to remain continent. With this approach, the risk of cancer developing at the point of connection of the bowel to the anus is small.
- Total proctocolectomy with permanent end ileostomy removes the entire colon, rectum, and anus. The end of the small intestine is brought through the abdominal wall to form a stoma. An external bag is required to manage stool output. This option is the most complete way to lower the risk for colorectal cancer, especially in people with an *APC* mutation.

Recommendations for Risk-Reducing Colectomy

If you have MUTYH-associated polyposis (MAP, an inherited mutation in both *MUTYH* genes) and your colon polyps can't be managed with colonoscopy alone, one of the surgeries listed above may be recommended. Your doctor may recommend risk-reducing total abdominal colectomy with ileorectal anastomosis or another option based on the number and distribution of the polyps in the colon and rectum.

If you have familial adenomatous polyposis (caused by a mutation in the *APC* gene), the National Comprehensive Cancer Network (NCCN) recommends a discussion of colectomy with your doctor as soon as your polyps are discovered. The type of colectomy depends on your medical history and preference, but given your high risk for rectal cancer, total proctocolectomy with permanent end ileostomy may be recommended. Colonoscopy alone rather than colectomy may be sufficient if you have a variation of FAP known as attenuated FAP and your polyp count is low.

If you have Lynch syndrome and you've been diagnosed with colorectal cancer, NCCN guidelines recommend consideration of a colectomy using one of the previously described procedures. This will not only treat your current cancer but prevent a new diagnosis.

If your doctor advises colectomy, it's important to understand what it involves, what to expect after surgery, and how to best prepare. A cancer genetics expert can help you understand how colectomy will affect your risk for future colon cancer. A colorectal surgeon can explain the potential risks and long-term effects of different colectomy procedures. If you choose a surgery that preserves your rectum or anus, you may still need to have regular screenings to be sure that cancer doesn't develop in the remaining tissue.

Risks of Colectomy

Before your surgery, be sure to discuss the risks of potential complications, some of which can be serious, with your surgeon:

- infection
- internal bleeding
- hernia
- delayed healing
- leakage from the colon into the abdomen

- damage to nearby organs
- pneumonia and other lung complications
- bowel obstruction
- blood clots in the lungs (pulmonary embolism) or the legs (deep vein thrombosis)
- dehydration with electrolyte abnormalities

Recovery after Colectomy

You'll need up to three weeks to recover from a colectomy, depending on your health and the type of procedure you have. You'll stay in the hospital for three to four days after a laparoscopic colectomy. You'll need another three to four days after your first post-op bowel movement before you can begin to eat normally again.

A low-fiber diet is recommended for up to a month after surgery to reduce the amount and frequency of stools and to promote healing. During this time, your bowel movements may be more frequent and looser than you're used to until you begin eating solid foods. Try not to strain, and be sure to stay well hydrated with up to 10 glasses of liquid every day. Your health care provider will give you tips to help your recovery.

Total Gastrectomy to Reduce the Risk of Stomach Cancer

If you have hereditary diffuse gastric cancer (HDGC) syndrome due to an inherited mutation in the *CDH1* gene, you have a high probability of developing stomach cancer before age 40. Cancers that are caused by *CDH1* mutations are diffuse, meaning that they affect much of the stomach, and they don't form specific or easy-to-find tumors. This makes early detection unlikely. It's difficult to accurately assess the lining of the stomach, and even endoscopy often fails to detect precancerous or cancerous changes. Experts recommend risk-reducing total gastrectomy between ages 18 and 40 to address the high risk of stomach cancer. This particularly aggressive approach is critical if you have a *CDH1* mutation because gastric cancer can start in any part of the stomach. Gastrectomy (removing the stomach) is frequently used to treat stomach cancer, and it's the only effective way to prevent it.

Questions for Your Gastrointestinal Surgeon

- Which type of colectomy do you recommend for me, and why?
- How many of these surgeries have you performed in high-risk individuals?
- What are the benefits and risks of this surgery?
- What are the possible complications, and how likely are they to occur?
- How will you address these complications if they develop?
- How long will I be in the hospital?
- What should I expect during recovery, and how should I prepare?
- What long-term follow-up care or surveillance will I need?

Gastrectomy Procedures

Total gastrectomy is performed under general anesthesia in a hospital. It can be done laparoscopically with several small incisions or as an open gastrectomy, involving a single, larger incision in the abdomen or chest. Your surgeon will explain the benefits and limitations of each operation and help you decide which is best for you. You'll have less pain, a quicker recovery, and a somewhat shorter hospital stay if you have a minimally invasive laparoscopic or robotic-assisted laparoscopic total gastrectomy, which are as effective as open gastrectomy. These operations are best performed in medical centers with surgeons who are experienced and knowledgeable about the protocol and care required for individuals with HDGC syndrome.

During gastrectomy, the abdominal skin, muscle, and tissue are pulled aside to access the stomach. The stomach is detached from connecting arteries and veins, separated from the esophagus and the intestine, and removed. One end of the jejunum (the lower part of the intestine) is then cut clear, pulled upward, and stitched to the open end of the esophagus, where it previously joined with the stomach (figure 18.1). The lower end of the intestine is then attached to the duodenum, forming a digestive conduit that replaces the stomach. (A section of the small intestine is often folded over to create a pouch that somewhat replaces the stomach.) Before you can begin eating on your own, an x-ray will be taken to ensure that these newly joined areas don't leak.

FIGURE 18.1 Before (*left*) and after (*right*) total gastrectomy

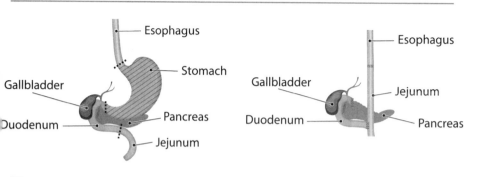

Risks of Gastrectomy

Complication rates are about the same for open and laparoscopic gastrectomies. Possible problems include

- internal bleeding
- infection at the incision site or in the chest
- damage to nearby organs
- blockage of the small intestine
- stricture (narrowing of the esophagus if scar tissue builds up)
- leakage where the esophagus and the small intestine are joined
- dumping syndrome (see "Dumping Syndrome" sidebar)
- hernia
- acid reflux
- diarrhea, nausea, and/or vomiting
- pneumonia, bronchitis, or other chest infection
- losing up to 20 percent of total body weight within six months of surgery
- malabsorption (the inability to absorb dietary nutrients)
- malnutrition, osteoporosis, and other conditions that may result from vitamin deficiencies

Recovery and Life after Gastrectomy

Total gastrectomy is a serious operation. The first few postoperative weeks can be difficult, and full recovery can take a long time. It's important to rest when you feel tired and to gradually increase how much you walk each day. It may take eight weeks or more before you can resume your routine activities and up to a year before your new digestive system fully heals.

After surgery, you'll spend a week or two in the hospital. Your abdomen and your incision will be tender, but pain medication will help you remain comfortable. For the first two or three days, you'll be fed intravenously or with a tube inserted into your small intestine to avoid infection and encourage healing. If no complications occur, you will then begin a liquid diet for a few days before beginning to eat lightly. Little by little, solid foods can be added back into your diet. Your doctor will give you specific instructions about what to eat after surgery.

While it might seem surprising, people can live well without a stomach. Yet eating and drinking in a more controlled way can be difficult. It takes planning, effort, and patience to change your preoperative eating habits and learn what your new system can and can't tolerate. It may take several months before your intestinal pouch expands and your system can handle a more normal diet. Initially, eating may feel more like a necessary chore than a pleasurable indulgence. You'll gradually be able to accept and enjoy more food, but you'll need to change what, when, and how you eat. Your body will continue to digest food, but in a much different way. Before surgery, food passed from your esophagus into your stomach, where it was digested before moving to the small intestine. After gastrectomy, food moves from the esophagus to the small intestine, where it is digested.

Even though eating may be uncomfortable, especially initially after surgery, and you won't be able to eat as much as you did before, your body still needs adequate calories and nutrition, particularly during the first months after surgery. Without a stomach, your body won't be able to directly absorb all the nutrients it needs from food. A nutritionist will help you develop a dietary plan to keep you healthy, which will include supplements to help prevent serious health conditions that can occur:

- Vitamin B_{12} deficiency can cause anemia, vision problems, depression, and other health issues. It commonly occurs a year or more after gastrectomy. Most people who have gastrectomy need B_{12} injections or supplements for the rest of their life.
- Lactose intolerance, the inability to digest lactose (the sugar in dairy products), may develop after gastrectomy.
- Osteopenia and osteoporosis, which weaken the bones, occur in some people after total gastrectomy because calcium, vitamin B_{12}, and vitamin D aren't easily absorbed.
- Iron deficiency anemia (when you don't have enough iron to carry oxygen throughout your body) causes fatigue and shortness of breath.
- Folate deficiency isn't common after total gastrectomy, but it sometimes develops when the body doesn't get enough folic acid, a B vitamin that helps to produce red blood cells.

Dumping Syndrome

After gastrectomy, uncomfortable symptoms may develop if your small intestine receives more food than it can easily digest. Dumping syndrome occurs when food enters the small intestine too quickly. The digestive tract responds by releasing excessive enzymes and sending fluid into the small intestine. Nausea, vomiting, abdominal pain and cramping, diarrhea, and feeling uncomfortably full from a small amount of food may occur within an hour of eating. Up to three hours after eating, you may sweat, feel weak or dizzy, or have an irregular heartbeat if your blood sugar falls or rises too quickly. Keeping a food diary can help you identify which foods cause problems. You can reduce or avoid uncomfortable side effects by changing the way you eat.

- Eat several small meals instead of too much at once.
- Take small bites, eat slowly, and chew thoroughly before swallowing.
- Eat a high-protein, low-carbohydrate diet.
- Avoid dairy products if they cause gas, bloating, or diarrhea.
- Avoid high-sugar and high-fat foods in the first three to six months after surgery.
- Avoid acid reflux by sitting up straight while you eat. Don't lie down soon after eating, and sleep with your upper body elevated.
- Drink liquids 30–60 minutes before or after you eat, rather than during meals.

Making the Decision

You may be conflicted between doing what is recommended to avoid potentially life-threatening stomach cancer and living without a stomach, which is scary and extreme. Like decisions about all surgeries, considering total gastrectomy should involve research so that you thoroughly understand how it's done, the permanent changes it will make to your body, and the dietary adjustments it requires. Your surgeon can put you in touch with previous total gastrectomy patients who are willing to share their experience. Ask whether they do or do not regret having the surgery, their experience with physical and emotional symptoms, and what they wish they had known before having the procedure. Another helpful resource is No Stomach for Cancer (www.nostomachforcancer.org), a supportive online resource for those who have had total gastrectomy.

— *My Story* —
Why I Chose Preventive Gastrectomy

My mom died in January 2018 of hereditary diffuse gastric cancer. She carried a *CDH1* mutation that we learned about only after her diagnosis. Unfortunately, we were unable to connect the dots in time to save her. All the information we would have needed to prevent her death existed before she developed the disease. The connection between *CDH1* mutations and diffuse gastric cancer was discovered more than 15 years before her diagnosis. Genetic testing was available and affordable. Preventive gastrectomy surgery was possible. And my mom had a cousin who died young of stomach cancer.

Payment and Insurance

Although federal law doesn't require coverage of risk-reducing gastrectomy or colectomy, most private health insurers cover these surgeries if you have an inherited genetic mutation that is linked to high cancer risk. You may be required to pay deductibles, copayments, and/or coinsurance. Some health plans, especially short-term and self-funded plans, may not consider risk-reducing surgery to be medically necessary, even for people with high cancer risk. If you're denied coverage for gastrectomy or colectomy, you can appeal the decision with a letter from your surgeon that describes the medical necessity based on your high-risk status and national guidelines for these procedures.

After my mom learned that she carried a *CDH1* mutation, word quickly spread in our family. Those of us who could potentially carry the mutation had genetic testing. My mom's two sisters, three of my cousins, and I tested positive for the mutation. In June 2018, I had my stomach removed. One aunt and two cousins had already done the same thing. It's been very challenging at times, yet I'm so grateful to have the option to avoid developing stomach cancer. I wish my mom had had the same opportunity. However, because of her, at least six family members, as well as future generations, have the option to avoid developing diffuse gastric cancer.

—*Jonathan*

Chapter 19

Factors That Affect
Cancer Risk

To achieve a healthy weight, follow a sensible, long-term strategy of maintaining an exercise and eating regimen that helps you gradually shed weight while keeping you satisfied and fit. Logging your food and tracking your exercise can help with this balance. Ask your doctor for a referral to a nutritionist or dietician if you need help getting started or maintaining a balanced diet.

Risk is the probability of something negative or harmful happening. When you drive your car, you risk getting rear-ended. Climb a ladder, and you risk falling off. We're all susceptible to cancer risk, although our risks are different. Having one or more risk factors, including an inherited mutation that predisposes you to cancer, doesn't necessarily mean that you're destined to have a cancer diagnosis—unless your lifestyle, your environment, and/or the aging process create irreparable damage that prompts cells to divide out of control and form tumors.

While your family history and inherited mutations influence the chance of having one or more cancers, many harmful lifestyle behaviors also contribute to cancer risk. You can't negate the effects of age, race, inherited mutations, and other risk factors for cancer that are beyond your control. You may not be able to offset all the effects of your environment either. Issues like where you live, your employment status, your access to health insurance and the effects of racism or other biases may affect your health and well-being. You can, however, choose to change your behaviors in ways that reduce the likelihood of a diagnosis. Smoking, for example, increases the odds of lung cancer. Stop smoking, and you decrease that likelihood.

Most cancers are caused by a combination of factors. The multistep evolution from healthy cell to malignancy usually takes several years, providing opportunities (especially while we're younger) to potentially lower inherited risk with intervening behaviors. Five well-studied behaviors impact cancer risk: nutrition, weight, physical activity, alcohol consumption, and smoking or other use of tobacco. These same factors can also affect prognosis and mortality.

Nutrition, Weight, and Physical Activity

Most confirmed data about the effect of lifestyle behaviors on the risk for disease, including cancer, can be summed up in just three words: nutrition, weight, and exercise. Over a lifetime, these closely related factors profoundly affect health, including the likelihood of developing and dying from cancer. These interrelated components are like the three legs of a stool. Managing all of them provides a balanced approach to limiting cellular damage that can progress to disease. Allowing any of these components to become unbalanced may tip the scale toward poor health and greater cancer risk.

About 60 percent of Americans have one or more preventable chronic diseases, many of which are related to poor eating patterns and physical inactivity.[1] According to the American Cancer Society, 18 percent or more of cancers in the United States and about 16 percent of related deaths are caused by poor diet, being overweight or obese, being sedentary, and drinking too much alcohol.[2] A healthy diet, controlled weight, and regular physical activity are essential for optimal health, regardless of gender, age, or genetic status.

Nutrition and Health Are Closely Related

No food or diet can completely protect you from cancer. While a cause-and-effect connection between most foods and cancer hasn't been made, the indirect relationship is clear. Your body needs essential nutrients to function optimally, and you need a strong immune system that can better repair genetic damage before cancer occurs. Research increasingly emphasizes the value of a high-fiber, primarily plant-based diet. For healthy eating, choose appropriately sized portions that are nutritionally robust (see "Inside the Smart Pantry" sidebar). Eat fruits and vegetables of different colors—the nutrients they provide are thought to work together to reduce cancer risk. Avoid or limit red meats

Inside the Smart Pantry

Build your diet around the following foods:

- lean proteins (skinless poultry, seafood, beans, nonfat dairy products)
- healthy fats (walnuts; flax; fatty fish; olive, peanut, and canola oils)
- high-fiber whole grains (cereal, bread, pasta, rice)
- nuts and seeds (almonds; walnuts; Brazil nuts; pumpkin, sunflower, and sesame seeds)
- a colorful variety of fresh, frozen, or canned fruits and vegetables

(for example, pork, beef, veal, and lamb) and smoked, cured, and processed meats (for example, ham, bacon, and salami), which may elevate the risk for colorectal, lung, pancreatic, and other cancers. Also limit heavily salted or sweetened foods and beverages, products made with refined white flour, fast food, and highly processed foods. Transitioning from the high-fat, high-calorie American diet to more nutritionally balanced meals can be challenging. The New American Plate (www.aicr.org) can help you change what you eat so that you get the balanced nutrition you need. It emphasizes satisfying foods that promote health, control weight, and reduce the risk for breast, prostate, colorectal, and other cancers, as well as many other diseases.

Are Any Foods Protective?

Research on the protective or harmful effects of certain foods frequently makes the headlines, only to be contradicted by other studies. It's difficult to investigate how diet affects cancer risk over a lifetime because researchers can't control the long-term diets of study participants, and when questioned, people often don't accurately recall what they've eaten over many years.

Changing your diet may improve your overall health and strengthen your immune system. Little is known, however, about whether and how diet may affect hereditary cancer risk. Some research suggests but doesn't prove that certain foods may offer protection against cancer.

- Soy foods don't appear to raise the risk for breast cancer and have been linked with lower risk in some studies.
- Whole-grain diets and limiting red meat are associated with lower colorectal cancer risk.
- Leafy green vegetables, fruits, dried beans and peas, and fortified bread contain folate, a B vitamin that has been linked to a lower risk for several types of cancer.[3]
- Broccoli, cauliflower, cabbage, brussels sprouts, bok choy, and kale have compounds that may help to protect against several types of cancer.
- Dairy products and high-calcium diets have been linked to lower colorectal cancer risk, although they may increase the risk for prostate cancer. Some studies link dairy products to breast cancer risk, while others don't.

Controlling Your Weight

Maintaining a healthy weight is one of the most important things you can do to boost your overall health and reduce your cancer risk. Yet 42 percent of American adults are obese, and nearly one in five children and youths between ages 2 and 19 are obese, which raises their risk for adult cancers.[4] Evidence consistently associates a high percentage of body fat with increased risk for ovarian, endometrial, colorectal, pancreatic, prostate, postmenopausal breast, and other cancers. Carrying extra weight may also promote the growth of some cancers in the following ways:

- creating chronic inflammation that may raise cancer risk
- increasing insulin levels that may help some cancers develop

- stimulating the production of estrogen, which may promote the growth of breast and endometrial cancers
- reducing immune function and increasing stress to cells that causes DNA damage
- increasing the likelihood of death from some cancers

Excessive weight results from a combination of eating too much, eating too many unhealthy foods, and not exercising enough. If you need to lose weight, don't waste your time on fad diets, which generally disregard the rudimentary rule of weight control—calories in, calories out. While you may initially lose pounds, the weight may return when your fad diet ends. To lose weight, you need to burn more calories than you eat. Maintaining a healthy weight means understanding what your body needs, in both moderation and balance, and making better choices about what you eat and drink. To achieve a

Calculating Obesity and Waist Circumference

You're considered overweight if your body mass index (BMI) is 25.0–29.9. You're considered to be obese and at higher risk for many chronic health conditions if your BMI is 30 or greater. You can use the calculator at the American Cancer Society (search for "BMI" at www.cancer.org) or calculate your own BMI: $703 \times$ weight in pounds $\div$ (height in inches)^2. The size of your waist is also important. A waist circumference of more than 35 inches in nonpregnant women and more than 40 inches in men means a greater likelihood of health issues.

Tips for Losing Weight and Staying Fit

- Learn about nutrition and what your body needs.
- Strive for a nutritionally balanced plate at every meal.
- Control portion size, especially of high-calorie foods.
- Choose wisely in the grocery store and when dining out.
- Keep a food journal of what and how much you eat and drink, and then see where you can make improvements.
- Focus on realistic weight loss goals, such as losing one or two pounds per week.
- Sit less and move more. Adopt a physically active lifestyle to maintain a healthy weight.

healthy weight, follow a sensible, long-term strategy of maintaining an exercise and eating regimen that helps you gradually shed weight while keeping you satisfied and fit. Logging your food and tracking your exercise can help with this balance. Ask your doctor for a referral to a nutritionist or dietician if you need help getting started or maintaining a balanced diet.

Physical Activity

Staying active throughout your life strengthens your heart and cardiovascular system, modulates hormone levels, and lowers risks for disease in unexplained ways. Combined with a sensible caloric intake, it's the most effective way to maintain a lifelong healthy weight. The combined data of over a million adults in the United States and Europe confirm that physical activity is associated with a lower risk of 13 cancers, including colon, breast, endometrial, kidney, bladder, and rectal.[5]

Any amount of exercise is good. Even small increases in moderately intense physical activity provide health benefits. Try to get 150–300 minutes of moderately intense aerobic activity or 75–100 minutes of vigorous aerobic activity per week. It's okay to break up your activity into several smaller increments as long as you sustain it for at least 10 minutes each time. Do resistance training at least twice weekly to improve the strength of your muscles and bones and to rev up your metabolism.

— EXPERT VIEW —

How Diet, Fitness, and Smoking Affect Surgery

BY MINAS CHRYSOPOULO, MD

Wounds need a lot of energy to heal well. People need a healthy diet before and after surgery. Protein, zinc, and vitamins A and C are crucial for wound healing. The importance of healthy nutrition is emphasized by the link between obesity and postoperative complications. Obese individuals have thicker fat layers with poorer blood supply. Their blood flow and the amount of vital nutrients and oxygen reaching their healing tissues are therefore less robust. They have much higher rates of infection, wound-healing problems, and hematomas and seromas compared to nonobese people. Staying well-hydrated before and after surgery—drinking 64 ounces of water a day and avoiding caffeinated beverages—is very important, as dehydration causes the skin and soft tissues to become dry, which inhibits healing.

Smoking also negatively impacts healing. Nicotine shrinks blood vessels, depriving tissues of the nutrients and oxygen required for healing. At best, this slows the wound-healing process; at worst, smoking can cause wounds to break down. (Many smoking-cessation products contain nicotine and increase the risk of healing problems.) Cigarette smoke contains carbon monoxide, which lowers the level of oxygen in the blood. Since oxygen is vital for healing, it's crucial to not smoke before and after surgery to decrease the risk of healing complications.

Finally, regular exercise before and after surgery (once cleared by your surgeon) boosts the immune system and is encouraged.

Tips for Staying Active

It's never too late to transform poor nutrition and sedentary habits into a healthy, fit lifestyle. Always discuss any new exercise program with your physician, especially if you're in treatment, recovering from surgery, or at risk for lymphedema.

- Exercise on most days.

- Begin slowly, gradually adding more time and effort as you become more fit.

- Pursue exercise you enjoy. Dance, hike, bike, swim, or whatever you like.

- Stay motivated by frequently changing your regimen and exercising with a friend.

- Minimize the time you spend sitting. Prolonged periods of sitting are linked to high blood pressure, obesity, and other health concerns. Standing and moving require more energy and burn more calories.

- Incorporate more exercise into your normal routine. Walk to lunch instead of driving, or use the treadmill as you watch TV.

- Make a commitment to fitness. Momentum is a powerful force.

Alcohol: An Unwise Choice

Alcohol is a known carcinogen that is particularly harmful when combined with smoking. How alcohol promotes cancer isn't completely clear, but it may help other harmful substances enter cells or reduce the levels of nutrients the body needs to defend itself from cancer. Although moderate drinking—a single drink a day if you're a woman and two drinks a day if you're male—appears to be heart-healthy, drinking alcohol in any amount increases cancer risk, particularly for breast, colorectal, liver, stomach, esophageal, and oral cancers. It may also raise a person's risk for prostate and pancreatic cancers and melanoma. (One drink is 12 ounces of beer, 5 ounces of wine, or 1.5 ounces of 80-proof distilled spirits.)

Even moderate drinking can increase the risk of breast cancer. According to the American Cancer Society, women who regularly have even a few drinks per week, especially those who don't get enough folate, raise their breast cancer risk. The more you drink, the higher your risk, and all forms of alcohol damage healthy cells. If you choose to drink, do so occasionally, rather than regularly, and in moderation. Less is better.

Smoking and Tobacco Products

The harmful effects of cigars, cigarettes, and other tobacco products can't be exaggerated. They contain carcinogens that can damage nearly every organ in the body and substantially raise the risk for cancer in the mouth, esophagus, kidney, bladder, pancreas, colon, and other organs. A burning cigarette creates 69 known cancer-causing chemicals. Secondhand smoke, the smoke breathed out by smokers and discharged from the burning end of cigars and cigarettes, is also harmful. Thirdhand smoke, the residual nicotine left by tobacco smoke that clings to clothing and other surfaces, may also be toxic.

About half of all Americans who smoke die because of it, more people than all of the combined deaths related to alcohol, car accidents, guns, and illegal drugs.[6] Smoking is responsible for about 80 percent of lung cancer deaths and about 30 percent of all cancer deaths in the United States.[7] If you're a smoker and you develop cancer, smoking can interfere with your treatment, promote infection, and delay healing. If you use any kind of tobacco, ask your doctor about medications that can help you quit or use the American Lung Association's smoking-cessation program (www.lung.org).

— *My Story* —

I Did Everything Right, and I Still Got Breast Cancer

At 33, I was shocked to be diagnosed with breast cancer. I didn't drink or smoke. I had been a vegetarian for almost 10 years and had exercised and followed recommendations for protecting myself. I breastfed my baby for over six months. My diagnosis made more sense when I later learned I had an inherited mutation. My genes were a stronger influence than my lifestyle. Although I lived a healthy lifestyle as an adult, as a teen I drank, smoked, and ate high-fat fast foods. I was overweight then and didn't exercise much. If I had known about my genetic destiny at age 16, I like to think I would have made better choices about my health. I'll never know for sure, but I believe my healthy lifestyle as an adult may have saved me from a worse prognosis. It certainly helped me get through treatment with fewer side effects. You're never too young to live a healthy life.

—*Susanne*

Other Lifestyle and Behavioral Risk Factors

Your lifestyle influences your genetic predisposition. You may not be the master of your fate if you have an inherited gene mutation, but you can certainly sway the outcome in your favor. It's in your best interests to do everything you can to avoid substances and behaviors that can cause genetic damage and to maximize your body's ability to repair the damage that does occur.

The Importance of Healthy Sleep

Sleep is essential. We can't function properly without it. Sleep affects the immune system, metabolism, and nearly every other part and function of your body. While you sleep, your body is busy repairing cells and recharging your mind and body, so that you can be mentally alert and physically healthy. At the same time, toxins are removed from pathways in your brain that facilitate learning and concentration, and create new memories.

Despite the many influences that can keep us awake, most adults need seven to nine hours of nightly sleep. Getting too little REM sleep—the deep stage of sleep where repairs are made—for too long can have serious consequences. Sleep deprivation can reduce cognition, cause mood shifts and lapses in attention, and leave us open to disease. Try these suggestions to establish good sleep habits and ensure you get the sleep you need:

- Go to bed at about the same time every night, and get up at about the same time each morning.
- Create a quiet, dark, sleep-friendly bedroom with a comfortable temperature.
- Resist using electronic devices, including TV and cell phones, within an hour of bedtime.
- Avoid alcohol, caffeine, and large meals close to bedtime.
- Exercise during the day, rather than just before you go to bed.
- Meditate to quiet your mind or relax in a warm bath before going to bed.
- Get up if you can't fall sleep after 15–20 minutes. Read, listen to music, or relax in some other way until you feel sleepy.
- Ask your doctor if any of your medications may be interfering with your sleep.
- Talk to your doctor if you need help with chronic insomnia or other sleep problems.

Combating Stress, Anger, and Anxiety

Stress is a part of life. Short-term anxiety, the kind you feel when you're stuck in traffic, is usually resolved when the source goes away, and it doesn't impact your overall health. Chronic worry, stress, or anger can affect your sleep, digestion, and concentration, and negatively impact your physical and emotional well-being. It's helpful to recognize and accept that you can't control everything that happens to you or around you.

Although it's not always easy, you can act to alleviate stress and stay positive. Deep breathing for several minutes is one way to instantly relieve intense negative feelings. Physical activity, meditation, yoga, and tai chi may also reduce symptoms of stress or anxiety. If you experience chronic stress or anxiety, talk to your doctor about anti-anxiety medications or a referral to a mental health professional who can treat these issues.

Environmental Exposures

Life in the twenty-first century involves exposure to innumerable pollutants, pesticides, and chemicals in our air, water, food, home, and workplace. Consider the total amount of chemicals in all of the skin care, beauty, cleaning, and other products that we ordinarily use every day. Many of these products contain known carcinogens that contribute to cell damage that can accumulate in the body and lead to cancer. (Despite internet rumors, radios, televisions, cellular phones, microwave ovens, power lines, and underwire bras haven't been found to affect cancer risk.) With a bit of awareness and planning, you can reduce your exposure to potential environmental toxins.

- Limit exposure to ultraviolet light from the sun, which can lead to melanoma and other skin cancers. Wear sunscreen and protective clothing when outdoors; avoid tanning beds and sun lamps.
- Wear protective gear if you're exposed to asbestos, formaldehyde, wood dust, or other harmful chemicals in the home or the workplace.
- Avoid being outdoors when air pollution is high, and avoid exercising in high-traffic areas. Air pollution is associated with a greater risk of cancer in the digestive system and increased mortality for breast, lung, liver, and pancreatic cancers.[8]
- Have wells on your property tested for arsenic and other chemicals, especially if they are your primary source of drinking water.
- Read labels and follow directions carefully when you use paint, cleaning products, or other chemicals. Substitute less toxic substances whenever possible.
- Have your home tested for radon, the biggest risk factor for lung cancer after cigarettes.
- Nighttime exposure to artificial light reduces the production of melatonin, a hormone that may lower cancer risk. Several studies found that female nurses and other women who work night shifts have higher rates of breast cancer.

— THE **FORCE** PERSPECTIVE —

Social Factors That Affect Health Outcomes

In addition to diet and lifestyle, other factors may affect your risk for cancer, your treatment options, and your chance of survival. Although you may not be able to change some of these factors, being aware of them can help you find resources to overcome them. In the United States, race and ethnicity affect the risk, prognosis, and overall outcomes for certain types of cancer. Researchers are studying the causes of these differences to determine how to improve health outcomes for all people. Some differences may be due to genetics.

These different outcomes may also be due to societal factors. Systemic racism has been linked to health disparities. People from certain groups don't always have equal access to the information, resources, or income they need to receive optimal health care. Similar disparities have been documented in people who have physical and mental disabilities and in those who live in low-income communities or rural areas. Any or all of these issues can affect health outcomes.

Although you may not be able to control all of the risk factors that affect your health, being aware of how your background puts you at risk for certain cancers may allow you to practice increased screening and prevention. You might not be able to change the community where you live, but you can work with local elected officials, organizations, and agencies to help overcome barriers, increase resources, and improve health outcomes.

———————

Part IV
Treatment
Choices for
Hereditary
Cancers

We treat cancer to prolong and improve the quality of life for individuals. Some slow-growing cancers may never pose a risk to health or life. Other cancers may be too advanced or people may be too sick to benefit from treatment. Certain treatments may be effective against cancer but may cause long-lasting or serious side effects (chapter 29). Sometimes, treating cancer might do more harm than good.

We live in an age when doctors and people with cancer are no longer constrained by the limitations of a single approach to treatment. For most cancers, an array of therapeutic alternatives is available. First-line therapy is expected to be the most effective; one example is surgery followed by chemotherapy. For early-stage cancers, first-line therapy may be enough to ensure that the cancer never returns. But if that initial course of treatment stops working, if its side effects are intolerable, or if the cancer recurs or grows, a second-line treatment, perhaps with another chemotherapy, a targeted therapy, or a combination of drugs, provides a different approach. If a second-line treatment fails, a third- or fourth-line treatment, if available, can then be tried. The number of available treatments continues to increase for many cancers, so several lines of therapy are often possible.

Local therapies, such as surgery and radiation, treat the tumor site and nearby lymph nodes. Systemic therapies treat the entire body to prevent or treat metastasis (the spread of cancer) beyond the tumor site. These broader treatments include chemotherapy and other drugs that target hormones or other tumor features or encourage the immune system to find and destroy cancer cells. Systemic treatments can be categorized by when and how they're used.

- Neoadjuvant therapy is used to shrink a tumor before surgery, evaluate the effectiveness of a treatment before surgery, or allow time for genetic testing, which can influence treatment decisions.

- Adjuvant therapy is given to kill any lingering cancer cells after a tumor is removed.

- Maintenance therapy is used to keep cancer from returning or to extend the period between treatment and recurrence.

- Treatment for advanced cancers may stop, continue, or change based on how a cancer responds. The goal is to shrink tumors, prevent cancer from advancing, reduce symptoms, extend survival, and improve the person's quality of life.

New and improved cancer testing and treatments, including biomarker testing, robotic-assisted surgery, precision radiation, targeted therapies, and immunotherapy, are increasingly used to treat numerous cancers and help people live longer and live better. And the arsenal of cancer treatments continues to grow. Medical discoveries begin with research that often culminates in a clinical trial. Regardless of the stage or type of your cancer, there is likely to be a clinical trial enrolling people like you. These research studies may provide you with access to the latest technology and high-quality care.

We still don't know all of cancer's secrets. But now, more than ever before, we have a deeper understanding of how cancers develop and progress. With advanced testing, doctors can see the unique genetic makeup of the tumor cells that result from thousands of mutations, which accumulate as a tumor develops and grows. These changes in cancer cells and the surrounding tissue allow doctors to customize treatment accordingly. This personalized approach is known as precision medicine. It's a giant leap beyond treating all cancers in the same way.

The chapters in this part focus on treatment options for hereditary cancers, which may be the same or different than the treatments for sporadic cancers, depending on

- the type of cancer

- the stage of cancer

- your age and health

- the biological characteristics of the tumor(s)

- how aggressively the cancer grows

- the mutation you inherited

- whether the cancer is newly diagnosed or a recurrence

If you develop cancer, you may be advised to have genetic testing to see whether you have an inherited mutation (see chapter 3). Knowing whether you have an inherited gene mutation can guide your treatment decisions. A mutation may affect the type of cancer you develop, how the cancer behaves, and the options for treating it. In other situations, testing a tumor may find changes that suggest that an inherited mutation caused your cancer. In either case, it's ideal to speak with a genetics expert about what an inherited mutation means for you and your relatives. Your personal preferences also may influence your treatment decisions. So, it's important to understand as much as you can about your cancer, carefully consider your options, and work with your medical team to make decisions that are right for you.

Chapter 20

Identifying Tumor Characteristics That Inform Treatment Choices

Biomarker testing and targeted therapies shift cancer care away from the traditional one-size-fits-all regimen to more personalized medicine that customizes treatment for each individual.

Pathologists—doctors who perform lab tests to diagnose disease and cancer—look for telltale changes that identify cells as benign, precancerous, or malignant. When cancer cells are found, pathologists determine their origin and whether they're noninvasive or invasive. Cancer cells have changes that distinguish them from normal cells, and they cause changes in the surrounding tissue. These changes provide clues that help doctors detect cancer, identify its type and subtype, determine to what extent it affects the body, and decide how best to treat it. To be involved in decisions about your treatment, it's important that you understand this information, the test results about your general health, and whether you have an inherited gene mutation.

Staging and Grading Cancer

Pathologists assign a stage to each cancer based on where it began, whether it has spread, how it's likely to behave, and whether other parts of the body are affected. Staging occurs at different times after a diagnosis.

- Before treatment, newly diagnosed cancers are staged using the results of imaging tests, endoscopies, blood tests, and/or biopsies. Initial staging helps doctors to create a treatment plan and to estimate your prognosis—the expected chance of recovery. Staging can also help doctors decide the order in which chemotherapy, radiation therapy, surgery, or other treatments will be given.
- After surgery, the stage may change based on the size of the tumor, the involvement of lymph nodes, and the extent of spread, if any, beyond the organ where the cancer started.
- During treatment, cancers may be restaged to monitor response.
- After treatment, restaging can guide treatment decisions and aid in evaluating the prognosis for cancers that advance or return.

Understanding the stage of your cancer and what it means can help you take an active role in your treatment and care. Your doctor's office can give you a copy of your pathology report (a summary of the pathologist's findings regarding the nature of your cancer), which you can review and keep as part of your medical record.

TNM Staging

Although some staging categories differ, depending on the type of cancer, most cancer types are described with the TNM system.

T describes the size and location of the tumor:

TX: No information about the tumor, or it can't be measured.

T0: No evidence of a tumor, or it can't be found.

Tis: Cancer cells are confined to where they began (in situ cancer or precancer).

T1-4: This indicates the size of the tumor and to what extent it has spread into nearby tissue.

N clarifies to what extent the lymph nodes are involved:

NX: No information, or the nodes can't be assessed.
N0: Lymph nodes are clear of cancer.
N1-3: This indicates the location, size, and number of lymph nodes with cancer.

M describes whether the cancer has affected other parts of the body:

M0: No metastatic disease is detected.
M1: Metastatic disease is in one or more distant organs.

Once the TNM categories for your cancer have been established, they're combined into an overall stage that helps to establish your treatment plan:

Stage 0 means the questionable area is either preinvasive or in situ cancer that hasn't spread beyond where it began. Stage 0 diagnoses have the best prognoses.
Stage 1 is an early-stage small cancer that hasn't grown deeply into the surrounding tissue or spread to the lymph nodes.
Stages 2 and 3 are larger areas of cancer that are embedded more deeply into nearby tissue and may affect lymph nodes.
Stage 4 is advanced or metastatic cancer that has spread to distant organs, making treatment more challenging.

Grading Cancer

In addition to staging, pathologists also assign a tumor grade to each cancer. This information describes the degree of abnormality in the tumor cells, which tells treating physicians how quickly a tumor may grow and spread. Grading varies depending on the type of tumor.

Targeted Approaches to Treatment

Chemotherapy is effective against many cancers, but it's also cytotoxic, meaning that it's harmful to healthy cells. For some cancers, targeted therapies are a powerful and more effective alternative. They block specific genes and proteins that some cancer cells need to grow and survive. Compared to many chemotherapies, these advanced anticancer drugs are often less likely to harm healthy cells, which may cause fewer side effects. In some cases, combining two different targeted therapies or using targeted therapy with other types of therapy, such as chemotherapy or hormone therapy, is the most effective treatment option.

Targeted therapies stop cancer growth in different ways:

- by blocking receptors that are in or on cancer cells, so they can't bind to proteins that instruct the cells to accelerate division or growth (figure 20.1)
- by blocking the connection between cancer cells and the blood cells that fuel their growth
- by delivering radiation or chemotherapy directly into cancer cells
- by making cancer cells more visible to the immune system, so that immune cells find and destroy them
- by impairing the ability of cancer cells to repair DNA damage that occurs from chemotherapy and other treatments

Tumor Biomarker Testing

Every bit of information about a tumor adds to the understanding of its unique nature and may help to identify treatments with the best chance of succeeding. Biomarker testing (also called tumor testing or molecular profiling) and targeted therapies are a two-step approach to treatment. Testing detects proteins, gene changes, and other molecular vulnerabilities in tumors, while targeted therapies exploit these weaknesses. Biomarker testing and targeted therapies shift cancer care away from the traditional one-size-fits-all regimen to more personalized medicine that customizes treatment for each individual. This is especially meaningful if you've been diagnosed with advanced cancer, because biomarkers may help identify additional treatment options. It's important to talk to your doctor about biomarker testing of your tumor and to understand the results of your test. If testing finds a change for which there is no approved targeted treatment, you may be eligible for a clinical trial of a new targeted drug.

Biomarker testing can be useful during many different aspects of cancer care:

- early detection
- identifying specific targets for treatment

FIGURE 20.1 Targeted therapies block the proteins and growth factors that some cancers use to grow and survive

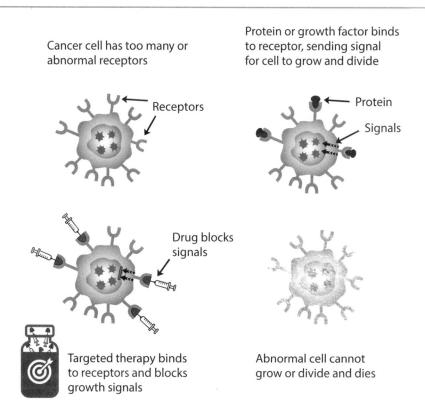

- monitoring response to treatment
- predicting which cancers are likely to return and need more treatment
- detecting a recurrence after treatment

DNA Damage Repair Genes

DNA damage repair (DDR) genes have numerous defensive mechanisms that control cell division and that repair damaged DNA to prevent cancer. Mutations in DDR genes impair a cell's ability to correct DNA damage, which may eventually lead to cancer. This explains why people who have an inherited mutation in a DDR gene have a greater cancer risk.

Questions to Ask Your Oncologist about Biomarker Testing

- Is an approved biomarker test available for the type of cancer I have?
- How accurate is the test?
- Will my insurance pay for it?
- Will I need to have a new biopsy to provide a sample of my tumor?
- How will the test results be used to make treatment decisions?

DDR genes benefit healthy cells, and they also benefit cancer cells by repairing the damaging effects of chemotherapy and other treatments. When tumor cells have difficulty repairing this type of DNA damage, targeted therapies may be given to deliberately disrupt alternative repair mechanisms that might fix treatment-related DNA damage in cancer cells. Mismatch repair genes and homologous recombination repair genes are types of primary DDR genes that recognize and repair errors that occur during cell division.

Mismatch Repair Genes, Microsatellite Instability, and Targeted Therapies

All five genes that are associated with Lynch syndrome—*MLH1*, *MSH2*, *MSH6*, *PMS2*, and *EPCAM*—are mismatch repair (MMR) genes. These genes correct a type of cell damage known as single-stranded DNA damage, which most often occurs when cells divide. When mutations occur in an MMR gene, the mismatch repair system doesn't work as it should. Uncorrected DNA

Biomarker Testing and Genetic Testing May Overlap

Tumor biomarker testing and genetic testing are used for different reasons, yet the results they provide sometimes overlap. If you have an inherited mutation and you've been diagnosed with cancer, your tumor will likely carry the same mutation. However, not all types of mutations can be detected using tumor biomarker testing so it will not find every inherited gene mutation, and it cannot be used to rule out an inherited mutation. Your inherited mutation may make you eligible for treatment with specific targeted therapies.

Biomarker testing can scan for many different mutations in tumors, most of which are acquired. Sometimes, biomarker tests find mutations that may be either inherited or acquired. In these cases, genetic counseling and genetic testing may be recommended to confirm or rule out that the mutation was inherited. (Read about the implications of an inherited mutation in chapters 5–7.)

Some cancer medications work equally well whether mutations are acquired or inherited. Having a mutation in your tumor may make you eligible for treatments with specific targeted therapies. For example, some advanced ovarian and prostate cancers are treated with PARP inhibitors, based on the presence of mutations that are found by tumor testing or the presence of inherited mutations that are found by genetic testing.

Testing for Tumor DNA in the Blood

Blood-based liquid biopsy (also called circulating tumor DNA testing) measures cancer cells or fragments of DNA that are released from dying tumors and enter the bloodstream. Less invasive, less painful, and less costly than a surgical biopsy, a liquid biopsy can be particularly useful for hard-to-access organs. It may be used to diagnose cancer, to monitor how a tumor responds to treatment, and to identify new mutations or other changes that develop in cancer cells. A liquid biopsy can sometimes find a recurrence before it is detectable by any other means.

While liquid biopsy may have several important applications, it's an evolving technology, and research continues into how and when a liquid biopsy can dependably guide treatment. This test may someday prove to be a reliable way to screen for cancer or to find cancer recurrence earlier.

errors accumulate every time cells divide and may eventually turn healthy cells into cancer cells.

Tumors with mutations in MMR genes are labeled MMR-deficient (dMMR). These tumors often have a high level of cellular abnormality known as microsatellite instability–high (MSI-H), which may be found during tumor testing. Tumors that are dMMR or MSI-H are more likely to respond to a type of immunotherapy known as an immune checkpoint inhibitor.

Your oncologist can tell you whether you're a candidate for these tests. MSI-H and dMMR tumors are frequently detected in colorectal and endometrial cancers. They're also common in people who have an inherited mutation in a Lynch syndrome gene, although not everyone with an MSI-H or dMMR tumor has Lynch syndrome.

HRR Genes and Targeted Therapies

Homologous recombination repair (HRR) genes, including *ATM*, *BRCA1*, *BRCA2*, *BRIP1*, *CHEK2*, *PALB2*, *RAD51C*, and *RAD51D*, repair a type of damage known as double-stranded DNA breaks. Cancers that can't easily repair this type of damage are known as homologous recombination deficient (HRD). HRD tumors can be identified with biomarker testing that looks for genomic instability or mutations in specific genes. Testing tumors for HRD may identify cancers that will respond to PARP inhibitors.

Insurance Coverage for Biomarker Testing

Most private health insurers pay for some biomarker testing of certain cancers if you meet established medical criteria. Coverage varies. Your oncologist can tell you whether a recommended bio-marker test is covered by your health plan and, if necessary, advocate on your behalf. If tumor testing suggests that you may have Lynch syndrome or another hereditary cancer syndrome, the cost of genetic counseling and testing for a related gene mutation is usually covered as long as you pay the copays, coinsurance, and deductibles that your plan ordinarily requires. Medicare and Medicaid generally view biomarker testing as a clinical diagnostic test and cover the related costs if all of the following requirements are met:

- You have recurrent, relapsed, treatment-resistant, or Stage 3 or 4 metastatic disease.

- You haven't previously had the same test for the same biomarkers.

- You want to seek further cancer treatment.

- The test is FDA-approved as a companion diagnostic test for a specific targeted therapy that also has FDA approval.

- Your oncologist orders the test from a specially certified laboratory.

- The test results provided to your oncologist specify treatment options.

Chapter 21

Treating Breast Cancer

If you have advanced or metastatic breast cancer, especially if it no longer responds to standard treatment, biomarker testing may also identify tumor abnormalities to guide further treatment decisions. New biomarker tests and targeted drugs are being developed as research progresses.

Breast cancer is more than one disease, and it has many different types and subtypes. Most breast cancer can be treated and cured when it's confined to the breast or the surrounding lymph nodes. Metastatic breast cancer that has spread beyond the lymph nodes to other organs is usually treatable, although it tends to come back at some point during or after treatment. Doctors use several sources of information to categorize breast cancer and decide how best to treat it. The treatment planning for breast cancer considers several factors, including

- cell type
- subtype, as determined by biomarker testing
- stage
- results of additional biomarker testing
- presence of an inherited mutation linked to breast cancer, as determined by genetic testing
- the number of and response to prior treatments

Cancer Type, Subtype, and Stage

After surgery or a needle biopsy confirms a diagnosis of breast cancer, a pathologist examines and categorizes the cancer cells according to their type and subtype. Staging determines the size of a cancer and whether it has spread from the breast to the lymph nodes, surrounding tissue, or beyond. This information allows your doctors to plan how extensive and aggressive treatment needs to be.

Staging breast cancer often includes a sentinel node biopsy to see if cancer cells have spread to the lymph nodes. In this procedure, a harmless dye or radioactive substance is injected into the breast tumor before surgery. One or two sentinel lymph nodes—the nodes in the armpit that are closest to the tumor—are then removed and examined. If these lymph nodes are free of cancer, no additional lymph nodes need to be removed. Sentinel nodes that contain cancer cells indicate that the cancer may involve additional lymph nodes or has spread beyond the breast. In this case, a more invasive axillary lymph node dissection may be needed. Limiting the initial removal of lymph nodes to just the sentinel nodes reduces the risk of lymphedema, a chronic swelling that often occurs when multiple lymph nodes are removed and the lymph system can no longer drain fluids in the arm (see chapter 29).

Stage 0 is preinvasive (DCIS).

Stage 1 is less than 2 centimeters and contained within the breast.

Stage 2 is a larger tumor that is confined to the breast or involves some axillary lymph nodes.

Stage 3 is a locally advanced tumor that has spread to the breast skin or chest muscle or involves several lymph nodes in the armpit or above or below the collarbone.

Stage 4 has extended to other areas of the body beyond the breast and lymph nodes. This stage is also known as metastatic breast cancer.

Biomarker Testing

All breast cancers are tested for cells that overexpress (have too many) receptors or have abnormal receptors on their surface, which may indicate the type of treatment needed.

- The HER2 protein can cause cancers to grow more quickly. HER2-positive breast cancers overexpress this protein.

- Estrogen receptors can make cells grow more quickly. Breast cancers that overexpress estrogen receptors are known as estrogen receptor–positive breast cancers.
- Progesterone receptors can also make cells grow more quickly. Breast cancers that overexpress progesterone receptors are known as progesterone receptor–positive breast cancers.
- Triple-negative breast cancers lack receptors for HER2, estrogen, and progesterone.

Depending on the type and stage of your cancer, additional biomarker testing may help with treatment selection. If you have early-stage breast cancer that is estrogen receptor–positive and HER2-negative, testing the tumor tissue from your lumpectomy or mastectomy can predict whether hormone therapy alone is sufficient to prevent a recurrence, thereby sparing you from chemotherapy. These tests include Oncotype DX, Breast Cancer Index, and MammaPrint. Your oncologist can determine if you're eligible for these tests and whether your insurance will pay for them. If you have advanced or metastatic breast cancer, especially if it no longer responds to standard treatment, biomarker testing may also identify tumor abnormalities to guide further treatment decisions. New biomarker tests and targeted drugs are being developed as research progresses.

Genetic Testing

Learning that you have a mutation before, rather than after, a breast cancer diagnosis increases the likelihood that you'll be diagnosed at an earlier stage and that you will survive.[1] But if you've been diagnosed with breast cancer and you haven't been tested, genetic counseling and genetic testing are strongly recommended if you meet certain criteria. Knowing that you have a mutation in a high-risk gene can make a difference in what you decide about treatment. You should consider testing if any of the following apply:[2]

- You have Eastern European Jewish (Ashkenazi) ancestry.
- A relative has tested positive for an inherited mutation associated with cancer.
- You have one or more relatives with breast, ovarian, pancreatic, or prostate cancer or melanoma.

- You were diagnosed with any type or stage of breast cancer, including DCIS, at age 50 or younger.
- You have cancer in both breasts or a new cancer in the same breast.
- You have been diagnosed with triple-negative breast cancer.
- You have estrogen or progesterone receptor–positive breast cancer and your doctor thinks you may be a good candidate for PARP inhibitor therapy (see "Options for Treatment" below).
- You have metastatic breast cancer.
- Biomarker testing of your tumor has indicated that you may have an inherited mutation.
- You have been diagnosed with male breast cancer.

Options for Treatment

Treating breast cancer almost always includes a local therapy (surgery or radiation) and one or more systemic therapies (chemotherapy, hormonal therapy, targeted therapy, or immunotherapy). Recommended treatments may be different if you test positive for an inherited mutation in a *BRCA1, BRCA2, PALB2,* or other gene (see chapters 5 and 7). If you have multiple treatment options, talk with your doctor about how each can reduce your risk for a recurrence or a new breast cancer in either breast. It's also important to understand and consider the potential short-term and long-term side effects of each treatment, some of which can be serious and impact your quality of life (chapter 29). Some treatments can temporarily or permanently affect your ability to become pregnant, so you should discuss your childbearing plans with your doctor before starting treatment. If you are sexually active, you should discuss contraception during treatment and when you can safely become pregnant. Some therapies can harm fetuses and should be avoided during pregnancy.

Surgical Procedures

Surgery to treat breast cancer may consist of breast-conserving lumpectomy (followed by radiation) or mastectomy. Both surgeries are typically accompanied by a sentinel node biopsy, and if that is positive may include an axillary dissection. Early-stage tumors that are smaller than 4 centimeters (about the size of a walnut) can be treated with lumpectomy and radiation or with mastectomy with similar survival rates. Mastectomy may be recommended for any of the following circumstances:

- Your tumor is larger than 4 centimeters. (Neoadjuvant chemotherapy or hormone therapy may shrink the tumor enough so that it can be removed with lumpectomy.)
- You have separate areas of cancer in different quadrants of your breast. (Lumpectomy may be possible when the areas are close together.)
- Your cancer is in your breast skin or chest wall.
- You're not a candidate for radiation.
- You're male.
- You have an inherited mutation in a gene that puts you at high risk for a second breast cancer.

Having a gene mutation that raises breast cancer risk doesn't necessarily preclude you from having a lumpectomy with radiation. However, if you're at high risk for another breast cancer diagnosis, you may wish to consider the possibility of bilateral mastectomy, which is more protective against future breast cancers in high-risk women. The National Comprehensive Cancer Network guidelines don't broadly recommend this approach for people with sporadic tumors because mastectomy doesn't improve survival, and their risk for another cancer in the opposite breast is low.

If you have an inherited mutation in a *BRCA1*, *BRCA2*, *PALB2*, *PTEN*, or *TP53* gene, you face a substantial risk for a second primary cancer in your remaining breast tissue. Less is known about how mutations in the *ATM*, *BARD1*, *BRIP1*, *CDH1*, *CHEK2*, *RAD51C*, *RAD51D*, or *STK11* genes affect this risk. For many women, removing both breasts reduces the concern about a new diagnosis. If you choose not to have both breasts removed, your remaining breast tissue should be screened annually with mammogram and MRI, ideally six months apart, and you should speak with your doctor about chemoprevention. Removing the remaining breast after mastectomy isn't typically recommended for men with mutations who develop breast cancer because their risk of a second diagnosis is low.

Radiation Therapy

Early-stage cancer is often treated with radiation therapy to lower the risk for a recurrence in the breast and surrounding tissue, especially if breast-conserving surgery is chosen. Radiation is usually given after surgery. When treatment includes chemotherapy, radiation is typically given when that treatment is completed. Radiation can be given by external beam radiation, which directs high-energy x-rays across the breast, or by brachytherapy, which is given in a single treatment during surgery using radioactive seeds that are placed near the tumor site after the tumor has been removed. Radiation may also be used to reduce tumor size and manage pain or other symptoms when metastatic breast cancer spreads to the bones, brain, or other organs. Radiation therapy is painless, and you'll feel nothing unusual during your treatment.

Hormone Therapy

Breast cancers that are estrogen receptor–positive and/or progesterone receptor–positive are treated with tamoxifen and/or an aromatase inhibitor, medications that block the effects of hormones on the cancer. Taken for 5–10 years, these hormone therapy medications reduce the risk of a recurrence or a new cancer developing in either breast. Hormone therapy may also be used to treat metastatic breast cancer either alone or in combination with targeted therapy.

Chemotherapy

Treatment with chemotherapy is standard for many types and stages of invasive breast cancer. Chemotherapy drugs can be given alone or together or can be combined with other therapies in regimens that are customized for each person. Chemotherapy is standard for almost all triple-negative breast cancers, which lack receptors for estrogen, progesterone, and HER2 and don't respond to standard hormone therapies and anti-HER2 targeted therapies.

Targeted Therapies and Immunotherapies

Numerous targeted drugs and immunotherapies are approved for treating breast cancer, primarily for people with a specific subtype, genetic test result, or biomarker test result. HER2-positive breast cancers are usually treated with anti-HER2 therapies that target HER2 receptors.

Several targeted therapies are also approved for treating estrogen receptor–positive and progesterone receptor–positive, HER2-negative early-stage and metastatic breast cancer, often in combination with hormone therapy. Targeted and immunotherapies are also approved for metastatic triple-negative breast cancer.

PARP inhibitors are targeted therapies that were specifically developed to treat breast cancers in people who test positive for an inherited *BRCA* mutation. These drugs block the poly (ADP-ribose) polymerase protein, which is used by cells to repair DNA damage. PARP inhibitors are especially effective at preventing cancer cells from repairing damage from chemotherapy. Two agents, Lynparza (olaparib) and Talzenna (talazoparib), are approved to treat metastatic breast cancers in people who have an inherited mutation in either *BRCA* gene. Lynparza may also be used after chemotherapy to lower the risk for a recurrence in early-stage triple-negative breast cancers or in estrogen/progesterone receptor–positive breast cancers that are high risk for recurrence.[3] Researchers are exploring whether PARP inhibitors might also prove beneficial for treating breast cancers in the following circumstances:

- as neoadjuvant therapy for people with *BRCA* mutations who have large tumors
- as part of combination therapy with an immunotherapy agent for people with *BRCA* mutations
- for people with inherited mutations in an *ATM*, *CHEK2*, *PALB2*, or other high-risk breast cancer gene
- for people with tumor biomarkers that indicate PARP inhibitor sensitivity

— *My Story* —
My Mutation Helped Me Decide
How to Treat My DCIS

My sister was diagnosed with Stage 3 ovarian cancer four years after her breast cancer diagnosis. Genetic testing showed that she had a *BRCA1* mutation. She encouraged our entire family to be tested, but I felt it would be something I would have to constantly worry about. But when my oldest daughter said that she wanted to know, I understood why I needed to be tested. At age 56, I tested positive for the same *BRCA1* mutation. My other sister and five of seven relatives also tested positive. Mastectomy seemed barbaric, and I opted for alternating mammograms and breast MRIs every six months. Then in 2016, my MRI showed DCIS. By then, I'd had time to reconsider surgery, and I decided to have a

Inherited Mutations May Affect Your Medical Options

Knowing your genetic status may be particularly relevant at different times during and after treatment for breast cancer.

- Learning that you have an inherited mutation may affect your treatment decisions about lumpectomy or mastectomy.

- If you have early-stage breast cancer (Stages 1, 2, or 3) and need systemic therapy, it may affect your eligibility to participate in a clinical trial.

- If you have metastatic breast cancer, it may affect your treatment options or eligibility to participate in a clinical trial.

- It may help your blood relatives understand their risk for cancer.

- An inherited mutation may put you at risk for a new cancer diagnosis and affect your options for risk management.

bilateral mastectomy with reconstruction. Four years later, I'm happy that I knew about my mutation, that I could be proactive, and that my three daughters and my son can do the same.

—*Lisa*

— *My Story* —

Battling Breast Cancer like
My Mother and Aunts

My family was devastated when my mother and three of her sisters passed away after battling breast cancer. They were so young, between the ages of 39 and 45. I was hoping to escape the same fate, but in 2010 I was diagnosed with triple-negative breast cancer, which was treated with a lumpectomy and radiation. Due to my family history, my oncologist recommended genetic testing, which revealed that I carry a *BRCA1* mutation. My sister also tested positive for a *BRCA1* mutation. My first reaction was "Why did I not know about genetic testing?" No one ever told me that it existed. Perhaps I could have prevented my diagnosis.

My oncologist prescribed eight rounds of chemotherapy, followed by double mastectomy and hysterectomy. I now feel empowered, and I can educate and support others. My volunteer work helps me to stay informed on advances in research. It gives me great peace of mind and great hope that my children and future generations will not have to face cancer.

—*Debbie*

— *My Story* —

An *ATM* Gene Mutation Caused
My Breast Cancer

Breast cancer was always a concern for me. I'm Ashkenazi Jewish. I have dense breasts. And my maternal first cousin passed away from breast cancer at the age of 41. I always did what I could to be on alert for breast cancer. I had annual mammograms for five years, always hearing the word "normal" after each one. Then, at the age of 44, I found a lump in my left breast during a self-exam. I couldn't believe it when I was diagnosed with Stage 3C breast cancer. I then had genetic counseling and multigene panel testing, which showed that I have an

Questions to Ask Your Oncologist about Breast Cancer Treatment

- What are my treatment options?
- What can I expect from each of these treatments?
- What are the benefits and risks associated with these treatments?
- What new therapies are available and appropriate for diagnosis and prognosis?
- Should I have biomarker testing to help guide my treatment?
- What is the chance that my cancer will come back after this treatment?
- Do I qualify for any clinical trials?

ATM gene mutation. I felt a sense of relief when I learned about my mutation. It provided a rational reason for why this was happening to me. While my cousin probably had the same mutation, she didn't have genetic testing, and we'll never know for certain.

My cancer was advanced, so there was little time to lose and a lot to do. I had a double mastectomy, chemotherapy, and radiation. Because I had multiple cancerous lymph nodes, I also participated in an immunotherapy clinical trial. With a husband and three sons, I was willing to do anything to give myself the greatest chance for survival. The same genetic information that can be scary and overwhelming can also be extremely empowering. This knowledge allows us to understand what we are facing and to act in an educated way.

—*Ellyn*

Follow-Up Care

After completing treatment, you'll need to be closely monitored for a recurrence, a new cancer, and any new or lasting side effects. Your doctor will personalize a follow-up schedule for you based on the type and stage of your cancer, the length of your treatment, and how long you remain cancer-free. Generally, posttreatment follow-up includes visits to your doctor every few months for three to five years after your initial treatment and then annually. It's important to keep all of these appointments.

Posttreatment screenings should include

- A baseline mammogram within the first year after surgery and then annually thereafter (if you still have one or both breasts).
- A 3D mammogram and breast MRI staggered six months apart for your remaining breast(s). (Mammograms aren't required after mastectomy.)
- A pelvic exam if you take tamoxifen and you still have your uterus. (Tamoxifen increases the risk for endometrial cancer, especially if you are postmenopausal.)
- A bone density test if you're taking Arimidex, Aromasin, or Femara. Periodic checks of your bone density are also recommended if you experience treatment-related menopause.
- All other recommended health screenings as recommended by your doctor.

Blood and imaging tests may be needed to check symptoms of recurrence or provide information about side effects that linger or develop after treatment. These tests aren't routinely recommended after treatment because they don't improve survival.

— EXPERT VIEW —

Treating Breast Cancer in Men

BY ANGELIQUE RICHARDSON, MD, PHD

Breast cancer is rare in men, and for that reason, it hasn't often been the focus of research.

Men tend to be diagnosed with breast cancer at a later stage than women are. This may be due in part to a lack of awareness about the risk in men. Like women, men are more likely to have cancer that is hormone receptor–positive. HER2-positive breast cancer is less common, but the frequency is somewhat higher in younger versus older men. Much of what we know about treating men is from research on women. Treatment is generally similar with a few notable differences. Men with breast cancer, even those with small tumors, typically undergo a mastectomy rather than breast-conserving surgery due to the small amount of breast tissue present. Men usually receive a combination of radiation therapy, hormone therapy, chemotherapy, and targeted therapy based on their HER2 status and other biomarker testing. For hormone receptor–positive disease, most men receive tamoxifen. Less often, aromatase inhibitors may be combined with drugs that block male hormones. This combination has more side effects than tamoxifen alone. Men who develop metastatic disease are ordinarily treated with the same therapies women receive. For hormone-positive cancers, the drug Ibrance (palbociclib) is specifically approved for use in men, although other CDK4/6 inhibitors may also be used.

All men who are diagnosed with breast cancer meet national guidelines for genetic counseling and testing. This is particularly important in metastatic cancer because men with a BRCA1 or BRCA2 mutation may benefit from PARP inhibitor therapy.

Chapter 22

Treating Gynecologic Cancers

Lynparza (olaparib), Rubraca (rucaparib), and Zejula (niraparib) are PARP inhibitors, targeted drugs for advanced and recurrent ovarian cancers. They're particularly effective in individuals with *BRCA* mutations, and they're used extensively in people with Stage 3 or 4 ovarian cancer.

Endometrial and ovarian cancers are the two most common gynecologic cancers associated with inherited gene mutations. Treatment for these cancers differs, depending on the type and stage of the cancer, the characteristics of the tumor, and whether you have an inherited mutation in a related high-risk gene. Although staging and prognosis for these cancers are different, some treatments are similar. Surgery, for example, is an important part of treatment for almost all individuals with ovarian or endometrial cancers. Minimally invasive surgery (using a laparoscope or robotic-assisted laparoscope) is an option for some gynecologic cancer surgeries, including hysterectomy, salpingo-oophorectomy, and removing cancerous tumors. Gynecologic surgery, however, permanently affects your ability to become pregnant. So, it's a good idea to talk with your doctor before treatment if you're concerned about preserving your ability to bear children. Ask for a referral to a fertility and reproductive specialist before your treatment so that you can learn what to expect from your treatment options. Additional information about fertility issues is provided in chapter 27.

Options for Ovarian, Fallopian Tube, and Primary Peritoneal Cancers

About 90 percent of sporadic and hereditary ovarian cancers begin in the epithelial cells that cover the ovaries and line the fallopian tubes. Peritoneal tissue contains similar epithelial cells. This chapter focuses on treatment for serous epithelial cancer that develops in any of these three areas. The term "ovarian cancer" refers to ovarian, fallopian tube, and primary peritoneal cancers, which are closely related and treated in the same way. The primary treatment for most types of ovarian cancer includes surgery and chemotherapy. Radiation is rarely used, although it may be given to destroy small areas of cancer that remain in the pelvis after surgery or to alleviate pain related to metastasis. Your treatment plan will depend on several factors, including

- the type, stage, and grade of your cancer
- the results of biomarker testing
- whether you have an inherited mutation
- whether your entire tumor can be surgically removed
- how your cancer responds to treatment
- the number of prior treatments and the therapies you've received (if you have recurrent or advanced ovarian cancer)

Genetic Testing

All individuals who have ovarian cancer should have genetic counseling and testing for an inherited mutation in a *BRCA*, Lynch syndrome, or other gene associated with ovarian cancer. Having a *BRCA* mutation can affect survival, yet in a good way. People with *BRCA* mutations who develop ovarian cancer tend to have a better treatment response and survive longer than those who don't have a mutation.[1] Less is known about ovarian cancer outcomes in individuals with other inherited mutations, although they also may have longer survival.[2]

If you test positive for an inherited mutation, knowing that information can help you make decisions about how you'll be treated.

- If you have a *BRCA* mutation, you may benefit from treatment with a PARP inhibitor.

- If you have a Lynch syndrome gene mutation, you may benefit from treatment with an immune checkpoint inhibitor, such as Keytruda (pembrolizumab).
- Your genetic test results may make you eligible for clinical trials.

Your genetic test results can also help you make medical decisions to prevent a new diagnosis of cancer or to detect it early. Additionally, your results can help your blood relatives understand their risk for cancer and make decisions about their own cancer screening and prevention.

Biomarker Testing

Biomarker tests look for changes that can guide treatment.

- CA-125 is a protein biomarker that may be elevated in the blood of people with ovarian cancer. The CA-125 test may be used to monitor the response to treatment of ovarian cancer.
- Mismatch repair deficiency / microsatellite instability–high (dMMR/ MSI-H) is a biomarker commonly found in tumors of people with Lynch syndrome. (It's rarely found in the ovarian cancers of people who don't have Lynch syndrome.) Tumors with this feature may respond to Keytruda (pembrolizumab), an immune checkpoint inhibitor that helps the immune system recognize and attack cancer cells.
- Gene mutations in the tumor may suggest how well treatment may work with a targeted therapy known as a PARP inhibitor.
- Homologous recombination deficiency (HRD) may also suggest treatment with a PARP inhibitor.
- Other biomarkers may identify your eligibility for clinical trials.

Types of Treatment

Most ovarian cancers initially respond to first-line treatment, which often produces full remission (also known as "no evidence of disease"). If your cancer comes back, your doctor may recommend a second-line treatment, which will likely include another course of chemotherapy and/or targeted therapy. A third-line treatment may be used if your second-line regimen doesn't produce the desired response. Ovarian cancer recurrence is common, even with full remission after initial treatment.

Surgery

Surgery is the primary method of staging and treating ovarian cancer. In most cases, the surgeon removes the ovaries, fallopian tubes, uterus, cervix, and omentum, a layer of fatty tissue that covers the stomach and intestines. Lymph nodes in the abdomen and pelvis may also be removed. Any fluid in the abdomen is checked for cancer cells. Larger or more advanced ovarian cancers require debulking, a more extensive surgical procedure to remove as much of the cancer as possible. Debulking is especially important when cancer has spread throughout the abdomen. Ideally, debulking leaves behind no visible cancer or tumors larger than 1 centimeter (less than one-half inch). Prognosis tends to be better when "optimal debulking" is achieved.

Sometimes, parts of the colon, bladder, or other abdominal organs must be removed to achieve the broadest possible debulking. More expansive surgery may be needed to remove the spleen, part of the liver, and other organs if they're also affected. Chemotherapy may be recommended to decrease the burden of disease before surgical debulking. A consultation with a gynecologic oncology surgeon is an important part of this process.

Generally, initial recovery from ovarian cancer surgery requires two or three days in the hospital and potentially longer, depending on the extent of the procedure.

Chemotherapy

For most people with ovarian cancer, the combination of surgery and chemotherapy produces the best outcome. Even when all visible cancer is removed, residual microscopic cancer is presumed to be present. Chemotherapy is given after surgery to kill these remaining cancer cells. Sometimes, chemotherapy is also given before surgery to shrink the tumor to facilitate a more successful and less risky surgical procedure. The decision to do chemotherapy first or surgery first should be made in consultation with a gynecologic oncologist.

Chemotherapy for ovarian cancer most commonly includes two drugs—usually a platinum agent (either carboplatin or cisplatin) and a taxane (most commonly, paclitaxel)—which are given in cycles over several months. Tumors that don't respond or initially respond but return within six months may require a different systemic treatment.

Targeted Therapies and Immunotherapies

Targeted therapies block specific genes and proteins that cancer cells need to grow and survive, while immunotherapies help the immune system to attack certain weaknesses in cancer cells. Genetic testing for an inherited gene mutation and biomarker testing of your tumor may help determine whether you're likely to benefit from one of these advanced therapies. A common targeted drug, Avastin (bevacizumab), cuts off the blood supply to the tumor. Avastin is often used in combination with chemotherapy and/or other targeted therapies.

Lynparza (olaparib), Rubraca (rucaparib), and Zejula (niraparib) are PARP inhibitors, targeted drugs for advanced and recurrent ovarian cancers. They're particularly effective in individuals with *BRCA* mutations, and they're used extensively in people with Stage 3 or 4 ovarian cancer. PARP inhibitors are typically used alone. However, Lynparza is approved for maintenance therapy in combination with Avastin.

Immune checkpoint inhibitors help the immune system recognize and attack cancer cells. Keytruda is for patients with dMMR/MSI-H tumors, which may be found in some ovarian cancers. These tumors are frequently seen in people with a Lynch syndrome gene mutation who develop cancer.

Treatment by Stage

Staging distinguishes between early-stage and advanced ovarian cancers. This is an important step because treatment approaches and prognoses are different. Most individuals with high-grade ovarian cancer of any stage are treated initially with both surgery and chemotherapy. Newly diagnosed people often have surgery followed by a course of first-line chemotherapy. Those who have large tumors or who aren't well enough for debulking surgery might be given chemotherapy before surgery. The regimen, timing, and type of chemotherapy and the addition of targeted therapies depend on your age and general health, the stage and grade of your tumor, how it responds to treatment, and other factors.

Early-stage ovarian cancer is confined to an ovary or fallopian tube (Stage 1) or the pelvis (Stage 2). Surgery and chemotherapy are usually recommended. However, some individuals with early, low-grade tumors may be treated with surgery alone. High-grade cancers—which include the majority of cancers in people with inherited mutations—usually require a course of intravenous chemotherapy. The exact regimen varies, depending on your age,

The Power of PARP Inhibitors

Following the discovery of the *BRCA1* and *BRCA2* genes in the 1990s, British researchers began exploring ways to improve treatment outcomes for people with breast and ovarian cancers related to inherited mutations in these genes. Although *BRCA* genes ordinarily fix DNA damage in cells, inherited mutations in these genes disable this capability. Tumor cells with mutated *BRCA* genes already have a deficient repair system, but the researchers found that *BRCA* genes use the poly (ADP-ribose) polymerase (PARP) protein as a backup repair system. This discovery led to the development of PARP inhibitors, a class of anticancer drugs that block the PARP protein and disable the remaining repair function. Damage then accumulates until the cancer cells can no longer divide, and they eventually die.

Researchers continue to explore the potential of these drugs for sporadic cancers and for cancers that develop from inherited mutations in *BRIP1*, *PALB2*, *RAD51C*, *RAD51D*, and other high-risk genes.

general health, and stage and grade of your cancer. Most of these early-stage cancers never return after treatment. Some types of ovarian cancer, such as endometrioid ovarian cancers and low-grade serous cancers, are responsive to hormonal therapies.

Most ovarian cancers are already advanced (Stage 3 or 4) by the time they're diagnosed. Treatments often include a combination of surgery to remove as much of the cancer as possible, chemotherapy, and targeted therapy.

If your initial course of chemotherapy produces a complete response (your cancer disappears) or a partial response (it shrinks), you then have two options. Either you can take a watch-and-wait approach with regular monitoring for any sign of recurrence, or you can start maintenance therapy to delay or decrease your chance of recurrence. Choosing the most effective maintenance regimen depends on several factors, including

- if you already took Avastin as part of your initial treatment
- how many lines of chemotherapy you previously received
- whether genetic testing shows that you have an inherited gene mutation
- whether your tumor is HRD-positive or has other specific biomarkers

Although the average five-year survival rate for advanced ovarian cancer is 17–40 percent, newer, less toxic targeted therapies are helping individuals live longer with fewer side effects and a better quality of life. More treatment options are in the research and development pipeline.

Follow-Up Care

After ovarian cancer, you'll need to regularly visit your doctor every two to four months for the first three years after initial treatment, and then every three to six months until your doctor suggests a different schedule. Each visit should include a physical examination, a pelvic exam, blood tests, and imaging tests to monitor for a recurrence. Signs that ovarian cancer has returned may include rising CA-125 levels, pelvic or abdominal pain, bloating, lack of appetite, trouble eating or feeling full quickly, unexplained weight loss, fatigue, urgency to urinate, and/or evidence of cancer on imaging tests. You should also have recommended screenings to identify any long-term side effects of treatment, and you should continue routine screenings for other cancers.

Treating Platinum-Resistant Ovarian Cancer

Platinum chemotherapy is a cornerstone of ovarian cancer treatment. Platinum-sensitive cancers respond to these chemotherapies and don't recur for six months or longer. After multiple courses of treatment, however, ovarian cancers that were initially platinum-sensitive can become platinum-resistant. They don't shrink when treated, or they initially respond but return within six months. Platinum-resistant cancers may also be less likely to respond to PARP inhibitors. The results of genetic testing and biomarker tests may open treatment options or clinical trials for people with platinum-resistant ovarian cancer.

— My Story —

Not Believing My Diagnosis, I Initially Refused Treatment

In early 2017 I developed bloating, filling up quickly when I ate, and I had an increasingly distended abdomen and persistent fatigue. I didn't visit my primary care physician until I began having abdominal pain. My doctor immediately suspected ovarian cancer, but didn't share that with me until a few days later when a CT scan showed lesions on my ovaries. I refused to believe I might have ovarian cancer, and I planned to refuse chemo. My doctor consulted with a gynecologic oncologist and ordered a paracentesis. This provided a tissue sample, which showed typical markers for high-grade serous ovarian cancer.

The oncologist called me into the office and told me that I had Stage 4, high-grade serous ovarian cancer. She proposed a treatment plan and asked me to consent to genetic testing. I said yes to testing and surgery but not to chemo. She responded that I'd live for maybe six months if I didn't have chemo. In the next couple of days, my common sense returned. I told my oncologist that I would follow through with her recommendations, and I started neoadjuvant chemotherapy the following week.

After first-line treatment, I was in remission for 10 months. After treatment when my cancer returned, I started on a PARP inhibitor, and I've been doing well for the last 18 months.

—*Tanya*

Options for Endometrial Cancer

Endometrial cancer is the most common cancer in the uterus, arising in the inner lining. It is associated with inherited mutations in about 3–5 percent of cases. Endometrial cancers are often divided into two categories. Type 1 is the most common: low-grade endometrial cancers that tend to be slow-growing and are less likely to recur or spread. Type 2 cancers are higher grade, tend to behave more aggressively, are more likely to spread, and have a poorer prognosis. Treatment and care decisions consider which therapies would be more effective for the type you have. These decisions also consider whether lymphovascular space invasion—cancer cells in the blood vessels or lymph vessels outside of the tumor—has occurred, which signals the need for more aggressive treatment.

The most common treatment plan for endometrial cancer begins with surgery, which usually includes removal of the uterus, cervix, ovaries, fallopian tubes, and some lymph nodes to stage the cancer. When certain higher-risk features are present, radiation to the pelvis or the top of the vagina is given to reduce the chance of recurrence. Systemic therapy may include chemotherapy and hormone therapy. Biomarker testing can help identify individuals with advanced endometrial cancers who may benefit from targeted therapy or immunotherapy.

Genetic Testing

Before you and your doctor decide on the best course of treatment, you may benefit from genetic counseling and genetic testing if you have any of the following circumstances:

- You have a blood relative with an inherited mutation in a gene that is linked to cancer.
- You were diagnosed with endometrial cancer before age 50.
- You were diagnosed with colorectal, stomach, ovarian, pancreatic, or urothelial cancer; a rare cancer; or multiple cancers.
- You have one or more close relatives who were diagnosed with endometrial, colorectal, stomach, ovarian, pancreatic, or urothelial cancer; a rare cancer; or multiple cancers.
- Biomarker testing shows that your tumor is dMMR/MSI-H.

If you test positive for an inherited mutation, that information can help you make decisions about how you'll be treated. If you have a Lynch syndrome gene mutation and have advanced cancer, you may benefit from treatment with an immune checkpoint inhibitor, such as Keytruda (pembrolizumab) or Jemperli (dostarlimab). Your genetic test results may make you eligible for a clinical trial.

Your genetic test results can also help you make medical decisions to prevent a new diagnosis of cancer or to detect it early. Additionally, your results can help your blood relatives understand their risk for cancer and make decisions about their own cancer screening and prevention.

Biomarker Testing

All endometrial tumors should be tested for dMMR/MSI-H, which may be a sign of Lynch syndrome. If your test is positive, genetic counseling and testing should follow to determine if you have an inherited Lynch syndrome mutation. Individuals with a tumor that has a positive dMMR/MSI-H test result may be candidates for immunotherapy, depending on the cancer stage or if the cancer has recurred. Additional biomarker testing may be recommended for the following situations:

- Tumor mutational burden (TMB) identifies a cancer that is likely to respond to the immune checkpoint inhibitor Keytruda.
- HER2 receptors that help tumor growth are overexpressed in about 3–5 percent of advanced endometrial cancers (particularly, high-grade serous endometrial cancers). These cancers may respond to off-label use of Herceptin (trastuzumab), a drug that targets the HER2 protein.

- Estrogen and progesterone receptor testing can help identify endometrial cancers that may respond to hormone therapy.

Treatment Strategies

Surgery

Surgery is the primary method of staging and treating endometrial cancer. Most often, it involves removing the uterus, cervix, ovaries, and fallopian tubes. Staging may also include a sentinel node biopsy, a procedure that involves injecting the cervix with a harmless dye during surgery. The dye travels to the one or two sentinel nodes in the pelvis that are closest to the tumor, which are then removed. If these nodes are free of cancer, no additional lymph nodes need to be removed. Sentinel nodes that contain cancer cells indicate that cancer has spread, and more extensive treatment may be needed. Larger or more advanced endometrial cancers may require a more extensive debulking procedure to remove as much cancer as possible.

Minimally invasive surgery is an option for most endometrial cancer surgeries. Generally, an overnight stay in the hospital is required, although some people go home the same day.

Radiation Therapy

Radiation is sometimes used after initial surgery to decrease the risk for recurrence. Radiation for endometrial cancer can be delivered using one or both of two different methods. A course of external radiation that directs high-energy x-ray beams to the pelvis is usually given five days per week for about six weeks. Alternatively, brachytherapy is a focused dose of radiation to the top of the vagina, where the uterus was removed.

In addition to being used for first-line treatment, radiation is also an option for recurrent endometrial cancer that hasn't previously been radiated and for reducing symptoms of advanced and metastatic cancers.

Chemotherapy

Chemotherapy is used for individuals with high-grade, early-stage endometrial cancer or advanced disease. Most often, this means a platinum agent in combination with a taxane, which are given after surgery to reduce the chance of recurrence. Sometimes, chemotherapy is given in combination with radiation.

Hormone Therapy

Several hormone therapies are used to treat select cases of early-stage and late-stage hormone receptor–positive endometrial cancers. If you have early-stage disease and can't safely have surgery or radiation, hormone therapy may be your primary treatment.

Targeted Therapies and Immunotherapies

Several targeted drugs and immunotherapies are used to treat advanced endometrial cancer. Targeted therapies include

- Avastin (bevacizumab)
- Lenvima (lenvatinib)
- Afinitor (everolimus)
- Herceptin (trastuzumab)

Immunotherapies include

- Keytruda (pembrolizumab)
- Opdivo (nivolumab)
- Jemperli (dostarlimab)

Treatment by Stage

Treatment for early-stage endometrial cancer usually includes a total hysterectomy to remove the uterus and cervix, salpingo-oophorectomy to remove the ovaries and fallopian tubes, and may also include the removal of lymph nodes. Surgery may be the only treatment needed for type 1 (low-grade, slow-growing) tumors. If additional treatment is needed, it may include radiation with external beam therapy or brachytherapy. Individuals who can't have surgery may instead undergo hormone therapy or radiation with external beam therapy, brachytherapy, or both. Postoperative treatment may include radiation and/or chemotherapy. Some young people with low-risk endometrial cancer may undergo treatment to preserve fertility. This approach involves hormone therapy and very close follow-up with multiple biopsies. It's important to speak with your doctor about the benefits and risks of fertility preservation after endometrial cancer.

Although some advanced endometrial cancers (Stages 3 and 4) are inoperable, treatment for these cancers usually includes surgery that removes the ovaries, fallopian tubes, uterus, and lymph nodes, as well as debulking if tumor spread is obvious in the pelvis or abdomen. This is usually followed by some combination of chemotherapy and radiation, depending on the extent of tumor spread.

Some palliative therapies, including radiation and surgery, may relieve symptoms in people with advanced cancer that progresses. Additional hormone, targeted, or immunotherapy treatments may be used, depending on the stage and grade, tumor subtype, number of prior treatments, and the results of biomarker testing.

Follow-Up Care

After initial treatment, you'll need to see your doctor every three to six months for the first three years. If you were treated for Stage 3 or 4 endometrial cancer or you had a high-grade tumor, your oncologist may recommend a CT scan of your chest, abdomen, and pelvis. Your doctor may recommend other imaging tests, depending on your circumstances. Each office visit should include a physical examination, a pelvic exam, and a check of the lymph nodes. A CA-125 blood test, other imaging tests, or a biopsy may be needed if you have any symptoms that might indicate a recurrence.

It's also important to follow through with recommended screenings to identify any long-term side effects of treatment and to continue the recommended screenings for other cancers. Endometrial cancer recurs most commonly at the top of the vagina, and recurrence is often accompanied by new vaginal discharge or bleeding. New symptoms should prompt a visit to your doctor, including a pelvic exam.

Questions to Ask Your Doctor about Gynecologic Cancer Treatment

- What type and subtype of cancer do I have?
- Should I have genetic testing before being treated?
- What treatment do you recommend for me, and why?
- What is my prognosis, and how will this treatment affect it?
- Will treatment affect my fertility?
- What side effects should I expect?
- Who will provide my treatment?
- Am I eligible for any clinical trials of other treatment options?
- Will I be able to become pregnant after treatment?

Chapter 23

Treating Gastrointestinal Cancers

Pancreatic cancer is a difficult cancer to detect early, and in most cases, it's already late-stage disease when diagnosed. However, diagnosis at earlier stages may become more common as new screening options become available for people with a high risk for this cancer.

If you develop cancer in your gastrointestinal tract, your treatment team may include a colorectal surgeon or a surgical oncologist, a radiation oncologist, and a medical oncologist who will coordinate your systemic therapies. This chapter describes treatment for hereditary colorectal, pancreatic, and gastric (stomach) cancers. Small bowel cancers (which are rare and treated in the same way as colorectal cancer) and anal cancers (which are typically due to the human papillomavirus rather than to inherited mutations) aren't addressed in this chapter.

Options for Colorectal Cancer

Colorectal cancer is treated with a mix of surgery, radiation therapy (more often for rectal cancers than colon cancers), chemotherapy, targeted therapy, and immunotherapy. Individual treatment plans are based on several factors, including

- cell type
- subtype

- stage
- biomarker testing
- genetic testing for an inherited mutation
- anatomic location within the large bowel

Biomarker Tumor Testing and Genetic Testing

All colorectal tumors, regardless of their stage or your age at diagnosis, should have biomarker testing for mismatch repair deficiency / microsatellite instability–high (dMMR/MSI-H), an abnormality frequently found in people with Lynch syndrome. Other biomarkers may be used to guide treatment for people with advanced colorectal cancer (see below).

If you have colorectal cancer, knowing that you have Lynch syndrome or an inherited mutation in another gene linked to colorectal cancer may help you and your relatives make health care decisions. Genetic counseling and genetic testing are recommended if you have colorectal cancer and meet any of the following high-risk criteria:

- A relative tested positive for an inherited mutation linked to cancer.
- One or more close relatives were diagnosed with endometrial, colorectal, stomach, ovarian, pancreatic, or urothelial cancer; a rare cancer; or multiple cancers.
- You have a history of numerous colorectal polyps.
- You were diagnosed with colorectal cancer before age 50.
- You were diagnosed with another primary cancer before or after your diagnosis of colorectal cancer.
- Biomarker testing of your tumor indicates that you may have an inherited mutation.

If you test positive for a Lynch syndrome gene mutation, you may benefit from treatment with an immune checkpoint inhibitor, such as Keytruda (pembrolizumab), Opdivo (nivolumab), or Yervoy (ipilimumab), though currently these agents are only approved for treating the colorectal cancer of people with advanced disease. If you test positive for a mutation in a different high-risk gene, you may be eligible for clinical trials of targeted therapies to treat hereditary colorectal cancer.

Treatment Strategies

Treatment for colorectal cancer primarily depends on the stage of the cancer. Staging considers the size of the tumor, how far it has grown into the layers of the wall of the colon or rectum, and whether it has spread into tissues or organs beyond its point of origin.

Surgery

Most early-stage colorectal cancers are treated with one of the following surgical procedures followed by chemotherapy, targeted therapy, and/or immunotherapy.

- Polypectomy removes small cancers that are inside polyps during a colonoscopy.
- Endoscopic mucosal resection ("resection" means the removal of tissue) removes polyps and the surrounding tissue during a colonoscopy so that larger polyps and some of the lining of the colon can also be removed.
- Segmental colectomy removes the cancerous area of the colon and a margin of healthy tissue (figure 23.1). This may be performed as a minimally invasive (laparoscopic) surgery or as an open surgery, depending on several factors. When it's not possible to join the remaining segments of the colon together, a temporary or permanent opening called an ostomy is created in the wall of the abdomen. The end of the bowel (the stoma) protrudes through this opening and carries stool into a colostomy bag worn on the outside of the body (figure 23.2). (Colectomy and ostomy are described in more detail in chapter 18.)

Surgery can also be used to relieve a blockage in the colon or improve bleeding, pain, or other symptoms. Surgery may not be an option if your tumor is too large or if there are too many tumors.

If you have an inherited mutation, more extensive surgery to remove your entire colon may more effectively address your high risk for a second colorectal cancer.

- Total abdominal colectomy with ileorectal anastomosis removes the entire colon while sparing the rectum. This surgery preserves bowel function, but it doesn't eliminate the risk for rectal cancer.

FIGURE 23.1 A segmental abdominal colectomy removes the cancerous area of the colon, and the remaining segments are then joined together

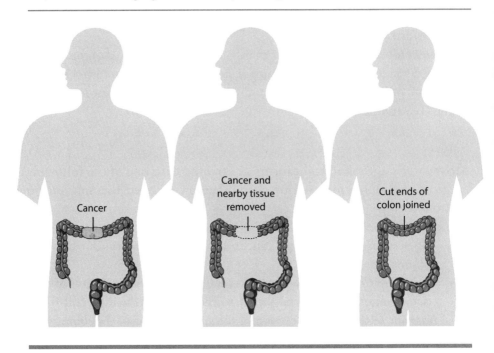

FIGURE 23.2 When it's not possible to rejoin the remaining segments of the colon, the end of the bowel is rerouted through an ostomy to carry waste into a colostomy bag

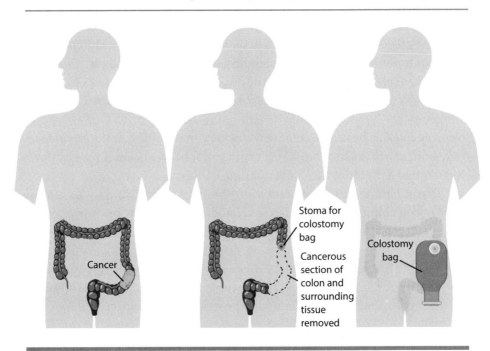

- Total proctocolectomy with ileal pouch and anal anastomosis removes the colon and rectum but spares the sphincter so that you retain bowel control. A portion of your small intestine may be used to create an internal storage pouch for waste.
- Total proctocolectomy with permanent end ileostomy removes the entire colon, rectum, and anus. This requires the creation of an ostomy, an opening made in the abdominal wall to facilitate waste removal to an external bag worn on the body.

In addition to the usual risks of general surgery—infection, delayed wound healing, fluid buildup at the surgical site, pain, and others—colectomy can cause uncommon but potentially serious complications, including

- internal bleeding
- hernia
- leakage from the colon into the abdomen
- damage to nearby organs
- pneumonia and other lung complications
- bowel obstruction
- blood clots in the lungs (pulmonary embolism) or the legs (deep vein thrombosis)
- dehydration with electrolyte abnormalities

Colectomy requires three or four days in the hospital. You can begin to eat normally a few days after your first post-op bowel movement. Overall recovery depends on your health and the type of procedure you have.

Chemotherapy

Chemotherapy may be given before surgery to shrink a tumor or after surgery to reduce the risk of recurrence. For colon cancer, this generally means 5-FU (5-fluorouracil), Xeloda (capecitabine), irinotecan, or oxaliplatin. For some colorectal cancers, combinations of chemotherapy are more effective, including

- 5-FU/LV: 5-FU and leucovorin, a drug that improves the effectiveness of chemotherapy
- CAPEOX: Xeloda and oxaliplatin

- FOLFIRI: 5-fluorouracil, irinotecan, and leucovorin
- FOLFOX: 5-fluorouracil, oxaliplatin, and leucovorin
- FOLFOXIRI: 5-FU, oxaliplatin, irinotecan, and leucovorin
- Lonsurf (combined trifluridine and tipiracil)

Radiation Therapy

Radiation therapy isn't routinely recommended for colon cancer, but it's often standard treatment for rectal cancers.

Targeted and Immunotherapies

Targeted therapies block specific genes and proteins that cancer cells need to grow and survive, while immunotherapies help the immune system to attack certain weaknesses in cancer cells. Genetic testing of your tumor for an inherited gene mutation and biomarker testing may help determine whether you're likely to benefit from one of these advanced therapies.

Immunotherapies may be used to treat advanced colorectal cancer. Keytruda (pembrolizumab), Opdivo (nivolumab), and Yervoy (ipilimumab) are immune checkpoint inhibitors that help the immune system detect and kill cancer cells in tumors that are dMMR/MSI-H. Keytruda is also used for cancers that have a feature known as high tumor mutational burden (TMB-high).

Targeted therapies, including Avastin (bevacizumab), Cyramza (ramucirumab), Zaltrap (ziv-aflibercept), and Stivarga (regorafenib), are used to slow the growth of advanced colorectal cancers. Several other targeted drugs and immunotherapies may be recommended, depending on tumor changes that are identified by biomarker testing:

- Tafinlar (dabrafenib) or Braftovi (encorafenib), which are usually combined with Mekinist (trametinib) or Mektovi (binimetinib)
- Herceptin (trastuzumab)
- Erbitux (cetuximab)
- Vectibix (panitumumab)

Treating Colorectal Cancer by Stage

Stage 0 is noninvasive and confined to the innermost layer of colorectal tissue. Some polyps that are found during colonoscopy may be Stage 0 cancers. These are sometimes called malignant polyps.

Stage 1 has grown into the superficial layers of the colon or rectum. The disease may have grown to, but not beyond, the muscle layer of the colorectum. Stage 1 colorectal cancers don't involve nearby lymph nodes. These early-stage cancers are usually treated successfully with surgery to remove the entire malignant area. The five-year prognosis for early-stage colorectal cancer is excellent—90 percent.

Stage 2 has grown through the muscle layer of the colorectum but doesn't involve nearby lymph nodes. Chemotherapy and radiation therapy are often recommended for Stage 2 rectal cancers. If you have early Stage 2 colon cancer and your tumor is dMMR/MSI-H, your prognosis may be better, and chemotherapy may not be necessary. The presence of high-risk features in a Stage 2 cancer, however, may indicate a potential benefit from chemotherapy. High-risk features are pathologic findings that suggest an increased risk that a Stage 2 cancer could spread (e.g., the invasion of tumor cells into blood vessels in the tumor specimen).

Stage 3 colorectal cancers affect one or more nearby lymph nodes but haven't spread to more distant locations in the body. Surgery to remove the cancer followed by chemotherapy is usually recommended for cancers in the colon. Chemotherapy and radiation are usually recommended before and/ or after surgery for most rectal cancers.

Stage 4 colon cancer is metastatic disease. It has spread to the peritoneum (the lining of the abdomen) or to distant organs and may affect distant lymph nodes. The five-year survival rate is lower than for earlier stages. Survival is improved when metastasis is confined to small areas in the lungs or liver, which can be removed by a surgery. Tumors in the liver may be destroyed with ablation (extreme heat or cold) or embolization (injecting materials that block blood flow to cancer cells). Radiation can temporarily reduce tumor size and relieve pain and other symptoms, but it's less likely to provide a cure. Radiation might be used to treat the lungs, bone, or other areas where colorectal cancer has spread.

Many of the same chemotherapy drugs that are used for early-stage colorectal cancers work well as treatment for metastatic disease. Chemotherapy can be given before surgery to shrink large tumors and after surgery to prolong survival. It is used alone or in combination with targeted therapies. Your individual treatment regimen will depend on whether chemotherapy is to be used for first-line therapy or a recurrence. If it's used for a recurrence, other considerations may include which drugs were used for your initial treatment, the elapsed time since that treatment, and your overall health. When one course of treatment stops working, another may be tried.

— *My Story* —

Thriving after My Experience
with Colorectal Cancer

The colorectal cancer in my family is due to Lynch syndrome. I was advised by my surgeon to have a full resection after my colorectal cancer diagnosis. I got a second opinion from my gastrointestinal doctor, who had also followed my brother, mom, and aunt through their colon cancers when they were alive. He agreed with the course of treatment and explained that I already had precancerous polyps on the other side of the colon. I opted for total resection.

I was mostly alone at the hospital because my husband was home with our babies. My closest friend was a pillar of strength for me. She was at the hospital before I arrived at the operating room, and she didn't leave me until I woke up 12 hours later. I was discharged three days later—10 years to the day of my mom's death from cancer. My recovery was ideal, with no complications, and I returned to work the following month.

Almost 5 years later, I feel great. I have scar tissue that caused some complications, and I am checked every year. Following Lynch syndrome guidelines, I had a total hysterectomy after having another baby.

—*Maria*

Follow-Up Care

Follow-up care for colorectal cancer focuses on finding a recurrence as early as possible and monitoring for long-term side effects. Your doctor will provide a customized plan and schedule for you, depending on the type and stage of your cancer, your treatment, and your risk for recurrence. Follow-up is especially important during the first five years after treatment when the risk of recurrence is greatest. Follow-up generally includes

- A physical examination.
- A carcinoembryonic antigen blood test, which looks for proteins that can indicate a recurrence.
- A CT scan of the chest, abdomen, and pelvis every 6–12 months for the first five years. This is typically recommended for individuals

who were treated for Stages 2 or 3 colorectal cancer. Routine CT imaging may not be recommended for individuals with resected Stage 1 colorectal cancer.

- A colonoscopy one year after your initial diagnosis. You should have a complete colonoscopy sooner if your entire colon wasn't evaluated when you were initially diagnosed—for example, if your tumor was blocking the colon. If colonoscopy at one year after treatment is normal, it's typically repeated every three to five years, depending on the findings. If you have an inherited mutation linked to colorectal cancer, your doctor may recommend an annual colonoscopy.

Options for Pancreatic Cancer

Pancreatic cancer treatment is determined by the stage of your disease and your overall health. Treatment may include surgery, radiation, chemotherapy, targeted treatments, and immunotherapy. This is a difficult cancer to detect early, and in most cases, it's already late-stage disease when diagnosed. However, diagnosis at earlier stages may become more common as new screening options become available for people with a high risk for this cancer. Because of the limited number of treatments available and the aggressive nature of pancreatic cancer, experts strongly recommend that anyone with pancreatic cancer consider participating in a clinical trial.

Tumor Staging

Pancreatic cancer can begin in exocrine cells, which release digestive enzymes, or in endocrine cells, which make insulin and other hormones that control blood sugar levels. Tumors in these cells behave differently, display different symptoms, and respond to different treatments. Most pancreatic cancers are adenocarcinomas that start in the ducts of exocrine cells. Pancreatic cancers of endocrine cells (often called neuroendocrine tumors or NETs) are treated differently than adenocarcinomas and aren't discussed here.

Pancreatic cancers are staged into one of four categories based on whether they're resectable, meaning that all or part of the cancer can be removed:

- Resectable cancers are shown by imaging to be completely removable with surgery and haven't spread to other organs.

- Borderline resectable cancers are shown by imaging to include some degree of involvement of nearby blood vessels, without spread to other organs.
- Unresectable cancers can't be removed by surgery because they significantly involve nearby blood vessels. This is locally advanced disease.
- Metastatic cancers have spread to other organs and can't be removed.

Genetic Testing for an Inherited Mutation

National guidelines recommend genetic testing for everyone with pancreatic adenocarcinoma. Genetic testing can inform your treatment options and your eligibility for clinical trials.

- An inherited mutation in a *BRCA1* or *BRCA2* gene may indicate that treatment with a platinum-type chemotherapy and maintenance therapy with a PARP inhibitor are the best options, depending on the stage of your cancer.
- An inherited mutation in a different high-risk gene may qualify you for participation in clinical trials of new targeted therapies.
- An inherited mutation in a Lynch syndrome gene may indicate that treatment with an immunotherapy agent could be effective, depending on the stage of your cancer.

Genetic test results also may help you make medical decisions to prevent a new diagnosis of cancer or to detect it early. Additionally, your results can help your blood relatives understand their risk for cancer and make decisions about their own cancer screening and prevention.

Treatment Strategies

Surgery

Pancreatic surgery is complex and precise, so it's critical to choose an experienced surgeon who can accurately assess your eligibility for a surgical procedure. The National Comprehensive Cancer Network recommends choosing a high-volume, multidisciplinary cancer center with surgeons who perform more than 15 pancreatic surgeries annually. Your surgeon will decide which procedure offers the best chance of entirely removing the cancer, considering its size and location. The following procedures may be performed as minimally invasive laparoscopic or robotically assisted operations, although not all medical centers have the required equipment and not all surgeons have the necessary skills:

- The Whipple procedure (pancreaticoduodenectomy) is most often performed for tumors in the head (the right side) of the pancreas. This surgery removes the head of the pancreas, part of the small intestine, the lower bile ducts, the gallbladder, and the surrounding lymph nodes.
- Distal pancreatectomy removes a tumor from the body or tail of the pancreas.
- Total pancreatectomy removes the entire pancreas, the gallbladder, part of the stomach and small intestine, the spleen, and nearby lymph nodes. This more extensive procedure is uncommon, but it is necessary when cancer has spread throughout the pancreas.

Be sure to talk to your surgeon before your procedure to understand the potential risks and side effects. All surgeries carry similar risks, including infection, bleeding, delayed wound healing, fluid buildup at the surgical site, and pain. Pancreatic surgery carries additional risk for more serious complications, including

- leakage of pancreatic fluid at the surgical site
- pus inside the abdomen
- small bowel obstruction
- inflammation of the abdomen
- diabetes
- difficulty digesting food

Recovery from pancreatic surgery is gradual. Unless complications occur, full recovery ordinarily takes about two months. The pancreas makes insulin and enzymes that are involved in breaking down food. These functions may be affected when portions of the pancreas are removed, leading to diabetes and digestive difficulty. You may need to take enzyme supplements and/or insulin, and you may be followed by an endocrinologist for the rest of your life. Consulting with a nutritionist can help you learn how to make necessary changes to your diet to improve digestion and ensure that you get the nutrients you need.

Radiation Therapy

Radiation therapy to shrink a tumor before surgery and/or to lower the risk of recurrence after surgery (sometimes given in combination with capecitabine, gemcitabine, or other chemotherapy) may be a part of treatment for all stages of pancreatic cancer. Radiation that is used at the same time as chemotherapy is called chemoradiation. If you're not a candidate for surgery, radiation therapy can stop tumor growth and relieve pain or other symptoms.

Chemotherapy

Chemotherapy for pancreatic cancer usually includes one or more of the following:

- 5-FU (5-fluorouracil)
- Gemzar (gemcitabine)
- Abraxane (nab-paclitaxel)
- Xeloda (capecitabine)
- oxaliplatin
- cisplatin
- irinotecan
- Onivyde (nanoliposomal irinotecan)

Treating Resectable and Borderline Resectable Disease

Surgery for early-stage pancreatic cancer with no evidence of metastasis may be the best option for long-term survival if your surgeon feels that the entire tumor can be removed. You may have several diagnostic tests to assess the size and borders of the area so that your surgeon can make the determination. If you have a borderline resectable tumor or if it's unclear that your entire tumor can be removed with clean margins, neoadjuvant chemotherapy may be prescribed to initially shrink the tumor. After surgery, you may receive several courses of chemotherapy or chemoradiation.

Treating Unresectable and Metastatic Disease

Treatment with a combination of chemotherapy agents is the primary approach when pancreatic cancer is too widespread to be removed by surgery. While chemotherapy doesn't cure metastatic disease, it can sometimes shrink tumors or temporarily slow their growth. If you have an inherited mutation in a *BRCA1*,

BRCA2, or *PALB2* gene, your doctor will likely prescribe FOLFIRINOX—a combination of leucovorin, 5-fluorouracil, irinotecan, and the platinum agent oxaliplatin—or they may prescribe Gemzar combined with cisplatin. These regimens generally improve response. If you have a *BRCA* mutation and your tumor responds or doesn't grow after 16 weeks of chemotherapy, you may benefit from maintenance therapy with the PARP inhibitor Lynparza for as long as your tumor remains stable and doesn't grow.

Surgery, ablation, and embolization are sometimes used to relieve symptoms related to limited metastases. Unfortunately, in most cases, diagnosis isn't made until pancreatic cancer has widely metastasized and can't be surgically removed. But even when a cancer is too widespread to be removed completely, surgery may be recommended to unblock or bypass a bile duct or the small intestine to improve jaundice and help you to feel better. A small, flexible plastic or metal tube called a stent may also be used to open a blockage to relieve pain.

Another pain-relieving option is a celiac plexus block. This stops celiac nerves that are damaged by pancreatic cancer from sending pain messages to the brain.

Targeted and Immunotherapies

If you have advanced pancreatic cancer, several targeted therapies, either alone or in combination with chemotherapy, might be beneficial. Tarceva (erlotinib) blocks proteins that promote tumor growth. Tarceva may be used in combination with the chemotherapy agent Gemzar as a first-line treatment for locally advanced, unresectable, or metastatic disease. Before deciding on a treatment plan, all advanced pancreatic tumors should be tested for biomarkers to help determine whether any of the following approaches may be effective:

- The PARP inhibitor Lynparza (olaparib) may be recommended if you have an inherited *BRCA1* or *BRCA2* gene mutation and your cancer didn't grow during four or more months of chemotherapy with a platinum agent.
- The immune checkpoint inhibitor Keytruda (pembrolizumab) may be of benefit if testing shows that your tumor is dMMR/ MSI-H, a characteristic that is uncommon in pancreatic cancer, but isn't unusual in people who have a Lynch syndrome–related

cancer. (Everyone who has a dMMR/MSI-H tumor should also receive genetic counseling and testing for an inherited Lynch syndrome gene mutation.) Keytruda is also used for cancers that have high tumor mutational burden (TMB-high).

- Additional biomarkers may identify your eligibility for clinical trials.

Follow-Up Care

Your after-treatment care depends on the type and stage of your cancer, how you were treated, and other factors. If you had surgery and you have no evidence of remaining disease, your doctor may want to see you every three to six months for the first several years. Follow-up visits to your doctor will include a physical exam, including feeling your abdomen and nearby lymph nodes. You may have CT scans or other imaging tests, and blood tests, including a test for CA 19-9, a biomarker used to monitor for recurrence.

Options for Gastric Cancer

The majority of stomach cancers are adenocarcinomas, which ordinarily start as small tumors in one section of the stomach and then grow and spread. People with Lynch syndrome or inherited mutations in *STK11*, *TP53*, and other genes may have an increased risk for gastric adenocarcinomas. Diffuse gastric cancer is a subtype made up of signet ring cells, which look different under a microscope. Instead of forming a solid tumor, these cells multiply and spread below the lining of the stomach, making them harder to detect early.

Up to 3 percent of all stomach cancers are hereditary diffuse gastric cancer (HDGC), which may be caused by an inherited mutation in the *CDH1* gene and other genes. HDGC tends to be aggressive, can affect much of the stomach, and is more likely to spread to other organs. Ideally, treatment should be managed by a gastroenterologist and a surgical oncologist who have considerable experience with HDGC. There has been minimal research on it, and there are limited treatment choices.

Staging stomach cancer is based on how many of the four stomach layers are involved and the number of lymph nodes affected. Generally, cancers that affect more lymph nodes are staged higher.

Biomarker Testing

All stomach cancers should be tested for mismatch repair deficiency / microsatellite instability–high (dMMR/MSI-H), an abnormality frequently found in people with Lynch syndrome. Biomarker testing that shows changes in HER2 receptors and/or the PD-L1 protein may help select the best treatment for advanced stomach cancer. Additional biomarkers may help identify your eligibility for clinical trials

Genetic Testing

If you've been diagnosed with gastric cancer, knowing that you have Lynch syndrome or an inherited mutation in a *CDH1*, *STK11*, *TP53*, or other gene is likely to influence your medical decisions. Genetic testing can also help you make medical decisions to prevent a new cancer or to detect cancer early. Additionally, your results can help your blood relatives understand their risk for cancer and make decisions about their own cancer screening and prevention. Genetic counseling and genetic testing are strongly recommended if you have gastric cancer and meet any of the following high-risk criteria:

- A close relative tested positive for an inherited mutation linked to cancer.
- One or more close relatives were diagnosed with breast (especially lobular), gastric, endometrial, colorectal, ovarian, pancreatic, or urothelial cancer; a rare cancer; or multiple cancers.
- You were diagnosed with diffuse gastric cancer before age 50.
- You were diagnosed with another primary cancer before or after your diagnosis of gastric cancer.
- You were diagnosed with diffuse gastric cancer at any age and have a personal or family history of cleft lip or cleft palate.
- Biomarker testing of your tumor shows that you may have an inherited mutation.

Treatment Strategies

Early-stage gastric cancers may be treated with a combination of surgery, chemotherapy, and radiation.

Surgery

- Endoscopic mucosal resection may be used to remove very early-stage cancers. An endoscope is passed through the mouth and into the stomach, allowing a gastroenterologist to see and remove the cancer. No incisions are required.
- A partial gastrectomy removes the portion of the stomach that contains the tumor with a margin of healthy tissue around it. Some gastrectomies may be performed using a laparoscope, which requires a smaller incision and allows a quicker recovery.
- A total gastrectomy (removal of the entire stomach) is recommended if you have HDGC. It's the same surgery that's recommended to reduce the risk of HDGC in people who have an inherited *CDH1* mutation (see chapter 18). This is the most effective way to prevent the cancer from growing and spreading and to improve survival.

Having a partial or complete gastrectomy can affect your body's ability to absorb vitamin B_{12}. Most people who have gastrectomy need B_{12} injections or supplements for the rest of their lives to maintain adequate levels of this important vitamin. Consulting with a nutritionist can help you learn how to make other changes to your diet to improve digestion and ensure that you get the nutrients you need after surgery.

Chemotherapy

Small, well-contained tumors may be treated with surgery alone, but most people with early-stage gastric cancer receive chemotherapy after surgery. Sometimes, neoadjuvant chemotherapy is given before surgery to shrink a tumor, which is then followed by surgery and additional chemotherapy. Common chemotherapy agents used for gastric cancer include 5-FU (5-fluorouracil), Xeloda (capecitabine), Taxol (paclitaxel), Taxotere (docetaxel), irinotecan, and oxaliplatin. In most situations, doctors will use a combination of two or more chemotherapies rather than a single drug.

When chemotherapy is combined with radiation, a single agent, often 5-FU or capecitabine, is used. Chemoradiation can be used for tumors that can't be completely removed with surgery.

Treating Stomach Cancer by Stage

When found early, at Stage 1 or Stage 2, the prognosis for gastric cancer after treatment is good. However, it's rarely detected so early. Gastric cancers in the earliest stages are often treated successfully with surgery, which removes the entire malignant area. However, depending on the location of the tumor, the invasion of different stomach layers, and the spread to lymph nodes, chemotherapy or chemoradiation may also be recommended.

Stage 3 is advanced disease that has spread to the deeper layers of the stomach, which may include the muscle wall and the outer layer, and affects nearby lymph nodes. Chemotherapy is typically given before and after surgery to remove the cancer.

Stage 4 gastric cancer has spread beyond the stomach to distant organs. Treatment is limited and less successful at this stage. The five-year survival rate is less than 20 percent. Treatment for metastasized stomach cancer often begins with surgery or chemotherapy—generally with 5-FU and other agents—and radiation to relieve symptoms and slow cancer growth. If your tumor is HER2-positive, you may be treated with Herceptin and chemotherapy.

The targeted therapy Cyramza (ramucirumab) may be given alone or with paclitaxel to slow or stop the blood supply to the tumor and also extend survival. After biomarker testing, the immunotherapy drugs Keytruda or Opdivo may be recommended for tumors that are dMMR/MSI-H or TMB-high, or that have the PD-L1 protein, haven't responded to prior therapy, and for which there are no other options.

Questions for Your Gastrointestinal Treatment Team

- What are my treatment options, including new therapies?
- What are the benefits and risks of these treatments?
- How do these treatments address my diagnosis and my high risk for a recurrence?
- What type of surgery, if any, do you recommend for me, and why?
- How many of these surgeries have you performed in high-risk individuals?
- What are the possible complications, and how likely are they?
- How will you address these complications if they occur?
- What should I expect during recovery, and how should I prepare?
- What long-term follow-up care or surveillance will I need?
- Do I qualify for any clinical trials?

Chapter 24

Treating Genitourinary Cancers

Information from genetic testing can guide treatment decisions. For example, individuals who test positive for an inherited mutation in *BRCA1* or *BRCA2* have a higher risk for a more aggressive form of prostate cancer and may want to discuss with their doctor whether to consider more aggressive treatment.

Options for Prostate Cancer

Many men develop prostate cancer at some point in their lives. Some have pronounced symptoms while others don't know that they have it. Many prostate cancers are slow-growing and not life-threatening, but some are aggressive and life-threatening if left untreated. Deciding whether and how to treat someone's prostate cancer depends on several factors:

- their age and expected lifespan
- their underlying health conditions
- the stage and grade of their cancer
- their priorities
- the urgency for immediate treatment, as identified by their doctor
- the likely side effects

Almost all prostate cancers are adenocarcinomas that develop in the prostate cells that produce a fluid found in semen. Doctors use clues from various tests to learn as much as they can about the cancer to recommend the best plan. For example, the Gleason score has been used since the 1960s to describe the appearance of prostate cancer cells from a biopsy and to help determine the aggressiveness of a cancer. Your pathologist assigns a grade from 1 to 5 to tissue from the two largest areas of cancer in the biopsy, and then combines these numbers to arrive at a score. Most prostate cancers are scored between 6 and 10. The newer Grade Group system provides similar information using different numbering. Doctors can estimate how likely a cancer is to grow and spread by considering the Gleason score and/or Grade Group, the results of a prostate-specific antigen (PSA) blood test, and the percentage of cancer reported in a biopsy sample.

- low/very low risk: Grade Group 1 (Gleason score up to and including 6)
- intermediate risk: Grade Groups 2 and 3 (Gleason score of 7)
- high/very high risk: Grade Group 4 (Gleason score of 8) and Grade Group 5 (Gleason score of 9 or 10)

Staging reflects if and where the cancer has spread beyond the prostate. Staging helps doctors plan the best treatment options and is based on the following information:

- the size of the cancer (tumor)
- whether the cancer has reached nearby lymph nodes
- whether the cancer has spread beyond the prostate and to other lymph nodes
- PSA levels at the time of diagnosis
- Gleason score

Genetic Testing

If you have prostate cancer, you may benefit from genetic counseling and testing for an inherited gene mutation if any of the following factors apply:

- A blood relative has an inherited mutation in a gene that is linked to cancer.
- One or more close relatives were diagnosed with breast, prostate, endometrial, colorectal, stomach, ovarian, pancreatic, or urothelial cancer; a rare cancer; or multiple cancers.

- You've been diagnosed with a localized prostate cancer that is Grade Group 4 or 5 and/or the cells have an appearance known as cribriform (when viewed through a microscope, they appear to have tiny holes) or intraductal features noted on the pathology report.
- You've been diagnosed with metastatic prostate cancer.
- You've been diagnosed with male breast cancer, colorectal, stomach, pancreatic, or urothelial cancer; a rare cancer; or multiple cancers.
- Biomarker testing of your tumor indicates that you may have an inherited mutation. This may include tumors that are mismatch repair deficient (dMMR), are microsatellite instability–high (MSI-H) (frequently found with Lynch syndrome), or test positive for mutations in *ATM*, *BRCA1*, *BRCA2*, or other genes.

Information from genetic testing can guide treatment decisions. For example, men who test positive for an inherited mutation in *BRCA1* or *BRCA2* have a higher risk for a more aggressive form of prostate cancer and may want to discuss with their doctor whether to consider more aggressive treatment. Whether other genes that are linked to prostate cancer also lead to more aggressive forms of prostate cancer is less clear. We need more research data.

Your genetic test results can also help you make medical decisions to prevent a new diagnosis of cancer or to detect it early and can help your blood relatives understand their risk for cancer and make decisions about their own cancer screening and prevention.

Types of Treatment
Surgery

Radical prostatectomy (figure 24.1) is a surgical procedure that removes the entire prostate. For individuals in the very low-risk and low-risk categories, lymph node removal may not be required. Often surgery can be performed using a laparoscope, which is less invasive. Nerve-sparing radical prostatectomy is an alternative for some people. It removes the prostate, but when possible it preserves the nerves on either side of the gland that enable erection. It's not an option for cancers that have grown into or are very close to the nerves or when nerves are tangled with the tumor.

In addition to the risks of general surgery—infection, delayed wound healing, fluid buildup at the surgical site, pain, and others—radical prostatectomy can cause potentially serious complications. Erectile dysfunction, urinary

FIGURE 24.1 During a radical prostatectomy, tissue is removed through an incision from the belly button to the pubic bone (*left*), a perineal incision between the scrotum and the anus (*center*), or several small laparoscopic incisions made manually or with robotic assistance (*right*)

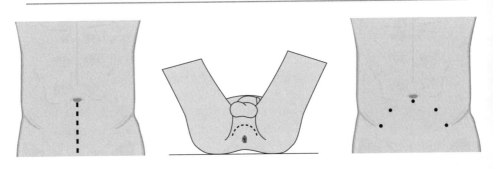

incontinence, urinary tract infection, internal bleeding, and narrowing of the urethra may occur, but in most cases these can be resolved with additional procedures. Prostatectomy requires an overnight hospital stay and 4–6 weeks of recovery at home. A urinary catheter remains in place for 7–10 days. It may take up to a year to regain full urinary control. Laparoscopic-assisted prostatectomy involves less pain, a shorter hospital stay, and faster recovery of urinary and bowel continence.

Radiation Therapy

Radiation can be used as a first-line treatment for early-stage prostate cancer to destroy malignant cells and reduce the risk of recurrence. External radiation directs high-energy x-ray beams to the prostate. This type of radiation destroys cancer cells but affects healthy cells as well. Some doctors inject a layer of gel between the prostate and rectum to protect these areas from radiation. Proton therapy, intensity-modulated therapy, and volumetric modulated arc therapy are more precise external-beam radiation technologies that target the tumor while reducing radiation to surrounding healthy tissues. Radiation is traditionally given five days a week for eight to nine weeks, although some accelerated regimens deliver higher doses in fewer sessions.

Brachytherapy uses seeds, which are placed directly into the tumor site during surgery and release radiation. They're left in place for one or two days before being removed, or they remain permanently and deliver consistent, low-dose radiation.

Cryotherapy

Minimally invasive cryosurgery—which despite its name isn't a surgical procedure—is an option for people who can't have surgery or radiation due to their
age or other health issues and for individuals with local recurrence after radiation. Ultracold gas is passed through needles inserted through the skin,
freezing and destroying prostate tissue, including cancer cells. This treatment
usually results in impotence. Focal cryotherapy targets only the tumor rather
than the entire prostate and reduces this risk, but the decision regarding whole
gland or focal cryotherapy depends on the extent of the tumor. Cryotherapy can
cause urinary incontinence and may damage rectal tissue.

New Ways to Find Prostate Cancer That Has Spread

Several tests, including PSA, MRI, CT, x-rays, and bone scans are
used to detect the spread of prostate cancer and to help stage it.
Sometimes, however, these tests fail to find metastatic disease. Newer
approaches—C11-choline-PET, Axumin-PET, and PSMA-PET—use
a positron emission tomography scan to try to detect metastatic
spread earlier. PET scans use a small amount of a radioactive tracer
drug, which is injected before the scan. The tracer moves throughout the body and attaches to its target. PET scanners can then detect
areas where high amounts of the tracer are found, which may reflect
the presence of cancer. By using these radioactive tracers, doctors
may detect metastatic prostate cancers earlier and plan treatment
using this information.

Hormone Therapy

Prostate cancers rely on testosterone, a type of androgen, which is the primary hormone produced by the testicles. Androgen deprivation therapy (ADT) is a standard treatment to lower testosterone levels so that most prostate cancer cells stop growing or die. ADT doesn't provide a cure, but it can reduce the size and limit the growth of prostate tumors, sometimes for years, by suppressing hormones. Candidates for ADT include individuals who

- can't have surgery or radiation therapy
- have rising PSA levels after previous treatment
- have advanced or high-risk prostate cancer
- have cancer that has spread beyond the prostate

Prostate cancer is treated with several types of ADT, which work in different ways. Luteinizing hormone–releasing hormone (LHRH) agonists, including the following, block the production of testosterone:

- Lupron, Viadur, Eligard (leuprolide)
- Zoladex (goserelin)
- Trelstar (triptorelin)
- Vantas (histrelin)

Luteinizing hormone–releasing hormone (LHRH) antagonists, including Firmagon (degarelix) and the oral agent Orgovyx (relugolix), also block the production of testosterone.

Anti-androgens slow prostate cancer growth by binding and blocking androgen receptors on cancer cells. Anti-androgens are typically given in combination with LHRH agonists or LHRH antagonists. Anti-androgens include

- Casodex (bicalutamide)
- Eulexin (flutamide)
- Xtandi (enzalutamide)
- Erleada (apalutamide)
- Nubeqa (darolutamide)

The androgen-synthesis inhibitor Zytiga (abiraterone) suppresses hormone production by the adrenal glands to further lower testosterone and is usually used with prednisone (a steroid drug that reduces side effects).

Orchiectomy is a surgery that removes the testicles. Orchiectomy is also considered to be a hormone therapy because removing the testicles suppresses testosterone production in the same way as LHRH agonists or antagonists and doesn't require ongoing treatment with those medications. This procedure is used less commonly than the therapies above.

Prostate cancer that initially responds to hormone therapy can eventually become resistant. The development of castration-resistant prostate cancer (CRPC) then requires a new approach. The results of genetic testing and biomarker tests can suggest treatment alternatives.

Targeted Therapies and Immunotherapies

In some cases, genetic testing or biomarker testing for certain tumor changes can show which targeted treatments or immunotherapies may most likely work for metastatic prostate cancer. Tumors may also be tested for additional biomarkers to identify your eligibility for clinical trials of new treatments.

- Keytruda (pembrolizumab) helps the immune system detect and kill cancer cells. The likelihood of the immune system effectively targeting tumors increases if the cancer contains many mutations. For this reason, Keytruda may be used for prostate tumors that are deficient in DNA repair (also called dMMR or MSI-H), an abnormality that is frequently found in people with Lynch syndrome. It may also be used for cancers that have a feature known as high tumor mutational burden (TMB-high) and can't be treated any other way.
- Lynparza (olaparib) is a PARP inhibitor that is prescribed for people who have an inherited mutation or an acquired tumor mutation in a BRCA1, BRCA2, or ATM gene and whose cancer progresses after treatment with Xtandi (enzalutamide) or Zytiga (abiraterone).
- Rubraca (rucaparib) is a PARP inhibitor that may be recommended for individuals with an inherited mutation or an acquired tumor mutation in a BRCA1 or BRCA2 gene and whose cancer progresses after treatment with androgen receptor–directed therapy and taxane-based chemotherapy.
- The Provenge (sipuleucel-T) cancer vaccine helps the immune system attack prostate cancer cells that progress after hormone therapy. This can be beneficial for people who have CRPC and do not have cancer-related pain or other symptoms.

Treating Early-Stage, Low-Risk Prostate Cancer

Early-stage prostate cancers frequently fall into the very low-risk or low-risk category, also referred to as Grade Group 1 cancers. These cancers are confined to the prostate, grow slowly, and often show no symptoms. At this stage, you have three primary options: observation (watchful waiting), active surveillance, and treatment. Your doctor will recommend an option based on your age, general health, and other factors.

Watchful waiting is an approach that delays treatment and includes minimal surveillance using PSA tests and digital exams unless symptoms change. It's an option for you if you

- have a life expectancy of fewer than 10 years
- have a low-grade cancer and want to defer treatment until necessary
- prefer not to have treatment or have other health problems that preclude treatment

Active surveillance is an option if you have early-stage, low-risk disease confined to the prostate. You will be monitored closely with PSA testing once or twice per year, annual digital rectal exams and MRIs, and sometimes annual prostate biopsies. If monitoring indicates that the cancer may be growing or spreading, additional testing such as a CT scan and lymph node biopsy may be performed. If you have low-risk or intermediate-risk disease and have a life expectancy of more than 10 years, biomarker tests such as Decipher, Oncotype DX Prostate, Prolaris, and ProMark may predict the aggressiveness of a cancer and may help you decide between active surveillance and treatment. If you choose active surveillance, any concerning change of the cancer status or symptoms often results in discussions about more definitive treatment.

Early-stage cancers that remain in the prostate but have a higher Grade Group or PSA may be treated with surgery or radiation and, in some cases, hormone therapy. Individuals who choose to have surgery or radiation usually remain free of disease for many years or the remainder of their lives.

Locally advanced prostate cancer is disease that extends beyond the prostate into the bladder, rectum, or other nearby tissue but doesn't involve lymph nodes or distant organs. Tumors at this stage are often high grade or have a high PSA level. The outlook for this stage remains reasonable, although recurrence is more likely than with less advanced disease. Treatment choices include external beam radiation with hormone therapy, external beam radiation and brachytherapy with hormone therapy, or radical prostatectomy, possibly with lymph node removal or with radiation and with or without hormone therapy. Clinical trials are an option before, during, or after treatment (at any stage). People who are older or have other medical concerns may choose observation, cryotherapy, hormone therapy, or external beam radiation.

Stage 4 prostate cancer has spread into nearby or distant lymph nodes, bones, the bladder, the rectum, or other parts of the body. It is rarely cured, but treatment can relieve symptoms and control tumor growth as long as possible to improve your quality of life. Five-year survival at this stage is 45–50 percent with the use of newer therapies, such as abiraterone or enzalutamide.

Many treatment alternatives may be tried, depending on the severity of your symptoms, expected side effects, and your personal preference. If you have Stage 4 prostate cancer, your treatment plan will depend on several factors, including the results of biomarker testing and genetic testing for an inherited mutation, the types of therapy you previously received, and how your cancer responds to hormone treatment. Your treatment might include hormone therapy alone or with surgery, chemotherapy, or external beam radiation. The following options might also be considered:

- Androgen receptor–targeted therapy can improve the effectiveness of standard hormone therapy.
- Xofigo (radium 223 dichloride) delivers radiation directly to areas of bone metastases.
- Transurethral resection of the prostate (TURP) may be recommended to remove a painful obstruction in the prostate and part of the prostate gland until a comprehensive treatment plan is developed.
- External radiation with or without hormone therapy may relieve bone pain.
- Bisphosphonate drugs, including Xgeva (denosumab) and Zometa (zoledronic acid), relieve bone pain and prevent fractures.

Follow-Up Care

After treatment ends, you should be monitored for a recurrence and long-term side effects, especially urinary and sexual dysfunction. Individual follow-up care is based on the type and stage of cancer, the length of treatment, and how long you remain cancer-free. Prostate cancer can come back years after treatment is completed, so it's important to keep all recommended screening appointments. For most individuals, follow-up includes

Monitoring the Spread and Severity of Prostate Cancer

Doctors use different imaging procedures to monitor and measure the extent of prostate cancer.

- Transrectal ultrasound measures the size of the prostate gland.

- MRI shows whether cancer has spread beyond the prostate into nearby tissues or organs.

- Bone scans show whether cancer cells have reached the bones.

- Computed tomography (CT) helps to monitor tumor growth.

- Some positron emission tomography (PET) scans can better characterize whether the cancer has recurred and the location of the spread. This is most helpful if there is a concerning rise of PSA after surgery or radiation, but CT and bone scans show no detectable cancer. Different types of PET scans are used, including C11-PET, Axumin-PET, and PSMA-PET. FDG-PET is often used for other cancer types, but it's not as informative for prostate cancer.

- Doctor visits every 3–6 months in the first couple of years after treatment. If there are no signs of recurrence, doctor visits every 6–12 months for the next three years are recommended.
- PSA testing every six months for the first five years and then annually thereafter. More frequent testing may be advised when the risk of recurrence is high.
- Digital rectal exams (if you still have your prostate and your PSA test is elevated).
- Other lab work, imaging tests, and bone scans as indicated by your symptoms.

Options for Bladder, Renal Pelvis, and Ureter Cancers

Cancers of the bladder, renal pelvis, and ureter share the same type of cells and develop similar cancers, but treatment may differ. Almost all bladder cancers and most ureter cancers are urothelial carcinomas that start in the cellular lining of the urinary tract. They can be either papillary (finger-shaped) or sessile (flat), and either noninvasive or invasive. Like other cancers, bladder tumors are graded according to the likelihood that they'll grow, spread, and recur. Low-grade tumors may recur, while high-grade tumors are more likely to do so.

Treatment for Bladder Cancer

Treatment for most bladder cancers includes some type of surgery, depending on the stage of the cancer and your tolerance for long-term side effects. For some patients, radiation with chemotherapy can be used instead of surgery. In some cases, additional treatment with chemotherapy or immunotherapy is needed. Individual treatment plans depend on the type and grade of cancer, whether it's been treated previously, your overall health, and your personal preference.

Surgery

Early cancers are usually removed with transurethral resection of a bladder tumor (TURBT). In this procedure, a surgeon inserts a resectoscope with a small wire loop at the end through the urethra and into the bladder. The loop scrapes away the cancerous tissue and cauterizes (seals off) the blood vessels to stop bleeding. Cauterization can also be done with electric current, a process known as fulguration. This reduces the chance of infection and inadvertent injury to the bladder. TURBT may be repeated to remove any tumor tissue that may remain after the first procedure.

Cystectomy is the removal of all or part of the bladder. Radical cystectomy, which is standard care for muscle-invasive disease, removes the entire bladder, lymph nodes that are close to the bladder, and sometimes nearby tissues and organs as well. For men, this may mean removing the prostate and urethra. For women, it may mean removing the uterus, fallopian tubes, ovaries, and part of the vagina. When the bladder is removed, urine is diverted through an ostomy (an opening made in the abdominal wall) and collected in a bag worn on the outside of the body. Sometimes, an internal storage pouch for urine can be made with a part of the intestine, eliminating the need for an external bag.

Bladder surgery can result in infection, delayed healing, discomfort, and other common side effects of surgery. Cystectomy or urinary diversion can also lead to urine leaks and problems with emptying the bladder. Unless a nerve-sparing cystectomy is performed, erectile dysfunction is likely. Some people may experience a loss of sexual sensation and/or the ability to orgasm if nerves in the pelvis are damaged or cut. The location and size of the tumor and your surgeon's experience with the procedure can affect the likelihood and severity of side effects.

Talk to your surgeon about alternatives for keeping all or part of your bladder and how each method will affect your prognosis and quality of life.

Radiation

Radiation therapy may be given to destroy cancer cells that remain after TURBT or in combination with chemotherapy to treat cancer that is localized to the bladder. In the case of advanced bladder cancer, radiation may also be used to relieve pain, bleeding, and other symptoms of metastasis in the bone, brain, or other organs.

Chemotherapy

Chemotherapy for bladder cancer may be given as systemic or intravesical treatment. Systemic chemotherapy is the traditional type of chemotherapy, which circulates throughout the body to treat cancer cells in the bladder and those that may have spread outside of the bladder. Unlike traditional systemic chemotherapy, intravesical chemotherapy is local treatment given directly into the bladder through a catheter inserted through the urethra. The drugs must come into contact with cancer cells to destroy them.

Intravesical chemotherapy is used most often with early-stage bladder cancers. Some types of intravesical chemotherapy contain a gel that stays in the kidneys for several hours to destroy cancer cells. Traditional systemic chemotherapy is often given for invasive bladder cancers to treat any cancer cells that may have spread beyond the bladder. It may be given as a single agent or as a combination of drugs, and usually includes a type known as platinum chemotherapy.

Immunotherapies and Targeted Therapies

Like chemotherapy, immunotherapy for bladder cancer may be given as an intravesical treatment directly into the bladder or systemically. Intravesical treatment is typically used for bladder cancers that have not yet invaded the bladder wall. Common intravesical immunotherapies include the bacillus calmette-guerin vaccine and interferon (Roferon-A, Intron A, Alferon). Systemic immunotherapy agents, known as immune checkpoint inhibitors, may be used to treat certain bladder cancers, including

- Advanced cancers that are MSI-H/dMMR. This is particularly important for people with Lynch syndrome, who tend to have cancers with these biomarkers.
- Advanced bladder cancers that test positive for a biomarker known as PD-L1.
- The cancers of people who are not eligible for platinum chemotherapy.
- Non–muscle invasive bladder cancers that have become resistant to BCG therapy in individuals who are not candidates for cystectomy.

Common immune checkpoint inhibitors include

- Tecentriq (atezolizumab)
- Bavencio (avelumab)
- Imfinzi (durvalumab)
- Keytruda (pembrolizumab)
- Opdivo (nivolumab)

Targeted therapies are also used to treat bladder cancers. Balversa (erdafitinib) is recommended for muscle-invasive bladder tumors that have a mutation in the fibroblast growth factor receptor (FGFR) gene. Padcev (enfortumab vedotin-ejfv) and Trodelvy (sacituzumab govitecan-hziy) are targeted therapies that may be used to treat tumors that no longer respond to platinum chemotherapy and immunotherapy.

Treatment by Stage

Non–Muscle Invasive Bladder Cancers

About 75 percent of bladder cancers that are caught early are treated successfully by removing the entire cancerous area, sometimes followed by chemotherapy or immunotherapy that is delivered directly into the bladder.

Stage 0 bladder cancers include low-grade (slow-growing) papillary tumors and high-grade (more aggressive) carcinomas in situ, which develop in the inner lining of the bladder. Almost all bladder cancers at this stage are cured, but a carcinoma in situ is more likely to recur. These cancers are usually removed with transurethral bladder tumor resection.

Stage 1 cancers have breached the inner lining of the bladder and spread into the connective tissue. These cancers are addressed with TURBT and fulguration, primarily to determine how far the cancer has spread. At this stage, high-grade and sometimes even low-grade cancers that aren't treated further often return. For this reason, a second TURBT is usually performed several weeks later to confirm that the staging is accurate. If that procedure removes the entire cancer, intravesical BCG or chemotherapy is then administered. If some cancer remains after TURBT, additional intravesical BCG may be given, or a cystectomy, the removal of all or part of the bladder, may be done.

High-grade tumors are more likely to recur without additional treatment, which usually involves another TURBT followed by several weeks of intravesical immunotherapy. Treatment with the systemic immunotherapy Keytruda may be recommended if the tumor doesn't become smaller. Cystectomy may be required if some of the cancer remains. Radiation with or without chemotherapy may be an option when a health condition precludes cystectomy, although the likelihood of a cure is then reduced.

Muscle-Invasive Bladder Cancers

Stage 2 bladder cancer has spread into the thick muscle wall of the bladder. The five-year survival rate at this stage is 50–60 percent. TURBT is performed first, primarily to determine how far the cancer has spread. Sometimes, chemotherapy is given before cystectomy and is designed to treat any cancer cells that might have spread beyond the bladder; chemotherapy that is given before surgery is easier to tolerate and increases the cure rate. Radical cystectomy, which is standard care for muscle-invasive disease, is then performed to remove the entire bladder, lymph nodes that are close to the bladder, and sometimes nearby tissues and organs as well.

Radiation therapy may be given to destroy cancer cells that might remain after TURBT. Radiation may also be used with chemotherapy as definitive treatment for muscle-invasive bladder cancers if the tumor is relatively small or is not extending out of the bladder. Systemic chemotherapy may be given as a single agent or a combination of drugs.

Stage 3 is advanced bladder cancer that has spread through the muscle wall to the fatty layer of tissue surrounding the bladder and prostate, or the bladder, uterus, and vagina; to one or more regional lymph nodes; and/or to lymph nodes in the pelvis. Prognosis is considerably poorer for this type of bladder cancer; the five-year survival rate is 25–50 percent. Individuals may still benefit from chemotherapy and radiation or surgery as described above.

Stage 4 bladder cancer has spread into the abdominal wall, to lymph nodes beyond the pelvis, and/or to other parts of the body. After TURBT to determine how much of the muscle wall is affected, systemic chemotherapy with cisplatin or carboplatin is usually recommended. Cancers that recur after chemotherapy may respond to targeted or immunotherapy. Clinical trials may offer new treatment options for recurrent advanced cancers.

Follow-Up Care

Follow-up screening is especially important because the risk for bladder cancer recurrence, even years after treatment, is high compared to other types of cancer. As a bladder cancer survivor, you also have a higher risk for a second, unrelated cancer in the kidneys, pancreas, prostate or vagina, lungs, or elsewhere. Smoking is a risk factor for most of these cancers and many others. If you smoke, quitting will reduce your chance of having cancer again.

Your doctor will personalize a follow-up care plan for you, depending on the type and stage of your cancer, the length of your treatment, and how long you remain cancer-free. It's important to keep all of the recommended appointments so that any recurrence can be found and treated as soon as possible.

Treatment for Renal Pelvis and Ureter Cancers

Urothelial cancers that develop in the renal pelvis (the lining of a kidney) or the ureters (the tubes that connect the kidneys to the bladder) are known as upper tract urothelial cancers (UTUCs). If you have an inherited mutation in a Lynch syndrome gene, you have a higher-than-average chance of developing UTUC. You may need an MRI; scans of your lungs, abdomen, and pelvis; and/or a bone scan to stage the cancer.

Grading is similar to what is used for bladder cancer: low-grade tumors are slow-growing and don't usually spread beyond the renal pelvis or ureter. High-grade tumors grow faster, and they recur and metastasize more often. Treatment options are more limited for these cancers.

Surgery is standard for most cases, sometimes with neoadjuvant chemotherapy, which is given prior to surgery. Because the area is small and hard to target, radiation is used only in situations when nearby tissue can be left unharmed. Treatment is categorized as local, regional, metastatic, or recurrent.

Treating Early-Stage Disease

Stages 0, 1, and 2 are local disease that is confined to the renal pelvis or a ureter.

- Stage 0 develops in the inner lining of the renal pelvis or a ureter. This stage includes noninvasive papillary carcinoma and carcinoma in situ, a flat tumor on the inside lining of the renal pelvis or ureter.
- Stage 1 has grown beyond the lining and into the layer of connective tissue.
- Stage 2 has grown into the muscle beneath the inner lining of the renal pelvis.

Most renal pelvis cancers at these stages are treated with surgery, depending on the location of the tumor and whether the other kidney is healthy.

- Nephroureterectomy removes the entire affected kidney, the associated ureter, and the bladder cuff (the connecting tissue between the bladder and ureter). As long as your remaining kidney works well, having just one kidney shouldn't adversely affect your quality of life or health. Dialysis, a procedure that mechanically filters blood, would be needed, however, if your remaining kidney were to fail. If you've already lost a kidney or you have kidney problems, a clinical trial that is testing segmental resection of the renal pelvis but preserves the remaining kidney function may be your best treatment option.

- Segmental resection of a ureter removes only the portion of the ureter that contains cancer and a margin of surrounding healthy tissue. The ends of the ureter are then rejoined to preserve normal urinary function.

Treating Advanced or Metastatic Disease

Systemic treatment for advanced or metastatic urothelial cancer of a ureter or renal pelvis is similar to those for bladder cancer. Treatment for Stage 3 regional cancer (which has spread to the functional part of the kidney or into the surrounding fatty tissue) or Stage 4 cancer (which has spread to lymph nodes or elsewhere in the body) is similar to treatment for Stages 3 and 4 bladder cancers. Clinical trials also provide treatment for recurrent or metastatic cancers, and participation is strongly encouraged.

Follow-Up Care

After treatment for local renal pelvis or ureter cancer, you'll need continued surveillance to monitor for a recurrence. This is standard posttreatment care for most cancers, but it's especially important for renal pelvis cancer, which is more likely to reappear as metastasis. For early-stage cancer, surveillance usually includes a physical examination, urine and blood tests, and regular cystoscopies for the first year or two after treatment. You might need these same tests every three to six months for three years if you had a late-stage cancer. These visits should continue at least yearly throughout your life.

Questions to Ask Your Oncologist about Genitourinary Cancer Treatment

- What is the stage and grade of my cancer?
- What other tests should I have before I decide on treatment?
- What is the goal of my treatment?
- What are my treatment options?
- Will these treatments cure my cancer?
- What is the risk of my cancer coming back?
- How much will these treatments improve that risk?
- What should I expect during recovery?
- What risks and long-term side effects are likely?

Chapter 25

Treating Melanoma

For metastatic melanoma . . . targeted therapies and immunotherapies now provide dramatically improved treatment, enhanced quality of life, and extended survival.

Melanoma is the most aggressive and dangerous kind of skin cancer, and people with certain inherited mutations are more likely to develop it. While it's far less common than basal cell and squamous cell skin cancers, melanoma more often spreads and is deadlier when it does. However, when detected and treated early enough, melanoma is relatively easy to cure. Treatment options are similar for the four main types of melanoma, even though a more aggressive approach is needed when it returns, advances, or metastasizes.

Most melanoma is superficial spreading melanoma, which begins in the outer layers of skin. Nodular melanoma is frequently already deep into the dermis by the time it's identified. It's more likely to ulcerate (break through the skin) and spread and tends to have a poorer prognosis. Acral lentiginous melanoma is the most common type among dark-skinned people and tends to have a poorer prognosis because it's usually detected later. Lentigo maligna melanoma grows slowly and is usually found in older adults who have extensive sun damage to their skin. A fifth type, ocular melanoma, is rare, behaves differently, and may require different treatment.

Options for Melanoma in the Skin

Genetic Testing

If you're diagnosed with melanoma, your dermatologist or oncologist may recommend genetic testing for an inherited gene mutation that is linked to melanoma if your family medical history includes any of the following:

- three or more melanomas, especially before age 45
- three or more blood relatives on the same side of the family with melanoma or pancreatic cancer
- one or more of a mole-like tumor known as a melanocytic *BAP1*-mutated atypical intradermal tumor, a close relative of melanoma in the eye, mesothelioma (cancer related to asbestos exposure), and meningiomas or astrocytomas (types of brain tumor)
- one or more Spitz nevus moles that affect children and adolescents

Information provided by genetic testing may help you to more confidently make medical decisions to prevent a new diagnosis or detect it early. Additionally, your results can help your blood relatives understand their risk for cancer and make decisions about their own screening and prevention.

Biomarker Testing

If you have advanced or recurrent melanoma, testing a sample of your tumor for certain changes can determine whether you would benefit from treatment with targeted therapy or immunotherapy.

- Tumors that have a V600E or V600K mutation in the *BRAF* gene may respond to a targeted drug known as a *BRAF* inhibitor.
- Tumors with mutations in the *C-KIT* gene may respond to other targeted drugs.
- Certain changes may show that you're eligible for clinical trials of new melanoma treatments. Depending on the study type, you may be able to join before, during, or after your treatment.

Treatment Options

Surgery and systemic therapy are the primary treatments for melanoma. Radiation may be given to destroy small cancerous areas that remain after surgery or to alleviate pain related to metastasis. Targeted therapies and immunotherapies are generally more effective than chemotherapy, although some chemo drugs may be used in an attempt to shrink advanced tumors after other treatments have been tried. While treatment for the four main types of skin melanoma is similar, individual treatment plans and prognoses depend on several different factors, including

- the thickness and location of the tumor
- whether the tumor is ulcerated (develops an open wound)
- how rapidly the cancer cells divide
- the extent of spread to the lymph nodes and other areas of the body
- whether the cancer has mutations in the *BRAF* gene
- your age and overall health

Surgery

Surgery with a wide local excision (WLE) is the primary treatment for most melanomas. Removing a melanoma is critical because, left untreated, malignant cells that spread to organs can be lethal. WLE procedures remove the area of melanoma and a wide margin of surrounding healthy tissue (figure 25.1). The width of the margin depends on the location of the melanoma and how far it has penetrated the layers of skin. Ideally, WLE removes all traces of melanoma that remain after biopsy, minimizing the chance of recurrence. However, some cancer cells may remain even when the surgical margin appears to be clear. If untreated, these residual cells can divide and cause a recurrence.

Depending on the thickness of the melanoma, surgery may also include a sentinel lymph node biopsy, a procedure that involves injecting the tumor with dye or a radioactive substance before surgery and then removing the one or two lymph nodes that are closest to the melanoma and take up the dye. If these nodes are free of cancer, no additional lymph nodes need to be removed. Sentinel nodes that contain cancer cells indicate that cancer has spread and may require the removal of additional lymph nodes or systemic treatment.

WLE is ordinarily performed as outpatient surgery under a local anesthetic. You'll be awake, but you won't feel any pain. WLE incisions are ordinarily

FIGURE 25.1 A wide local excision removes the melanoma and a margin of surrounding healthy tissue

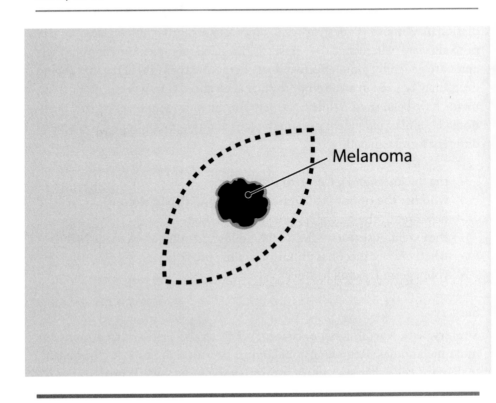

stitched closed, and the stitches are removed in 10–14 days. A skin graft—a layer of skin transferred from somewhere else on your body—may be required to close very wide incisions. Postoperative discomfort is ordinarily managed with an over-the-counter pain reliever, and most patients feel better after a few days.

Radiation Therapy

Radiation isn't typically the main treatment for melanoma, although external beam radiation therapy and proton radiation therapy may be used to kill cancer cells that can't be completely removed with surgery or that have spread to the lymph nodes or beyond. Radiation reduces the likelihood of recurrence, but it doesn't improve survival. Radiation can also reduce pain and other symptoms of advanced melanoma, especially in the bones or brain, and shrink the size of lymph nodes or skin nodules.

Mohs Surgery for Melanoma

Mohs surgery (also called Mohs micrographic surgery) is more precise than WLE and causes minimal scarring. It's standard treatment for other skin cancers but has limited use for Stage 0 melanomas, particularly lentigo maligna melanoma, which is confined to the top layer of the skin.

The Mohs procedure progressively removes one thin layer of skin at a time, which is immediately checked for cancer cells. In this case, the surgeon also acts as the pathologist. If cancer cells are found in one layer of tissue, another thin layer in the same area is then removed and examined. This layer-by-layer excision and examination continues as many times as necessary until a layer of skin is entirely clear of cancer cells. Some cancers can be completely removed in the first layer, while others require repeated attempts.

Chemotherapy

Chemotherapy may sometimes shrink areas of metastatic melanoma. However, targeted drugs and immunotherapies tend to be more effective, so chemotherapy is usually used only when other therapies fail. Chemotherapies that are used for melanoma include DTIC (dacarbazine) or its oral equivalent, Temodar (temozolomide). Cisplatin, Paraplatin (carboplatin), Taxotere (docetaxel), Taxol (paclitaxel), and Abraxane (nab-paclitaxel) may be used alone or in various combinations.

When clusters of metastatic melanomas are confined to an arm or a leg and can't be surgically removed, high doses of chemotherapy can be delivered with isolated limb infusion (ILI) or isolated limb perfusion (ILP). During ILI, chemotherapy is directed through a catheter that is placed into the artery and vein that feed the tumor. A tourniquet stops blood circulation in the limb so that the medication is concentrated where it's needed and doesn't affect the rest of the body. The drugs are flushed from the limb after 30–40 minutes, and blood flow is restored. ILP is a similar procedure that introduces heated chemotherapy for 60–90 minutes before it's flushed from the limb.

ILI and ILP are performed under general anesthesia and require a hospital stay of three to seven days. Both procedures may cause swelling, redness, and sometimes blistering of the skin on the affected limb for several weeks or longer. These specialized procedures are only available at some melanoma centers and should be performed by surgeons who are experienced in these techniques.

Targeted Therapies

Several targeted therapies have proven beneficial for the treatment of advanced, metastatic, and inoperable melanomas. *BRAF* inhibitors and *MEK* inhibitors may help slow tumor growth. About half of melanomas have one of two *BRAF* mutations known as V600E and V600K, which stimulate tumor growth. Combining a *BRAF* inhibitor, like Tafinlar (dabrafenib), Braftovi (encorafenib), or Zelboraf (vemurafenib), with a *MEK* inhibitor, like Mekinist (trametinib), Cotellic (cobimetinib), or Mektovi (binimetinib), significantly prolongs survival and is standard treatment for advanced tumors with these biomarkers.

These drugs may also be used for inoperable tumors that have these biomarkers. Mekinist and Tafinlar are also prescribed adjuvantly when lymph nodes are affected.

C-KIT inhibitors, including Gleevac (imatinib) and Tasigna (nilotinib), target cells that have biomarker changes in the *C-KIT* gene, which occur more often in acral lentiginous and mucosal melanoma. These drugs have limited efficacy.

Immunotherapies

Your doctor may suggest immunotherapy to help slow tumor growth and help you live longer. You may be treated with one or more of the following therapies to stimulate your immune system to recognize and attack melanoma cells.

Immune checkpoint inhibitors, including Keytruda (pembrolizumab), Opdivo (nivolumab), and Yervoy (ipilimumab), may be used adjuvantly when lymph nodes are affected and for inoperable or metastatic melanoma. Opdivo is sometimes prescribed with Yervoy. These drugs don't require biomarker testing.

Imlygic (talimogene laherparepvec or T-VEC) is a genetically engineered virus that is injected directly into the tumor to kill cancer cells and stimulate an immune response against melanoma that has spread into the skin or lymph nodes. No biomarker testing is required.

Proleukin (aldesleukin) and IL-2 are synthetic versions of the interleukin-2 protein, which are sometimes used to boost the overall growth and activity of immune cells, especially lymphocytes (white blood cells), which attack and kill cancer cells.

Treatment by Stage

Staging a melanoma based on the following characteristics helps your doctors plan the best treatment for you:

- the thickness of the tumor as measured from the surface of the skin to the deepest part of the tumor
- whether the tumor is ulcerated (has broken through the skin)
- whether melanoma cells are found in the lymph nodes
- whether the lymph nodes are matted (joined together)
- whether small groups of satellite or microsatellite tumor cells have spread to tissue near the primary tumor or to lymph vessels
- whether melanoma cells have spread to other parts of the body

Stage 0 is confined to the epidermis, the upper layer of the skin. This stage is melanoma in situ. It's the easiest stage to treat and cure, usually with a wide local excision.

Stage 1 is present in the epidermis and the dermis. The tumor may be less than 2 millimeters thick without ulceration or less than 1 millimeter thick with ulceration. A melanoma that grows from the epidermis to the deeper layer of the dermis can enter the subcutaneous fat beneath the skin, the bloodstream, or the lymph vessels and then metastasize to other parts of the body. Almost all melanomas at this early stage are treated successfully with surgery, which may include sentinel node biopsy.

Stage 2 is thicker and also confined to the skin. WLE, often with sentinel lymph node biopsy, is usually adequate treatment.

Stage 3 has spread to nearby lymph nodes or tissue and is more likely to come back, even after surgery. If the entire area of melanoma can be removed, targeted therapy or immunotherapy typically follows to slow growth and lengthen survival. Adjuvant options for delaying or preventing recurrence include Opdivo, Keytruda, and Tafinlar with Mekinist. Melanoma at this stage is considered to be advanced, and the five-year survival rate when it reaches the lymph nodes is 64 percent.

Stage 4 has spread to distant areas of the skin, lymph nodes, liver, brain, or other organs. This is metastatic melanoma. Targeted therapies and immunotherapies now provide dramatically improved treatment, enhanced quality of life, and extended survival. Treatment options may differ but usually involve targeted therapy, immunotherapy, surgery, or radiation to treat affected lymph nodes and relieve symptoms. If one treatment fails or stops working, another may be tried. Your treatment plan will be developed based on your age and health, how quickly the melanoma is growing, the number and locations of metastases, the results of biomarker testing, and your personal preferences.

Some patients experience no related symptoms, while others have multiple symptoms that affect their functionality and quality of life. Radiation may control a limited number of brain metastases, which is one of the most common complications of melanoma at this stage. Surgery, targeted therapies, and immunotherapies may also be helpful. Five-year survival is 25 percent when melanoma reaches distant organs. If you're diagnosed with advanced or metastatic melanoma, you may want to consider participating in clinical trials of new agents.

Follow-Up Care

Follow-up care is especially important during the first five years after your treatment, which is when the risk of recurrence is greatest. The National Comprehensive Cancer Network (NCCN) guidelines for follow-up are based on the stage of melanoma. Monthly self-examinations of the skin and lymph nodes and annual exams by a health care provider are recommended after treatment for all stages of melanoma. The frequency of clinical examinations and imaging tests to check for recurrence will vary, depending on the stage of melanoma and the time since you completed treatment.

Treating Recurrent Melanoma

Recurrent melanoma can develop in the same area of the skin months or years after treatment if any remaining cancer cells grow. Small melanomas in the same area can be treated with another wide local excision and lymph node dissection, if necessary. Systemic drugs that weren't included in your initial treatment may be beneficial, and isolated limb perfusion may be used for recurrence in an arm or a leg. Radiation may relieve bone pain or other painful symptoms. The prognosis of recurrent melanoma depends on the extent of the metastases.

Options for Ocular Melanoma

The treatment for melanoma in the eye considers the location, size, and spread; your age and overall health; and other factors. Because treatment can damage eye tissue and affect vision, the quality of your eyesight in the opposite eye is also considered, as are your personal preferences regarding side effects. The goal of treatment is to preserve your eye and vision, but that isn't always possible.

If you're diagnosed with ocular melanoma (OM), it's important to learn as much as possible about the disease, your prognosis, your treatment choices, and possible side effects and complications. Talk with your doctor about all of your options, including whether the suggested treatments will cure your melanoma, if they will preserve your eye, and how they might affect your eyesight. Ask whether you need to be treated right away or if it's safe to take a wait-and-see approach, especially if you don't have symptoms and the tumor isn't growing. Getting a second or even third opinion is a good idea before deciding on a treatment plan.

Treatment Options

Although ocular melanoma can often be treated with radiation therapy, in some cases it requires surgery.

Surgery

Different surgical procedures may be recommended to treat ocular melanoma, depending on the size and location of the tumor. Surgery may involve removing the tumor and some of the healthy tissue of the eye surrounding it. Enucleation, removal of the entire affected eye, is likely to be recommended for very large or painful tumors, when the optic nerve is affected, or when your vision is greatly diminished or absent.

Vision cannot be restored after enucleation. However, after surgery a temporary implant may be put in place and attached to the eye muscles, so that it moves like a natural eye. A permanent, realistic-looking artificial eye that is customized to match your other eye can be fitted after a full recovery, usually in 10 weeks. Enucleation is generally a safe outpatient procedure, but it may produce a temporary mild headache, a droopy eyelid, and/or itching in the eye socket.

Radiation Therapy

Various types of radiation damage melanoma cells so that they stop growing or die and the tumor shrinks. Brachytherapy is the most common type of radiation used for ocular melanomas, especially for small- or medium-size tumors. In brachytherapy, radioactive seeds are arranged on a plaque, a gold disk that is placed on the eye directly over the tumor. The plaque gives off constant radiation to the eye before it's removed in four or five days. The gold helps to protect sensitive tissues in the eye from radiation damage. Fluid leakage from an irradiated tumor may require repeated treatment.

Alternatively, proton radiation with a thin beam of radioactive particles can be delivered externally to the eye over several days. The depth of penetration is customized for each tumor. Given daily, usually for one week, this type of radiation minimizes damage to the surrounding eye tissue.

Chemotherapy

Standard chemotherapy drugs aren't typically used to treat ocular melanoma, although chemotherapy eye drops are sometimes used.

Treatment for Local, Regional, and Metastatic OM

Unlike most cancers, ocular melanoma often isn't formally staged, and how tumor characteristics affect prognosis isn't well understood or defined. Tumors are categorized as local, regional, or metastatic.

Local OM is confined to the eye. For a very small melanoma, your doctor may recommend removal with a laser or a wait-and-see approach that closely monitors you for disease progression. For many people, this means avoiding treatment for several years. The five-year survival at this stage is 85 percent. Small local melanomas may also be treated with surgery, radiation, photocoagulation (minimally invasive laser treatment), or transpupillary thermotherapy laser treatment.

Regional ocular melanoma has spread beyond the eye to nearby tissues or, less frequently, the lymph nodes. The same treatments that are used for local OM may be used effectively at this stage. For medium-size tumors, surgery and radiation are equally effective, although surgery is sometimes required after radiation. Radiation is normally the treatment of choice for larger tumors; laser treatment or surgery may be necessary if malignant cells remain after radiation. Enucleation is generally recommended for large melanomas that can't be radiated. The five-year survival for regional OM is 71 percent.

Metastatic ocular melanoma has invaded other parts of the body. No treatments are approved specifically for this stage, and it cannot be cured, which underscores the importance of finding and treating OM early. Systemic therapies, such as the chemotherapy, targeted drugs, and immunotherapies that are used for melanomas of the skin, aren't as effective for OM, which is more likely to metastasize. Half of the people with OM develop metastatic disease within 15 years of their original diagnosis.[1] The factors that influence whether ocular melanoma spreads distantly are not entirely clear, although tumors that are large, well supplied by blood vessels, and/or have an overlying orange pigment appear to do so more often.

Many cases of metastasis develop in the liver, and the related treatment focuses mainly on slowing tumor growth and managing symptoms. Local therapies such as hepatic perfusion (high-dose chemotherapy delivered directly to the liver) or embolization (a procedure that injects an agent into an artery to deliver concentrated doses of treatment while reducing or blocking blood flow to a tumor) may improve survival. Chemotherapy, immunotherapy, and/or radiation may be used for embolization treatment. Clinical trials are looking into new ways to treat this disease. The five-year survival is 13 percent.

Follow-Up Care

Follow-up is extremely important after treatment for ocular melanoma. Many experts recommend twice-yearly physical exams by your doctor and a complete ophthalmic oncology exam at least annually for the rest of your life. Your follow-up care should also include periodic visits to an experienced medical oncologist, who can recommend the blood tests and scans you need to detect any signs of recurrence or metastasis as soon as possible. Your treating physician will provide a list of recommended blood work and scans based on the type and stage of the melanoma, your treatment, and your age and overall health. This testing may include ultrasound or MRI imaging of the liver at least annually, since that is the primary site of OM metastasis.

— *My Story* —

I Had Ocular Cancer, but My Sight Was Saved

Every year I went to the eye doctor and had my eyes examined as part of an annual visual exam. One year, my ophthalmologist found something in my eye near the optic nerve and referred me to an ophthalmologic oncologist. I was shocked to find that I had melanoma in my eye. I was a healthy 50-year-old. I never considered myself at high risk for cancer. I was scared, but my ophthalmologic oncologist was a world-class expert who inspired confidence. At the time, he was pioneering a new type of brachytherapy that involved implanting a gold plaque with radioactive seeds to treat uveal melanoma. He encouraged me to get a second opinion. That doctor wanted to remove my eye. I decided to go with my first oncologist and his radiation technique to save my eye.

During the procedure, he placed a plaque with radiation seeds on the back of my eye. I didn't feel anything unusual. After five days, the implant was removed, and I went home. My only other treatment was two outpatient sessions of laser to protect my vision. Eventually, I did lose some of the vision in the center of my eye, but I still have peripheral vision and can do all of the same activities I could do before cancer. Twenty-five years later, I'm doing well. I still see my eye cancer specialist annually for follow-up visits, and I've remained cancer-free.

My first cousin had breast cancer at age 33 and has a *BRCA2* mutation. I haven't had genetic testing, but I'm considering it.

—Jack

Part V
Living with
Inherited
High Risk

If you are someone who has inherited a high risk for cancer—even if you've never had a diagnosis—you face unique issues that most other people will never encounter. The day-to-day and long-term emotional and physical challenges of having an inherited gene mutation or hereditary cancer can be difficult to understand and deal with. It's hard to have to make decisions about actions to protect your present and future health. Whether you're a previvor, a person in treatment, or a long-term survivor, you may struggle with issues that require tough decisions. In these final chapters, you'll find suggestions for coping with many of these issues, including

- sexual health and intimacy
- fertility, pregnancy, and family planning
- treatment-induced early menopause
- immediate and long-term side effects of treatment
- finding support

Chapter 26

Regaining Sexual Health and Intimacy

Your sexual life may not be the same as it was before, and it may require some effort, but you needn't live a life without sex or intimacy because you've had cancer or a risk-reducing procedure to prevent it.

Saving your life is the primary goal of cancer prevention and treatment. Sometimes, though, it comes at a high price. Regardless of your age, gender, sexual orientation, or partner status, intimacy and sexual health are often important elements of overall health and quality of life. When life throws us a curve—like being at high risk for cancer or being treated for it—and disrupts our normal lives, sexuality and sensuality are often the first casualties. Emotional upheaval and the aftermath of treatment may change the way you feel about your body, your sensuality, and ultimately your ability to be sexually satisfied, especially if you had similar issues before treatment.

For many cancer survivors, intimacy and sex after treatment can be awkward, painful, or impossible. Surgery, radiation, chemotherapy, and hormone therapy can directly or indirectly impact sexual function. While these treatments may effectively address cancer, they may also damage nerves and blood vessels, create scar tissue, disrupt the balance of sex hormones, and remove organs. The most common problems related to sex and intimacy during or after treatment involve a change in body image, pain or discomfort during sexual activity, changes in arousal, reduced sexual drive, and erectile dysfunction. Sexual dysfunction can result from different issues and may require a multidisciplinary approach.

Body Image

Cancer treatments may change your appearance, sometimes drastically. Whether temporary or permanent, hair loss, dry skin and hair, weight changes, scarring, and other visible remnants of treatment may erode your confidence and your self-image. You might be fearful that your partner will no longer find you attractive if you're missing your breasts or if you're dissatisfied with your reconstructed breasts. If you're a man who has been treated with hormone therapy, you might be concerned that your breasts are growing larger or embarrassed that your testicles have shrunk. Perhaps you're self-conscious about having an ostomy and worry about how your partner will react to this change.

Don't assume that you're undesirable if your partner doesn't initiate intimacy. Your partner may be afraid of hurting or embarrassing you or may be reluctant to push for intimacy when you're tired, stressed, or not in the mood, especially if you're emotionally distant. These feelings are natural, but left unresolved they can undermine your sense of self-worth. As a result, you may feel awkward, shy, or ashamed about the way you look and dread the thought of being naked or intimate.

— *My Story* —

I Was Nervous about My Partner's Reaction

When I woke up after my bilateral mastectomy, I was bandaged and had no idea what the surgery site looked like, nor did I want to know. Before surgery, my doctor had told me I would have scars, swelling, and four drains hanging out of me. The day after the surgery, he came to visit me in the hospital and said that he needed to remove my bandages to examine me. I asked my partner to look [at my body] for me. I sat upright while the doctor slowly unraveled the bandages, staring not down at my chest but into my partner's eyes. I could see and feel him taking it all in. I was impatient and asked him what he thought and to describe what my chest looked like. All he could say was "You are so beautiful and so sexy." I cried, and my heart was overwhelmed with gratitude.

It took me about a week to feel strong enough for intimacy, but when it happened I felt so empowered knowing that I am not my breasts. I am still the same playful, silly, feminine, loving gal that I was before surgery.

—Staci

What You Can Do

- Focus on becoming more comfortable with your posttreatment self. Take time to explore your own body to see what kind of touch feels pleasant or uncomfortable.
- Practice positive self-talk: "I'm the person I've always been," "I am strong," "I am loved." Words are powerful, and they can reinforce or change how you feel about intimacy.
- Give yourself time to adjust and become comfortable with your body after treatment.
- Wear lingerie or a light robe or turn off the lights until you become more comfortable in your skin.
- Take intimacy slowly. Focus on the interactions that make you feel most comfortable and are most satisfying, like touching, hugging, or kissing.
- Experiment with a new hairstyle, different clothing styles, or makeup that enhances the way you feel.
- Wear a scarf, wig, or hairpiece if you're uncomfortable about hair loss.
- Exercise, meditate, learn tai chi or yoga, or find other ways to improve fatigue and mood and promote calmness, which can directly affect your self-esteem.
- Consider joining a support group or speaking with a mental health professional about the way you feel.

Coping with Pain

After months of treatment, intimacy and physical pleasure may be the last thing on your mind, especially if it's painful. While lingering pain is a common side effect of many treatments, in some cases, it remains even after recovery. Chemotherapy and radiation can damage sensitive mucous membranes in the mouth, vagina, anus, and penis. Pelvic radiation can burn skin, damage ovaries and testicles, and turn soft tissue thick and less elastic. Chemo and hormone therapy can dry vaginal tissue and weaken the pelvic floor, and surgery can reduce the size and length of the vagina, potentially making intercourse uncomfortable or painful. You may sometimes experience genital pain during sex, and ejaculation may hurt if the urethra or prostate becomes irritated from treatment. Neuropathy from treatment can affect the genitals, making arousal more challenging. Neuropathy in your fingers might make touching your partner feel different.

What You Can Do

- Ask your doctor about a vaginal moisturizer to treat dry or atrophied tissue.
- Use a water-based, lubricating gel, like K-Y Jelly or Astroglide, before penetration. Refrain from penetrative sex if you have genital pain or soreness.
- Delay intercourse until you're aroused and your vagina is fully expanded.
- Try a new sexual position if what you're used to is uncomfortable or painful.
- Speak with your doctor about treatment for dyspareunia (vaginal dryness or pain during sex).
- Ask your doctor about vaginal dilators to improve vaginismus, an involuntary contraction or clenching of the pelvic floor muscles, which can make penetrative sexual activity very painful. This condition may result from pelvic radiation or treatments that lower estrogen levels. Using dilators may help you practice relaxing the pelvic floor while expanding the vagina.
- See a physical therapist who specializes in pelvic rehabilitation and can teach you to relax your pelvic floor muscles through exercise and manual manipulation.
- Talk to your doctor about ways to relieve treatment-related pain. Ask for a referral to a pain specialist if necessary.

Reduced Sexual Desire

Even though some aspects of treatment may be difficult, you may be comfortable in your body and effortlessly slip back into the closeness and intimacy you experienced before your diagnosis. For some people, however, it's not that easy. It may be difficult to feel sexy when you're fatigued, anxious, or depressed about your situation, or when you're trying to cope with vaginal dryness, hot flashes, and other signs of premature menopause. Erogenous zones that have little or no sensation may leave you less than enthusiastic. Or you may be numb in some areas and hypersensitive in others.

Oophorectomy, hysterectomy, prostatectomy, and other treatments for below-the-belt cancers may create issues that affect libido; treatments for other cancers may create problems as well. Many individuals experience long-term sexual dysfunction after treatment for breast, gynecologic, or prostate cancers, with the greatest impact resulting from the most common treatments: surgery, radiation, hormone therapy, and chemotherapy. Hormone treatment can be especially damaging to libido and sexual functionality because it reduces or blocks the very substances that rev up our sexual engines. Surgery may leave painful scarring or may damage sensation in sensitive tissues, while chemotherapy and radiation may cause tissues to atrophy. Medications for nausea, pain, depression, and insomnia may also negatively impact sexual function.

All of these treatments can take a physical and emotional toll on your sensation, mood, and the fundamentals that produce and affect libido. That doesn't necessarily mean that your desire and responsiveness are gone forever.

What You Can Do

- Speak with a gynecologist, urologist, or another doctor who specializes in sexual medicine, or a sex therapist as soon as unmanageable problems develop.
- Consider vaginal estrogen treatment if you were treated for a cancer that wasn't estrogen-sensitive. Unlike estrogen pills or patches, vaginal applications stay in place and don't circulate through the body. When vaginal tissue becomes healthier and sexual activity is no longer painful, you may notice that your interest in intimacy improves.
- Consider using a vibrator if you have difficulty reaching orgasm. Not only can this be pleasurable, but it can also help you understand what feels good while enhancing arousal and desire.
- Talk to your doctor about ways to manage menopausal symptoms.
- Ask your doctor about medication that may improve your libido.

Erectile Dysfunction

Various treatments for prostate cancer, including surgery, radiation therapy, and hormone therapy, may diminish your sexual function. Pelvic radiation may damage the nerves or blood vessels that are involved in achieving an erection. People who are treated with antihormone medications may experience a significantly reduced sex drive. Common problems are loss of libido, erectile dysfunction (an inability to achieve or maintain an erection), and impotence (inability to achieve an erection or orgasm). Dry ejaculation—an orgasm that occurs without releasing semen—isn't dangerous and doesn't preclude having sex. It's important to take a proactive approach to sexual recovery.

What You Can Do

- Talk to your doctor about penile rehabilitation, which uses various strategies, including medication such as Viagra or Cialis, to promote blood flow to the penis and improve erectile function.
- If oral medications don't work, don't give up. Consider using sexual aids, such as an erection ring or a vacuum erection device (also called a penis pump), which can help you maintain an erection.
- Speak with a urologist about other options, including penile injection therapy or an inflatable surgical implant. Ask for a referral to a therapist who specializes in sexual dysfunction.

— EXPERT VIEW —

Addressing Sexuality for Men

BY SHARON BOBER, PHD

Many people are aware that preventive procedures and cancer treatments related to inherited mutations may affect female sexuality. However, men with inherited gene mutations, especially mutations related to prostate, pancreatic, breast, and colon cancers, may also face issues of sexual dysfunction, body image, and intimacy. Although television commercials and magazine ads attempt to reduce the stigma of erectile dysfunction, this kind of marketing underscores the notion that male sexual health only involves the capacity to get an erection. Yet men who are treated for breast cancer may also struggle with changes

Questions to Ask Your Oncologist or Urologist

- Will my treatment affect my ability to have a normal sex life?

- If side effects occur, how long will they last?

- Is it safe for me to have sex during treatment?

- What can I do about my lack of sexual interest?

- What can I do to make sex less painful or uncomfortable?

- What can I do to minimize the effect of treatment on my sexuality?

- Could any of my existing health conditions or medications affect my low libido or sexual dysfunction?

- May I have a referral to a sexual therapist or a medical professional who deals with these issues?

in body image, and they may feel a loss of body integrity or fear that they are less attractive to their partners. Men in my practice often speak about feeling embarrassed if they need to use some kind of erectile aid, so they avoid physical touch with a partner because they don't want to "start something they can't finish." Partners may then wrongly assume that this distance is because they are no longer desirable. This often leads to avoidance of physical closeness. Both partners may feel sad and frustrated but also feel stuck and alone regarding sexuality and intimacy.

Individuals who undergo treatment for prostate cancer face significant changes in sexual function that go beyond the capacity to get or maintain an erection. In addition to erectile dysfunction, those who are treated with androgen deprivation therapy commonly experience a loss of libido, hot flashes, mood changes, and decreased energy. These side effects may affect both the cancer survivor and their sexual partner. For example, one of the most frustrating concerns after prostate cancer treatment is that drugs like Viagra (sildenafil) and Cialis (tadalafil) often do not work, and some people may feel "doubly damaged."

If you're bothered by treatment-related changes in body image, self-esteem, or sexual function, it's important to become educated and identify experts who are knowledgeable about effective options for treating your sexual dysfunction. By using counseling and concrete strategies to help cope with physical, emotional, and relationship factors, sexual recovery is possible. Couples that can communicate about what's happening and discover how to expand their range of giving and receiving pleasure are more likely to experience satisfying intimacy, even if the sexual interactions are different than they were before preventive procedures or cancer treatment.

Rebuilding Intimacy

Sometimes, couples give up if they don't know how to talk about problems of intimacy or how to improve their situation. Partners who seem distant or uncaring may be fearful or distressed by a medical issue that they can't control and can't fix. Communication is key. Although talking about bedroom issues can be challenging, sharing how you feel and what you want is the first step toward restoring a mutually satisfying sex life. Talk openly with your partner, who probably shares your anxiety but may not volunteer opinions or feelings until prompted. Express your feelings, and encourage your partner to do the same. Your tone and attitude make a difference.

Intimacy is more than just sex. It's touching, trusting, sharing, and caring deeply. If your precancer intimacy routine isn't possible or no longer works, experiment to reinvigorate your sex life. Encourage your partner to touch your neck, inner thigh, breast, or penis with light, medium, and deep touches to see what feels good and what doesn't. It can take time, effort, and patience to rekindle your intimacy and get your love life back on track. Your sexual life may not be the same as it was before, and it may require some effort, but you needn't live a life without sex or intimacy because you've had cancer or a risk-reducing procedure to prevent it. There are ways to counteract or circumvent the toxic effects of treatment. Any issues can be resolved if you and your partner are willing to discuss and share the experience. You can regain a meaningful love life; you just might need to go about it differently. Though you and your partner may need a new perspective, sex and intimacy can still be meaningful.

What You Can Do

- Encourage your partner to be a willing participant in solving your shared sexual dilemma. Although it's your body, the life disruptions caused by cancer and treatment affect you both, and resolution means addressing these issues together.
- Keep an open mind, and don't be afraid to explore new ways to feel satisfied.
- Direct your partner's attention to the areas where you feel touch, instead of where you don't.
- When you're not in the mood for intercourse, concentrate on enjoying each other in other ways.
- Kiss, cuddle, and caress, and see what happens. Remember that your brain is the most powerful sexual organ you have. Sexual pleasure doesn't require penetration.
- Give yourself time to adjust to your new circumstances and to restore your sexual health.
- Work toward being comfortable in your posttreatment body, and let nature take its course.
- Consider individual and/or couples counseling.

Looking for Help

Don't wait for your medical team to ask if you're having problems with body image, sex, or intimacy, because chances are that won't happen. Medical school doesn't prepare physicians to confront or handle issues of sexuality, and doctors may be uncomfortable, dismissive, or simply without the time to talk about sex. However, it's still important to tell your doctor if you're having any issues. Broach the subject, and be as straightforward as possible about your concerns.

If your doctor can't help, ask for a referral to a sexual guidance counselor or therapist who has expertise in cancer-related intimacy issues so that you may receive the care you need. Other options for information and support are online and in-person support groups, patient blogs, and sexuality workshops, which may be offered by hospitals and medical centers.

Chapter 27

Effects of Prevention and Treatment on Fertility

Assisted reproductive technology may provide options for you to conceive your own biological children in the future, even if you become infertile from the effects of surgery or other treatment.

If you're diagnosed with cancer during your reproductive years, it's important to know that your ability to have children may be compromised by some cancers and some treatments. (Some preventive procedures also affect fertility.) This is particularly true if your cancer is caused by an inherited mutation because you're more likely to be diagnosed at an earlier age before you've completed having children. For some people, this means not being able to conceive or carry a baby to term. For others, it means being unable to produce enough healthy sperm to fertilize an egg. Infertility can be a tough pill to swallow if you look forward to having biological children.

The American Society of Clinical Oncology and NCCN guidelines recommend that oncologists discuss options for fertility preservation with individuals before cancer treatment, but that doesn't always happen. If the ability to have biological children is a concern or it might be in the future, it's important to talk with your doctor to get a clear understanding of how medical procedures or medications might affect your fertility and family planning. Ask about options to preserve your fertility before you commit to cancer treatment or a prevention plan. You may want to request a referral to a fertility or reproduction specialist who can help you make decisions about these issues. Additionally, some treatments may harm fetuses, so before you start treatment, let your oncologist know if you might be pregnant.

Preserving Fertility in Women

Some preventive measures and cancer treatments can affect your fertility by damaging or removing reproductive organs, including

- cancer that damages the ovaries, fallopian tubes, uterus, or cervix
- surgery that removes the uterus, ovaries, or fallopian tubes
- radiation treatment to the pelvis or abdomen that damages the ovaries
- chemotherapy and hormone therapy that interrupts or stops reproductive hormones
- targeted agents and immunotherapies that can cause premature ovarian failure, although less is known about their long-term effects on fertility

Surgery

To conceive and deliver a baby naturally, you need one healthy ovary (with enough eggs), at least one healthy fallopian tube, and a healthy uterus that can support the baby until it's born. Surgery that scars or removes any of these organs can affect your ability to have a child.

- Bilateral oophorectomy (removal of both ovaries) causes early menopause, and the ovaries no longer produce eggs. You may still be able to conceive if only one ovary is removed.
- Bilateral salpingectomy (removal of both fallopian tubes) prevents eggs from moving from the ovaries to the uterus.
- Bilateral salpingo-oophorectomy (removal of both ovaries and both fallopian tubes) prevents the ability to conceive.
- Hysterectomy (removal of the uterus) ends menstrual periods and the ability to carry a baby to term.

Radiation Therapy

Pelvic radiation can temporarily or permanently damage the ovaries, the uterus, and/or the blood veins that support the uterus, increasing the risk of miscarriage and premature birth. Radiation delivered to the breast or elsewhere shouldn't affect your ability to have a baby, although it can destroy the ability to produce milk and breastfeed.

In some cases, ovarian shielding (placing a protective cover on the outside of the body over the area of the ovaries and other parts of your reproductive system) can reduce the harmful effects of radiation to these organs. Ovarian transposition is another way to protect the ovaries and eggs during radiation. It's a surgical procedure that repositions the ovaries beyond the radiation field to reduce their radiation exposure. This doesn't always work, and a better option, if possible, is to have eggs or embryos frozen before any radiation treatment (see "Preservation Procedures" below).

Chemotherapy

Chemotherapy is a powerful and effective way to kill cancer cells, but sometimes it also targets healthy egg and sperm cells, which are necessary for reproduction. Some chemotherapies cause early menopause and permanent infertility. Others temporarily stop menstrual periods; although periods usually return within six months or so after you stop receiving chemotherapy, your fertility may be reduced. The extent of reproductive damage depends on your age at treatment, the type of chemotherapy drugs used, and the total dose. Some chemotherapy drugs can result in premature ovarian failure while others reduce the ovarian reserve, the set number of eggs that you have at birth. Women are born with about 2 million eggs, but that number steadily declines as you age. Some types of chemotherapy further reduce your egg supply, making it more difficult to become pregnant. (Your doctor can order a test to evaluate your ovarian reserve.) Other chemotherapies can lead to temporary or permanent menopause. Your ovaries no longer have eggs or have only poor-quality eggs that can't be fertilized. Chemo is less likely to affect fertility in younger people, who have more higher-quality eggs than older individuals do.

Alkylating chemotherapy drugs, including Cytoxan (cyclophosphamide), are most likely to cause infertility, especially at high doses. Platinum-based and other chemotherapy drugs can also cause damage. Anthracycline drugs, including Adriamycin (doxorubicin), Cerubidine (daunorubicin), Ellence (epirubicin), and Idamycin (idarubicin), are more likely to affect reproductive organs and damage the heart muscle when given at higher doses. Ordinarily, this kind of damage can be managed. However, the heart, lungs, kidneys, and other vital organs may be unable to support the physiological demands of pregnancy and delivery. (The heart must work up to 50 percent harder during pregnancy to support both you and your fetus.) For some people, ovarian suppression with an injectable gonadotropin-releasing-hormone agonist (for example, leuprolide or goserelin) shuts down the brain signals that tell the ovaries to make estrogen and progesterone. This may temporarily protect the ovaries during chemotherapy, but not all experts agree that this protects fertility in premenopausal individuals.

Preservation Procedures

Assisted reproductive technology (ART) may provide options for you to conceive your own biological children in the future, even if you become infertile from the effects of surgery or other treatment. ART is an umbrella term for fertility treatments that preserve your eggs or embryos. These procedures provide an effective backup plan if you experience early menopause or otherwise become infertile.

If you need an oophorectomy or chemotherapy that may reduce or eliminate your fertility, your eggs or embryos can be frozen before treatment. This is the most effective approach to have your own biological children. Egg and embryo freezing involves taking hormone injections for 8–12 days to stimulate your ovaries to make multiple eggs. Your eggs are then harvested and immediately frozen with liquid nitrogen, which suspends most cellular activity and keeps the eggs from aging. When you're ready to become pregnant, your healthy eggs can be thawed and fertilized in a laboratory with sperm from your partner or a donor in a process called in vitro fertilization. After several days, the fertilized eggs develop into embryos and can be implanted into your uterus.

Alternatively, harvested eggs may be fertilized by in vitro fertilization, and the resulting embryos can be frozen. When you're ready to become pregnant, the embryos can be transferred to your uterus. This procedure is a viable option if you're able to defer your treatment for at least two weeks.

Ovarian tissue freezing is an experimental option if your chemotherapy or radiation can't be delayed for the two to three weeks required for egg freezing or if you can't undergo hormonal stimulation to retrieve eggs or embryos for freezing. This procedure begins with surgical removal of a sample of your ovarian tissue, which is then frozen until you complete your treatment. The thawed tissue is then transferred back into your body. If it begins to function normally, it may release an egg that may be fertilized naturally or collected for in vitro fertilization.

Pregnancy after Cancer

Many individuals are able to have a healthy, natural pregnancy after cancer treatment, although some are more likely to experience treatment-related side effects that affect conception or pregnancy. Generally, pregnancy after cancer is believed to be safe. It doesn't increase your risk of recurrence or affect your baby's health. Although pregnancy raises levels of estrogen, research shows that even people who become pregnant after treatment for early-stage estrogen receptor–positive breast cancer aren't at greater risk for recurrence. Depending on your genetic predisposition, your risk for recurrence, and the type of cancer for which you were treated, your doctor might advise waiting to conceive until your risk of recurrence or your side effects reach an acceptable level.

Deciding when to try to have a baby is a personal decision between you and your partner. If you're a cancer survivor, however, it's wise to talk to your oncologist, obstetrician, or fertility specialist about when it's safe to conceive and carry a baby. Doctors typically recommend waiting two years or more after all treatment is completed to allow damaged reproductive organs to heal.

— *My Story* —
The Hardest Decision

I was engaged when I tested positive for a *BRCA1* mutation. At 31, I was approaching the age when my risk increased. Oophorectomy was recommended when I was done having children; I was unsure what to do about my breasts. I finally made up my mind, and after my wedding, I had both breasts removed. It was the hardest decision I've ever made. I wanted to become pregnant, but I was concerned about screening, particularly at a time when increased estrogen could spike my risk, and early cancer (which could be very aggressive) would be difficult to find. It was a risk I wasn't willing to take.

Questions to Ask Your Doctor about Cancer Treatment and Fertility

- Will my cancer or treatment cause premature menopause or otherwise affect my fertility?

- How can I preserve my fertility before treatment?

- Will any of my treatments create problems during pregnancy, labor, and/or delivery?

- After treatment, how will I know if my fertility has been affected?

- How long should I wait before trying to conceive?

- Will becoming pregnant affect my risk of recurrence?

- Will trying to have a child change my follow-up care plan?

- Should I talk with an obstetrician or a fertility specialist who has experience with cancer survivors?

- What emotional support resources do you recommend?

I don't regret my decision. I was sad when I couldn't breastfeed. I was aware that breastfeeding is best for newborns and creates a strong mother-child bond. But feeding times were still special, and bonding was solid. My children are almost 4 and 2 now, and they're healthy. I feel confident that I'm doing everything within my power to make sure that I will be here for them for a long time.

—*Kendra*

Preserving Fertility in Men

Cancer and related treatment can affect your ability to make healthy sperm and produce children. Infertility occurs when an individual can no longer make sperm, when their sperm count is low, or when sperm are damaged by treatment.

Surgery and Radiation

Surgery that removes the prostate creates infertility by eliminating the ability to make or ejaculate semen. Individuals who have a testicle removed but still have one that functions may be able to produce a child. (A semen analysis performed after treatment can assess sperm production.) Sperm production is permanently lost when both testicles are removed.

Radiation therapy aimed at or near the testicles may also cause infertility by damaging DNA in cells that produce sperm. Lower doses may temporarily stop sperm production, but it may restart two or three years after treatment. Higher doses are more likely to result in permanent infertility. Radiologists can sometimes protect your fertility by using radiation shielding (covering the testicles with lead-lined shields to minimize exposure to harmful radiation of the groin or pelvis). Intensity-modulated radiation therapy, which is a precisely focused type of radiation, is another option for minimizing exposure.

Chemotherapy

Some individuals who have chemotherapy experience infertility, depending on the type and number of drugs used and the total dose given. In some cases, regimens may be changed to protect your fertility. Cyclophosphamide alone and high doses of platinum-based cisplatin and oxaliplatin can damage sperm cell production and the production of testosterone by the testicles. Sometimes, the dose can be adjusted so that it's still effective while reducing the chance of infertility.

The risk is greater when treatment includes two or more alkylating chemotherapy drugs or a combination of chemotherapy and radiation. Individuals who are treated with certain chemotherapies may take medication that makes the testes dormant before treatment so that they're less likely to be damaged. Sperm cells that are damaged by chemotherapy may sometimes repair themselves and produce healthy sperm within a year or two after treatment. An oncologist can determine when it's safe to have children.

Preservation Procedures

Assisted reproductive technology is an option to preserve your ability to produce children after treatment when sperm counts are low, sperm quality is poor, or sperm are absent in the semen.

- Sperm banking before treatment freezes and indefinitely stores your sperm for future use, just as eggs may be frozen. If you later decide to have children, your sperm can be thawed and used to inseminate your partner directly or to fertilize your partner's eggs using in vitro fertilization. The resulting embryo can then be transferred to your partner's uterus.
- Testicular sperm extraction surgically removes, freezes, and stores healthy sperm cells from a small sample of testicular tissue for later in vitro fertilization.
- Electroejaculation involves positioning over the prostate gland an electrical probe, which emits a mild electrical current to stimulate ejaculation to obtain a semen sample. Healthy semen that is obtained this way may then be used for in vitro fertilization or frozen and stored until needed.

Other Parenting Alternatives

If you're unable to have your own biological children, you can fulfill your wish for parenthood in other ways, even though this may not be your first choice. A fertility specialist can explain the benefits and limitations of using donor sperm, eggs, or embryos or using one of the following options:

Questions to Ask Your Doctor about Fertility

- Can my treatment cause infertility?
- Are there other recommended cancer treatments that might not affect my fertility?
- Will my fertility return after treatment?
- What fertility preservation procedures do you recommend?
- After treatment, how will I know if my fertility has been affected?
- How long should I wait before trying to have a child?
- Should I speak with a fertility specialist?
- What emotional support resources do you recommend?

- If pregnancy is unsafe or impossible after cancer treatment, you might consider a gestational carrier. This individual will be implanted with your embryo, which has been fertilized with the sperm of your partner or a donor, and then carry and deliver your child. Babies born through this method will carry genes from you and your partner (or sperm donor).
- If it's not possible to use your own eggs, another option is to use an egg donor, whose eggs will be artificially inseminated with sperm from your partner or a donor. Babies born in this way will carry the genes of the egg donor and either your partner or the sperm donor. The egg donor may also serve as a gestational surrogate, carrying the fetus to term.

- If it's not possible to use your own sperm, artificially inseminating your partner with donated sperm is an option. Babies born this way will carry the genes of the sperm donor and your partner's genes.
- Whether you're a previvor or a cancer survivor, if you want to have children and can't become pregnant, adoption is a wonderful way to create or expand your family. Your doctor will need to provide an accurate assessment of your health and prognosis. Your genetic predisposition or cancer history, however, shouldn't preclude your approval as an adoptive parent.

Preimplantation Genetic Testing

Many people with inherited mutations have watched cancer devastate their family, and some people want to explore every option to lower the chance of passing their inherited mutation to their children. Preimplantation genetic testing (PGT) can be used during assisted reproductive technology to screen embryos for a parent's inherited mutation and genetic predisposition to disease or cancer. When embryos reach an adequate size after in vitro fertilization, one cell from each is removed and screened for inherited high-risk mutations. Any unaffected embryos can then be frozen and later implanted in you, your partner, or a surrogate. PGT is the only way to determine before pregnancy whether an embryo carries a genetic mutation.

Reproductive planning is deeply personal and individual. Whatever choices you make, know that others have been there, and you don't have to grapple with these decisions alone. FORCE has peer support volunteers who have considered these options and can share their perspective and experiences with you.

Paying for Fertility Treatments

Health insurance plans don't always cover fertility preservation or treatment for infertility. Some state laws require plans to cover fertility diagnosis or treatment, but coverage varies. You can find a list of state laws on the website of the National Conference of State Legislatures (www.ncsl.org). Some organizations offer financial aid for people who need assistance with coverage for these services.

Chapter 28

◥

Managing Menopause

> Whether to use hormones is a personal decision and requires discussion with health care providers who have expertise with preventing and treating hereditary cancer and dealing with the effects of menopause.

$\mathbf{M}$enopause is a natural transition when a woman's ovaries stop releasing eggs and making hormones, menstrual periods cease, and the overall level of circulating hormones—estrogen, progesterone, and testosterone—drastically decreases. Most individuals begin having symptoms of menopause a year or more before their periods end—usually between ages 45 and 55—as their estrogen levels fluctuate and gradually decline. This perimenopausal transition may last a few years until menstruation stops completely, signaling the end of fertility and the onset of menopause.

Some risk-reducing procedures and cancer treatments abruptly stop ovarian hormone production, bypassing the gradual transition of perimenopause and resulting in early menopause that occurs in days or weeks. For many people, the menopause experience means a variety of uncomfortable symptoms that may make life miserable. Others have only mild symptoms, and some have no bothersome effects at all. Some cancer treatments and procedures may cause early menopause:

- Oophorectomy removes the ovaries and causes immediate menopause.
- Radiation given in high doses to the pelvis may cause permanent damage to the ovaries and thus cause menopause.

- Hormone therapies, including tamoxifen and aromatase inhibitors, cause menopause-like symptoms that generally resolve when the medications are stopped. Lupron (leuprolide) and Zoladex (goserelin) are often given to suppress ovarian function in premenopausal women who have breast cancer, causing temporary menopause.
- Chemotherapy may damage ovaries and cause early menopause immediately or months after treatment, depending on the type and amount of the medication. These effects may be temporary or permanent. The younger you are, the less likely you will have early, permanent menopause from chemo.

Symptoms of Early Menopause

If you are premenopausal, the effects of early menopause may be more intense than the typical symptoms of natural menopause. Some symptoms are well tolerated and eventually decrease or disappear. Others may be managed with over-the-counter aids or nonmedical intervention. More persistent symptoms may require prescription medications, which may cause other side effects.

Hormone replacement therapy is the most effective way to relieve menopausal symptoms. It's recommended for many, but not all women. See your doctor if symptoms are severe or interfere with your quality of life. The menopause experience is different for everyone, and finding the right remedy is often a trial-and-error process.

Hot Flashes

Hot flashes—episodes of mild to extreme heat felt throughout the body—are the most common symptom of menopause. These uncomfortable bursts are sometimes accompanied by heavy perspiration, a flushed face, or a rapid heartbeat. Hot flashes often become less troublesome in time, but some people have them for years. They can be unpredictable and inopportune, occurring at work, in the car, or when you're out and about, so it's helpful to be prepared. Dress in layers. Notice whether spicy foods, alcohol, or caffeine trigger hot flashes so that you can avoid them. Combat night sweats (hot flashes while you sleep) by keeping your bedroom cool and well ventilated, or try tucking a Chillow, a cooling pillow, into your pillowcase. Regular yoga, acupuncture, and/or meditation may reduce the frequency and intensity of hot flashes. Hypnosis may also be helpful.

Estrogen replacement therapy is the most effective treatment for hot flashes (see "Replacement Hormones" below). Low-dose Paxil (paroxetine), a medication used in higher doses to treat depression and anxiety, is the only other FDA-approved medication for hot flashes. Used off-label, the antidepressant Effexor XR (venlafaxine) and the antiseizure medication gabapentin reduce hot flashes in some individuals. Some research suggests that the drug oxybutynin—which is currently approved for treating overactive bladder—may also decrease hot flashes.

Vaginal Dryness and Atrophy

After menopause, lubricating moisture in the vaginal walls is secreted less frequently, and vaginal tissues may atrophy, becoming thin and dry and making intercourse and even a Pap smear painful. Over-the-counter vaginal lubricants (K-Y, Astroglide, and others) may make intercourse more comfortable. Regularly applying vaginal moisturizers (Liquibeads, Replens, and others) may relieve dry tissues. Having sexual intercourse regularly may increase blood flow and also reduce vaginal dryness.

If symptoms persist, ask your doctor about a low-dose local estrogen cream, tablet, insert, or ring that releases small amounts of weak estrogen to the vaginal walls but minimizes absorption into the bloodstream. Intrarosa (prasterone/DHEA) vaginal tablets and Osphena (ospemifene) oral tablets are FDA-approved for treating painful intercourse due to vaginal dryness and atrophy.

Decreased Libido

Some people notice that they're less interested in sex after menopause when estrogen and testosterone levels decline. This is more likely to be the case when the ovaries are removed before menopause. The FDA hasn't approved any testosterone formulations for women. Some physicians prescribe compounded testosterone or a tablet that combines testosterone and estrogen.

If your doctor determines that low hormone levels, blood pressure medication, or another underlying physical issue aren't causing your lack of libido, it may be due to stress, depression, anxiety, or relationship issues. A sexual dysfunction expert can help you sort out these issues.

Fatigue

Individuals frequently report a lack of energy during menopause. A combination of factors, including stress, anxiety, and insomnia, can sap your energy. It may seem counterintuitive, but getting plenty of exercise may help you feel more energized. It may also decrease stress and anxiety and improve insomnia. Start slowly and gradually exercise more frequently and with more intensity. Eat well and address any problems that interrupt your sleep (see "Sleep Disturbances" below). If fatigue persists, talk to your doctor about medications that might be contributing to your tiredness, and ask about blood tests to rule out an underactive thyroid or other conditions that may be the cause.

Sleep Disturbances

Insomnia—not being able to fall asleep or stay asleep—is another common menopausal occurrence. You can improve your ability to sleep by reducing or eliminating alcohol and caffeine. Avoid naps or limit them to 30–40 minutes in the early afternoon. Don't eat, exercise, or use computers or other blue light electronics within two hours of bedtime. Read instead, take a warm bath, or do whatever makes you drowsy. Try to go to bed at the same time each night and wake up at the same time each morning, even on weekends. If you still need help to get deep and restful sleep, talk to your doctor about short-term medication or ask for a referral to a sleep clinic.

Weight Gain

After menopause, changing hormones shift the distribution of your weight to your abdomen. Your metabolism slows, and your body needs fewer calories. The trick to avoiding weight gain during this time is ample exercise and a balanced, reduced-calorie diet. Try for 45–60 minutes of brisk walking or other weight-bearing aerobic exercise at least five days a week and resistance exercise three days a week to retain muscle mass and increase metabolism.

Skin and Hair Changes

Having less estrogen reduces collagen, making your hair thinner and skin drier. You can improve both by staying hydrated, avoiding caffeine and alcoholic drinks, and eating enough fruits, vegetables, lean protein, and healthy fats, which contribute to skin and hair health from the inside. Generously use a sunblock with an SPF of 30 or higher every day, year 'round. Use mild cleansers and skin care products instead of soap. Keep your skin well moisturized throughout the day and before bed. Avoid smoking, which decreases circulation and blood flow to the skin. See a dermatologist for problems with thinning hair on your head, new facial hair, and deep wrinkles. There is more information about managing skin and hair changes in chapter 29.

Joint Pain

Aches, stiffness, and swelling around joints are common with the drastic hormonal changes that often occur during menopause. Maintaining a healthy weight, getting enough dietary calcium and vitamin D, and performing low-impact exercises, such as walking, swimming, or yoga, may help. Try ibuprofen or acetaminophen as often as recommended by the label. Acupuncture may give you relief from pain. Your doctor can determine whether your pain is a symptom of menopause, arthritis, or another condition and whether you might benefit from physical therapy and/or prescription medication.

Memory and Cognitive Changes

Many people with menopause experience temporary forgetfulness and brain fog as their hormone levels drop. If you find it hard to focus, forget words, or feel that you're losing your mental edge, engage your mind with daily reading, puzzles, or other brain-challenging activities. Keep notes and make lists of things you might forget. Eat nutritionally balanced meals and avoid alcohol. Getting enough sleep may also improve clarity and memory. Some research has shown that yoga, exercise, mindfulness, and cognitive training may also be helpful. Researchers are also studying whether Vyvanse (lisdexamfetamine), an FDA-approved stimulant for treating attention deficit hyperactivity disorder, improves memory in women after risk-reducing salpingo-oophorectomy.

Mood Swings

Sadness, anxiety, grief, anger. You may experience one or more of these feelings during the ups and downs of menopause. You may be happy one minute and irritable or crying the next for no apparent reason. These feelings are normal as long as they don't linger or interfere with your life. Understanding why you feel the way you do is the first step in managing emotional upheaval. A mental health professional can help you sort through your emotions and/or prescribe medication to regain your emotional balance.

Practice different relaxation techniques to see what works best. Take a few minutes each day to breathe deeply and quiet your mind. Sitting quietly with your eyes closed, slowly breathe in and out. Focus on your breath, and if your mind wanders, bring your attention back to your breath.

Urinary Incontinence

Without estrogen, the urethral sphincters (the muscles that control the flow of urine) thin and weaken, often causing urinary incontinence (involuntary leaking of urine). After menopause, you may find that you can't always control your urine as well as before. You may lose urine when you laugh, cough, or sneeze (stress incontinence), or you may not be able to get to the bathroom in time (urge incontinence). You may be embarrassed to seek help for urinary incontinence, but it can often be greatly improved or cured.

The first step is to see a doctor, who will perform a physical exam and analyze a sample of your urine. You may need a referral to a urogynecologist or a urologist (doctors who specialize in urinary conditions) or a pelvic physical therapist. In the meantime, maintain a healthy weight and don't smoke. Absorbent pads can help minimize the impact of accidents.

Kegel exercises can strengthen your pelvic muscles and help control leaks. When your bladder is empty, focus on the muscles that you squeeze to stop urine. Squeeze and hold for 10 seconds, relax, then repeat. Do three sets of 10–15 Kegels daily.

Replacement Hormones

For many high-risk individuals, replacement hormones provide welcome relief from menopausal symptoms and prevent osteoporosis. Estrogen-only therapy (ET) may be used by women who no longer have their uterus. Hormone replacement therapy (HRT), a combination of estrogen and progesterone, is used by those who have an intact uterus. HRT may include a synthetic version of progesterone called progestin. Testosterone may sometimes be added to hormone replacement.

Hormone replacement therapy was once routinely prescribed to alleviate symptoms of natural menopause. This practice mostly ended after the

Women's Health Initiative found that women who were given HRT (estrogen and progesterone) had a higher risk of breast cancer compared to women who didn't receive hormones. Although this was an important study, the participants represented a much older population than women who experience early menopause. Nevertheless, this research convinced some doctors to stop prescribing hormone replacement.

Other research has shown that low-dose hormone replacement appears to be safe and doesn't increase breast cancer risk in women who have a *BRCA1* or *BRCA2* mutation, haven't been diagnosed with cancer, had RRSO before menopause, and have intact breasts. While the risks of short-term hormone replacement are minimal for previvors after mastectomy and RRSO, replacing hormones isn't recommended if you're postmenopausal and you still have your breasts and ovaries. Because estrogen-only therapy slightly increases the risk for uterine cancer, it's prescribed primarily for women who have had a hysterectomy. If you still have your uterus, estrogen-progestin therapy is preferred to protect against uterine cancer.

Little is known about hormone replacement therapy after ovarian or endometrial cancer. Although scant evidence suggests harm, more research is needed to conclude that it is safe. Most oncologists don't prescribe hormones after breast cancer due to concerns that they could increase the risk for recurrence. When no other remedy restores quality of life, however, some oncologists may prescribe just enough low-dose hormones to alleviate symptoms for people who have had hormone receptor–negative breast cancer, bilateral mastectomies, and treatment that was completed at least three years prior. Oral estrogen may increase the risk for gallbladder disease and blood clots, particularly if you smoke; the risk is lower if you use an estrogen skin patch instead of a pill.

Limited hormone use may be appropriate for the high-risk population, given the following:

- Hormones may be safer for previvors after preventive mastectomy and oophorectomy.
- Research suggests that short-term use of low-dose hormones doesn't increase breast cancer risk in previvors with intact breasts who experience surgical menopause from RRSO.

If you've had estrogen receptor–positive breast cancer, the risks of taking hormones usually outweigh the benefits.

— THE **FORCE** PERSPECTIVE —

The Menopause Experience Is Personal

Whether to use hormones is a personal decision and requires discussion with health care providers who have expertise with preventing and treating hereditary cancer and dealing with the effects of menopause. When you experience symptoms of menopause, don't automatically assume that you need hormones. Try not to be influenced by other people's perception of what menopause is supposed to be like. Let your own experience determine whether you need some type of replacement hormones.

If lifestyle changes and nonhormonal treatments don't adequately manage your symptoms, speak to your gynecologist or ask your doctor for a referral to a physician with expertise in menopause who can help determine whether the overall benefits of hormone replacement therapy outweigh the risks for you. The North American Menopause Society's website (www.menopause.org) can help you find a menopause specialist near you.

Long-Term Side Effects

While most side effects of menopause are mild and eventually dissipate, some may last longer, affect health more seriously, and require medical monitoring.

Increased Risk for Heart Disease

The risk for heart disease, the leading cause of death in women in the United States, increases after menopause, regardless of your age. Your risk is higher if you experience early-onset menopause because you have years ahead of you without the protective effects of natural estrogen. Other risk factors include smoking, a sedentary lifestyle, diabetes, a waistline of more than 35 inches, high blood pressure, high cholesterol, and a family history of heart disease. Some research shows that estrogen replacement therapy that is started soon after early menopause begins may be protective against related heart disease.

Bone Loss

Natural or treatment-induced menopause accelerates bone loss, increasing the risk for fractures. Although we naturally lose some bone as we age, the

Bioidenticals and Compounded Hormones

Bioidenticals are hormones derived from animal, plant, or synthetic sources that are chemically identical to the hormones made by the body. Estradiol tablets (a form of estrogen), low-dose estradiol vaginal medications, and oral progesterone capsules are examples of FDA-approved bioidentical hormones. No evidence shows that bioidenticals are safer or more effective than commercial hormone preparations. Both are approved by the FDA and are prescribed to treat menopausal symptoms.

Some physicians consider compounded hormones to be safer or more effective than commercial preparations, yet little research compares these custom-mixed hormones to commercial hormone preparations. Compounded hormones are neither tested nor approved by the FDA. Nor are they regulated, so preparations may vary between pharmacists and from one prescription to the next. Neither the FDA nor the North American Menopause Society recommend custom-compounded products over well-tested, government-approved products for most women.

low levels of estrogen during menopause accelerate this loss. At age 65, you should have a baseline bone density scan with dual-energy x-ray absorptiometry (DEXA) to measure the calcium and mineral content of your hips and spine.

Doctors use DEXA results to assess and categorize bone mineral density in three ways. Normal thinning means your bone density is about the same as other women your age. Osteopenia refers to bone mass below normal levels compared to women your age. Left untreated, osteopenia can lead to osteoporosis, a serious condition that develops when bones lose more mineral density than your body can replace, become brittle and weak, and can easily break. Your doctor can explain how you can prevent or slow bone loss with adequate calcium intake and weight-bearing exercises. Your doctor may recommend one of the following medications if you're at elevated risk for osteoporosis:

- Bisphosphonates, including Actonel, Boniva, and Fosamax (all given orally) and Reclast (given intravenously), preserve bone density.
- Prolia (denosumab) given by subcutaneous injection in the doctor's office every six months blocks cells that are responsible for bone loss. It's also being studied to see whether it lowers breast cancer risks in people with an inherited *BRCA1* gene mutation.
- Raloxifene mimics the effects of estrogen. It is FDA-approved to prevent and treat osteoporosis.
- Parathyroid hormone creates new bone with daily use for 18–24 months. It doesn't protect against bone loss once you stop using it. Teriparatide (Forteo) is a synthetic form of this hormone for people with very low bone density.
- Low-dose, short-term hormone therapy may reduce your risk for osteoporosis.

— *My Story* —
I Have to Do What's Right for Me

As a previvor with a mutation, I had my ovaries and fallopian tubes removed at age 39. I began having hot flashes and night sweats, but they were bearable so I decided not to use HRT. Then six months after

Tips for Better Bone Health

- Don't smoke.

- Avoid or limit alcoholic beverages.

- Limit intake of cola drinks.

- Get the daily recommended amounts of calcium and vitamin D for your age.

- Determine whether any of your medications can affect bone loss.

- Perform weight-bearing or resistance exercise for at least 30 minutes a day, three days a week.

my surgery, I started vaginal estrogen for severe dryness caused by vaginal atrophy. A bone scan showed that I also had osteopenia; another scan the following year showed I was losing bone.

I preferred to try to increase my bone mass with diet and exercise instead of taking a bisphosphonate. But after researching the safety and benefits of hormones on bone, cardiovascular health, and menopausal symptoms, I decided to begin HRT more for my long-term health than my hot flashes and night sweats. After two years of using a combined estrogen-progesterone patch and vaginal estrogen, my bone mass increased. I'm young and active, and I want to stay that way. I'm not sure whether HRT or diet and exercise (or both) are responsible. I'm protecting my health the best way I can.

—*Eva*

Chapter 29

Side Effects and Other Quality-of-Life Issues

Regardless of your diagnosis, treatment, or prognosis, there is usually something that can reduce, manage, or eliminate side effects and improve your quality of life during or after treatment.

Risk-reducing procedures and cancer treatments save lives, but they may cause problems when they also affect healthy tissue or organs. These side effects may be mild or intense, temporary or long-lasting, depending on your age, overall health, and the type of procedure or treatment you have. Problems can vary from person to person, even among those who receive the same treatment. Most people don't experience all the possible side effects of a particular drug or procedure. The most common effects decline or resolve on their own as your body adjusts to a particular medication or treatment ends. This chapter addresses the common side effects of risk-reducing medication, surgery and cancer treatment. Side effects related to sexuality are discussed in chapter 26; those regarding fertility are included in chapter 27; and those related to menopause are covered in chapter 28.

When your doctor recommends a treatment regimen, ask about its potential side effects, if they can be prevented, and what can be done if they appear. For some treatments, you may decide that the risk of serious side effects outweighs the benefits. Report any uncomfortable or painful symptoms to your doctor, who may prescribe medications, change treatment doses, or substitute medications to reduce or eliminate side effects that interfere with your quality of life. It's important to speak with your doctor before skipping doses, changing your dosage, or stopping your therapy. You may need to try different approaches before finding one that minimizes or resolves your side effects. Regardless of your diagnosis, treatment, or prognosis, there is usually something that can reduce, manage, or eliminate side effects and improve your quality of life during or after treatment.

Summarizing Side Effects by Treatment

Chemotherapy

Chemotherapy causes side effects of different frequency and severity, depending on the specific drug. Common temporary side effects include hair loss, mouth sores, anemia, bleeding, a weakened immune system, nausea, vomiting, diarrhea, and loss of appetite. Taxanes, such as Taxol (paclitaxel) and Taxotere (docetaxel), and platinum chemotherapy (carboplatin and oxaliplatin) may cause neuropathy, nerve damage that can result in tingling, burning, or numbness. This is usually temporary but may persist in some people. Many of these effects can be managed with another medication or by changing how the medication is given. Long-term side effects may include early menopause, heart damage linked to Adriamycin (doxorubicin), and hearing loss caused by cisplatin. Copious intravenous fluids are given just before and after cisplatin to reduce the risk of possible kidney damage.

— My Story —

I Didn't Know That I Could Lose Partial Hearing from Treatment

In 2009 I started five rounds of chemotherapy for fallopian tube cancer. One of the drugs was cisplatin. The oncologist discussed short-term side effects of the treatment, including hair loss, a depressed immune system, and nausea. He didn't explain the long-term effects. Shortly after my chemotherapy was completed, I noticed a marked loss of hearing. I attributed it to genes because my mother had hearing difficulties. A few years later I finally saw an audiologist and found out that cisplatin was the likely cause of the type of hearing loss that I have.

When I requested payment for hearing aids from my insurance company, I was told that my claim wouldn't be reviewed because I didn't have a baseline hearing test before having cisplatin. I never knew that I needed a test because my oncologist didn't inform me that hearing loss was a side effect.

—*Ruth*

Radiation Therapy

Common side effects of radiation include fatigue and redness, irritation, or swelling at the treatment site. Other complications may develop, depending on the area of the body that is radiated. Radiation that disrupts lymph nodes can cause a condition known as lymphedema, which is a buildup of fluid in the limbs.

Radiating the pelvis may cause bladder irritation, urinary or fecal incontinence, or lymphedema in the legs. Very rarely, serious complications, such as a bowel blockage or a fistula (an abnormal opening between two organs, such as the bowel and the bladder), may occur and may require surgery to correct. Pelvic radiation may also narrow the vagina and dry vaginal tissues, making sexual intercourse painful. Vaginal narrowing that results from pelvic or vaginal radiation can be reduced by using vaginal dilators or with a type of physical therapy known as pelvic rehabilitation. Radiation to the pelvis may also lead to erectile dysfunction (see chapter 26).

Hormone Therapies

Hormone therapies for men and women are different and cause different side effects. In women, common side effects include hot flashes, sexual complications, fatigue, difficulty focusing, other cognitive changes, joint pain, weight gain, and increased body fat. Aromatase inhibitors and Faslodex can eventually weaken bones, which can be serious.

If your prostate cancer is treated with androgen deprivation therapy, you may experience erectile dysfunction, diminished libido, and hot flashes. Other organs that use androgens may also be affected, leading to increased body fat, fatigue, anemia, thinning of bones, fractures, and decreased muscle mass.

Targeted Therapies

Common side effects from targeted therapies include abnormal blood counts, allergic reactions, headaches, fatigue, shortness of breath, mouth and tongue sores, skin rashes, joint pain, muscle weakness, neuropathy, a change in how food tastes, decreased appetite, upset stomach, nausea, vomiting, and diarrhea. Targeted therapies may also cause birth defects, so it's important to use a reliable form of birth control during treatment.

Some of these therapies can increase the risk for a new cancer. PARP inhibitors, for example, have been linked to a small increased risk for a blood disorder known as myelodysplastic syndrome and the related cancer acute myeloid leukemia. Talzenna is linked to fertility problems in men, Lynparza may cause urinary tract infections, and Zejula may cause potentially serious high blood pressure. Rarely, Avastin and Lenvima may cause very high blood pressure, tears in the stomach or intestine, or a fistula. Targeted therapies may also delay wound healing, so they shouldn't be taken soon before or after surgery. Lenvima may cause a rare, reversible swelling of the brain. While you are taking this drug, any headaches, seizures, weakness, confusion, blindness, or change in vision should be reported to your doctor.

Several anti-HER2 agents may cause heart damage, so routine monitoring is important if you take these drugs. In addition to side effects that are common to targeted therapies, CDK4/6 inhibitors may also create lung inflammation and liver damage, which are more serious. Kisqali can cause irregular heartbeat, and Piqray may cause rare but serious lung inflammation, severe skin reactions, and high blood sugar levels.

Immunotherapies

Frequent effects from immunotherapies include abnormal blood counts, allergic reactions, headaches, fatigue, shortness of breath, mouth and tongue sores, skin rashes, joint pain, muscle weakness, neuropathy, upset stomach, nausea, vomiting, diarrhea, and appetite changes. Some immunotherapies may cause birth defects, so using a reliable method of birth control during treatment is important.

Side effects from immune checkpoint inhibitors are similar to those of targeted therapies. They may also cause rare but severe immune-mediated reactions in the colon, kidneys, liver, lungs, adrenal glands, pituitary gland, skin, thyroid, and pancreas (leading to diabetes), which may be treatable with steroids.

Proleukin (aldesleukin) and interleukin-2 are immunotherapies that are sometimes used to treat melanoma. These drugs may produce fever, chills, fatigue, aches, other flu-like symptoms, and reduced blood counts. High doses (which are administered in a hospital) may create an accumulation of fluid throughout the body and a strong feeling of being unwell.

Managing Immediate Side Effects

Fatigue

Fatigue is the most common side effect of cancer treatment. More than feeling tired now and then, fatigue is utter exhaustion, a complete lack of energy that limits your ability to feel and function normally, even if you've slept well. Cancer-related fatigue is so pervasive among people in treatment and survivors that the National Comprehensive Cancer Network (NCCN) publishes guidelines for doctors to acknowledge and manage it. Recommendations for improvement include increased physical activity (to boost energy levels, improve sleep, and promote mental health) and nutritional counseling. Acupuncture, relaxation therapy, yoga, massage, and mindfulness meditation may also help. Talk to your doctor about other factors that can sap your energy, including any underlying mental and physical health conditions that might contribute to fatigue.

Tips for renewing energy:

- Exercise daily. Physical activity, rather than complete rest, is the best remedy for fatigue. Being sedentary can cause or intensify your fatigue. Start slowly with short daily walks, gradually increasing their frequency, intensity, and length. It may be difficult at first, but the more you move, the more energy you'll recover.
- Eat whole grains, fruits, vegetables, lean proteins, and nutrient-dense, iron-rich foods.
- Resolve sleep issues so that you get the rest you need.
- Do more on days when you feel more energetic and less on days when you don't.
- Ask your doctor about psychostimulants, medications that rouse certain parts of the brain and may improve cancer-related fatigue.

- Consider emotional counseling, support groups, and stress management techniques. They may elevate your mood and strengthen your ability to cope with stress that may be affecting your energy.
- Accept that you may not be able to accomplish all that you did before treatment.

Low Blood Counts

Many cancer treatments, especially certain chemotherapies, reduce blood cell counts. Anemia is a lack of red blood cells, which may cause fatigue, dizziness, headaches, irregular heartbeat, or shortness of breath. *Neutropenia* is a similar decrease of white blood cells, which provide the body's primary defense against infection. If you have either condition, your doctor will focus on identifying and managing the cause and restoring your blood counts to healthier levels. If you are in treatment, your doctor may adjust your dose or change your medications.

If you become anemic, it's important to eat sufficient quantities of iron-rich foods (dark green leafy vegetables, beans, fish, and lean meat) or take iron, vitamin B, or folic acid supplements. Receiving a transfusion of red blood cells may also be helpful. Managing neutropenia often involves antibiotics to fight infection, medicines that stimulate the production of white blood cells, and in some cases, a bone marrow transplant.

Diarrhea or Constipation

Many people experience bowel changes during treatment. Chemotherapy, radiation, and gastrointestinal surgery may lead to loose and watery bowel movements (diarrhea). Persistent or severe diarrhea may result in the body losing more fluids than it takes in, causing dehydration and the loss of important minerals. Treatment-related diarrhea can be managed by drinking plenty of fluids (8–12 cups daily), eating several small meals throughout the day, eating foods that are high in potassium, getting enough (but not too much) sodium, and taking antidiarrheal medication as recommended by your doctor.

Constipation is the opposite problem. It's the inability to move the bowels, and it commonly occurs with pain medications. You can improve your regularity by staying hydrated, avoiding alcohol, being more active, and increasing the amount of fruits, vegetables, and high-fiber foods in your diet. If you still need help, ask your doctor whether a stool softener or processed fiber (Metamucil, Citrucel, and others) is safe to add to your daily diet or if you need a laxative to resolve the issue.

Hair Loss

Hair loss can be distressing because hair is such a visible part of an individual's persona. Many chemotherapies destroy rapidly growing cells, including hair follicles. However, not all chemotherapy drugs cause hair loss, and not everyone who receives chemotherapy loses their hair. Hair loss—on the head, arms, legs, face, and pubic area—may occur as soon as you start treatment or two to four weeks later. Hair often grows back in two to three months after chemotherapy ends.

Radiation may also temporarily eliminate hair in the treated area. Regrowth generally occurs within three to six months after radiation therapy is completed. Hair that regrows may be thinner, curlier, or straighter than it was. In time, it may return to how it was before treatment.

Tips for avoiding or reducing hair loss:

- Ask your doctor if a recommended treatment will likely cause hair loss and whether you're a candidate for any alternative treatments that don't result in hair loss.
- Ask your treatment center if scalp cooling, a cold cap for your scalp that minimizes hair loss from chemotherapy, is available. (Centers with these devices administer them for a fee, and they are worn before, during, and after each chemotherapy session.) A cold liquid is circulated through the FDA-approved DigniCap or Paxman cooling cap, narrowing blood vessels and reducing the amount of drug that reaches hair follicles. Other caps, which are filled with a cold gel, need to be replaced periodically as the cap thaws and the temperature of the gel increases. With this method, you're responsible for renting the cap and the refrigeration unit, applying the cap, and replacing it when needed. Scalp cooling can be pricey, and you won't know if it works until you try it. Your health insurance may cover a portion of the cost if your doctor provides a prescription for scalp cooling. The nonprofit organization HairToStay (www.hairtostay .org) may be able to help you pay for cold caps and scalp cooling.

- Consider cutting your hair short or shaving it to avoid having it come out later in clumps.
- Visit a wig shop (if you prefer to wear a wig until your hair grows out), where a professional can ensure a proper fit. Most health insurers pay for all or part of the cost of treatment-related wigs with a doctor's prescription. If you need financial assistance to pay for a wig, contact the American Cancer Society or visit EBeauty (www .ebeauty.com) for information about donated wigs.
- Use hats or scarves to protect your bare head from the sun. The Look Good Feel Better program (www.lookgoodfeelbetter.org) provides free information about selecting a wig, fitting turbans, and tying scarves.

Nausea and Vomiting

Several chemotherapy drugs, targeted therapies, and immunotherapies are likely to cause nausea and vomiting. Controlling these common, unpleasant effects will help you to feel better and prevent more serious problems, including weight loss, nutritional deficiencies, dehydration, and fatigue. Antinausea drugs, including Zofran (ondansetron), Aloxi (palonosetron HCl), and Emend (aprepitant), may be used alone or with a corticosteroid. FDA-approved Marinol (dronabinol) and Cesamet (nabilone) are prescribed less often. Notify your doctor if you can't keep fluids down or if you throw up for 24 hours or longer.

Tips to minimize nausea and vomiting:

- Breathe through your mouth when you feel nauseated.
- Eat several small meals rather than a few large meals.
- Avoid greasy, fatty, or strong-smelling foods, like onion and garlic.
- Season your food with ginger or drink ginger tea to settle your stomach.
- Choose cool or cold foods over warm or hot foods.
- Stay hydrated. If plain water doesn't appeal, add fresh citrus juice or try ginger ale.
- Suck on hard candy or ice.
- Don't lie flat for an hour or two after eating.
- Consider meditation, acupuncture, or hypnosis.

Appetite Problems and Weight Changes

Many people experience weight fluctuations during chemotherapy. You may feel more lethargic, exercise less, eat poorly, retain fluids, or take prescribed steroids to offset other side effects. All of these factors contribute to weight gain, as does treatment-induced menopause. While gaining a pound or two probably isn't significant, carrying extra weight is detrimental to your overall health and increases the risk for another cancer diagnosis.

Unlike many other side effects, weight gain doesn't automatically disappear after treatment. Good nutrition is important while you're being treated. Replace fatty snacks, fast foods, and restaurant takeout with properly proportioned, nutritious meals. Try keeping a food journal. Forgo dieting, and eat to give your body what it needs. A registered dietician or nutritionist can customize an eating plan that keeps you healthy and satisfied. Push yourself to be more active. Lose fat and build muscle with aerobic exercise and resistance training.

Cancer and related treatment may also cause weight loss. Surgery or radiation directed to the gastrointestinal tract can affect your ability to digest food and absorb nutrients. Chemotherapy and radiation may decrease appetite. It can be hard to eat when your appetite is gone and nothing tastes good. If you become underweight, add extra calories to your meals. Eat several small nutritionally balanced meals or snacks every two to three hours. If food doesn't appeal to you, try a nutritional meal replacement like Ensure.

Ask your doctor if your treatment medication could be causing your weight loss and if the dose can be adjusted. Request a referral to a nutritionist, who can help you adjust your diet so that you get adequate nutrition. If you continue to lose weight, your doctor may recommend steroid medications or megestrol acetate, a type of progesterone that may stimulate your appetite.

Bleeding or Bruising

Chemotherapy and targeted therapy reduce platelets, the cells that promote blood clotting, and may result in bleeding and bruising. Tell your doctor about bleeding that doesn't stop after a few minutes; bleeding from your mouth or nose; bleeding when you vomit; bleeding from your vagina (other than menstrual blood); heavier-than-normal bleeding during your period; urine that is red or pink; or stool that is black or bloody.

Tips to decrease bleeding and bruising:

- Avoid over-the-counter medicines that contain aspirin or ibuprofen. If your platelet count is low, ask your doctor for a list of other medicines that you should avoid.
- Limit or avoid alcohol.
- Check with your doctor before taking dietary supplements, which may promote bleeding.
- Take extra precautions to prevent bleeding or bruising. Brush your teeth gently, using a toothbrush with soft bristles. Wear shoes inside and outside. Use an electric shaver instead of a razor. Keep your skin and lips well moisturized.
- If you start to bleed, press down firmly on the area with a clean cloth until the bleeding stops. Use ice on areas that bruise.

Skin and Nail Changes

Some treatments produce mild to severe changes in the skin or nails. Certain chemotherapies may cause your skin to become dry or itchy, your skin may change pigment, and/or your nails may crack and darken. Areas of skin that are radiated sometimes become swollen or blistered, or you might look sunburned. Some people develop a moist reaction after radiation: painful, wet sores that become infected. Your doctor may prescribe specific medication to treat your skin while you're still receiving radiation.

Tamoxifen, targeted drugs, and immunotherapies may cause a rash, dry or blistering skin, and nail problems. Herceptin may thin and dry the skin.

Tips for dry or irradiated skin:

- Preventively moisturize your skin for a week or two before your treatment begins.
- Bathe or shower with lukewarm water and unscented baby soap or a mild cleansing cream.
- While your skin is still damp, gently rub in a fragrance-free cream or ointment, which moisturizes more effectively than lotion.
- Keep your skin well moisturized throughout the day and before bed.
- Try not to rub or scratch itchy skin. Your doctor can prescribe a soothing topical medication.

- Protect your skin with an SPF 30 or higher sunblock that protects against UV light.
- Stay hydrated, avoid caffeine and alcoholic drinks, and eat fruits, vegetables, lean proteins, and healthy fats, which contribute to skin health from the inside.
- Avoid smoking, which decreases circulation and blood flow to the skin.

Herceptin and some chemotherapy may cause nails to become brittle, darken, or lift from the nail bed. These effects can't typically be avoided, but you can take steps to otherwise protect your nails during treatment:

- Keep your nails short. Don't file any spots or grooves that appear. Wear gloves when you wash dishes, and try to keep your hands dry and well moisturized.
- Prevent dry cuticles with a generous application of cuticle cream or a moisturizer that doesn't contain alpha or beta hydroxy acid.
- If you polish your nails, use a formaldehyde-free product.
- Avoid artificial nails during treatment. If you have professional manicures or pedicures, bring your own sterilized tools to protect against infection.
- Let your doctor know right away if you develop signs of infection or inflammation.

Mouth Sores

Cancer-related sores that develop in the soft tissues of the mouth—lips, tongue, gums, the floor or roof of your mouth—can be mild to severely painful. Sometimes, they make it difficult to talk and eat. Unmanaged mouth sores may extend into the esophagus, making it hard to swallow and even breathe. These painful sores may develop as a result of chemotherapy—Adriamycin (doxorubicin), cisplatin, 5-FU (5-fluorouracil), and others—radiation therapy to the head or neck, targeted drugs, and some immunotherapies. Your doctor may recommend medicines that coat your mouth or numb the pain.

Tips to prevent or reduce mouth sores:

- Don't smoke before or during treatment.
- Swish cold water or ice chips in your mouth during the first 30 minutes of treatment to reduce the risk of mouth sores.

- Eat a produce-rich diet.
- Avoid alcohol, acidic and spicy foods, and other foods and beverages that may further irritate your mouth.
- Drink through a straw. Slowly eat small pieces of food.
- Rinse your mouth several times a day with a saline solution or a non-alcohol mouthwash to reduce discomfort.

— EXPERT VIEW —

Integrative Medicine and Hereditary Cancer

BY DILJEET SINGH, MD, DRPH

Integrative medicine is the health philosophy of using all available tools to help people achieve their best health outcomes. It emphasizes that these approaches to care be considered in combination with standard-of-care treatments when they are available. People diagnosed with cancer and those at high risk may benefit from integrative medicine combined with oncology. Nutrigenomics (how diet affects gene expression) and epigenetics (inherited modifications of gene expression) show that what we eat and how we live may influence how our genes behave. These studies support the use of Mediterranean and anti-inflammatory dietary approaches to cancer prevention.

Integrative oncology focuses on the innate healing abilities of our bodies and the tools we have to support these abilities. Integrative medicine includes biologically based practices (diet, dietary supplements, herbs), mind-body medicine (guided imagery, hypnosis, meditation, stress management, social support), manipulative or body-based practices (massage therapy, reflexology), energy medicine (acupuncture, Qigong, Reiki, yoga), and whole-system approaches (Ayurveda, traditional Chinese medicine, homeopathy). Although no studies of lifestyle modification specifically focus on people with inherited gene mutations, data from other populations tell us that aspects of our lifestyle, including diet, exercise, stress management, social support, and sleep habits, all have a tremendous impact on our overall health and well-being.

Adherence to a healthy diet and regular physical activity, along with individualized approaches to stress management and sleep, are the first essential steps in an integrative approach to optimal health for high-risk people. If you are interested in integrative therapy, you can

Palliative Care

Palliative care is specialized medical attention that focuses on making life easier for you and your family while you're being treated. Unlike hospice care, which is an end-of-life service, palliative care may benefit anyone with cancer of any stage. This specialized care is especially supportive if you have metastatic disease. The American Society of Clinical Oncology recommends palliative care for everyone with advanced cancer within eight weeks of diagnosis. It can make your life a lot easier as you go through different therapies.

As your health care team continues to treat your cancer, your palliative team focuses on relieving your emotional, psychological, and physical side effects—pain, fatigue, nausea, loss of appetite, trouble sleeping, anxiety, stress, and other problems. Your team may include a doctor who specializes in palliative care, a nurse, a social worker, physical or speech therapists, a nutritionist, and/or a household aide. Palliative care provides a range of therapies and services beginning at the time of diagnosis and continuing throughout treatment, including

- relieving your pain, fatigue, and other physical and emotional side effects

- helping you understand your treatment options to make the best medical decisions

- working with you, your family, and your doctors to ensure that you receive the medical, social, emotional, and practical support you need

- assisting your navigation through the health care system and health insurance coverage

Health insurance usually pays for some palliative services that are provided by medical professionals, but it doesn't always pay for nonmedical services, such as an aide who helps with meals or takes you to doctor appointments. Your health insurance company or your palliative care team can determine what your coverage includes. Medicare Part B may cover some palliative care. In some states, Medicaid also covers some palliative care treatments and medications. It's a good idea to request a schedule of copays or fees for which you'll be responsible before you agree to receive services.

request a referral. The Society for Integrative Oncology (www
.integrativeonc.org) has a directory of members that can be searched
by name, location, or expertise.

Long-Term Effects of Prevention and Treatment

While many side effects resolve on their own and don't usually last long beyond treatment and recovery, others remain or develop months or years later.
These may be more serious, may require medical intervention, or may never
go away.

Fatigue

Debilitating cancer-related exhaustion often lasts for years after treatment.
This is more likely to be the case if you have advanced disease or if you're treated
with a combination of therapies. Fatigue often occurs when radiation or toxic
anticancer drugs disrupt the normal functions of healthy cells or reproductive
and thyroid hormones. It's important to tell your doctor if you experience persistent fatigue. Tests can look for underlying causes, which can often be treated
with medication. Research consistently supports aerobic exercise (swimming,
walking, biking) combined with resistance training as a way to overcome fatigue and increase energy (see "Managing Immediate Side Effects" above).

Chronic Pain

Short-term discomfort from some treatments can be expected after surgery
and during recovery. Chronic pain is different. It remains or develops after
treatment is over. Finding relief for persistent pain can be frustrating, especially when pain seems to affect every movement you make. You should always
talk to your doctor if you have unrelenting pain that disrupts your normal
life because left untreated, it can reduce your functionality, interfere with your
sleep, and weaken your physical, emotional, and psychological well-being.
It's important that you not ignore your pain, try to tough it out, or believe
that nothing can be done to help you.

While pain can't always be eliminated, it can usually be improved so that
you feel better. A combination of oral medications, anesthetic skin patches,

physical therapy, therapeutic massage, acupuncture/acupressure, and other integrative therapies (see "Expert View: Integrative Medicine and Hereditary Cancer") often works well. Routine exercise prompts your body to release endorphins, which block pain signals to the brain and may make your pain more tolerable. If your pain is debilitating, a combination of short- and long-acting opioids may be beneficial. Radiation may reduce pain from bone metastases.

You may need to consult with a pain specialist and go through a trial-and-error process to find a solution that works. Common long-term pain related to cancer and treatment includes the following:

- Arthralgia (joint pain and stiffness) may develop when estrogen levels decline, which may be caused by aromatase inhibitors or chemotherapies that cause early menopause. Arthralgias also develop when cancer spreads to the bone. Corticosteroids and nonsteroidal anti-inflammatory drugs, including ibuprofen, may reduce inflammation-induced pain, although you should ask your doctor if it's safe to take them long term. Reducing the dosage of a treatment drug often reduces these symptoms. If an aromatase inhibitor is causing your arthralgia, your doctor may recommend a different one. The antidepressant drug Cymbalta (duloxetine) may improve some arthralgias. Applying ice or heat may be a short-term remedy. Acupuncture, yoga, or therapeutic massage reduces joint pain and improves functionality for some people. Modest walking, bicycling, swimming, and resistance training with light weights may safely relieve pressure in your hips and knees.
- Neuropathy (nerve pain) may result from taxane and platinum chemotherapies. These medications may injure or irritate nerves, causing pain, numbness, burning, or pins-and-needles tingling. Radiation and tumors that press on sensitive nerves may also cause neuropathy. Severe neuropathy may affect simple, everyday functions, such as walking or getting in and out of bed. It may cause numbness in the feet that hinders mobility and increases the risk of falling. Anticonvulsants or antidepressants like Cymbalta (duloxetine), which alter chemical signals in the body, may be more effective than conventional painkillers. Using a battery-operated *transcutaneous electrical nerve stimulation (TENS)* unit that delivers low-voltage electrical impulses under the skin is another option. If your pain is severe, ask

your doctor about an implantable pump that delivers potent pain medicine directly into your spinal fluid. Yoga, neurofeedback, and other mind-body approaches may limit pain by refocusing the brain, changing how pain signals are perceived. These techniques may also help you manage depression, stress, and negative emotions, all of which can intensify pain. Nerve-blocking medications or the destruction of rogue nerves may resolve severe pain that doesn't respond to other treatments.

- A significant number of individuals who have mastectomy experience a sharp, burning, or shooting pain in the mastectomy scar, underarm, chest wall, or shoulder long after they've healed. This chronic postmastectomy pain syndrome is a type of neuropathy that results from severing sensory nerves in the chest. Postmastectomy pain syndrome may be difficult to diagnose because it can be mistaken for ordinary postsurgical pain. Acupuncture and massage may provide temporary relief. Antidepressants that calm damaged nerves may be a longer-lasting solution. A neurologist can make a correct diagnosis and prescribe the best path forward. It may also be helpful to consult with a pain specialist.

Lymphedema

Removing or radiating lymph nodes creates a lifetime risk for lymphedema, chronic swelling that develops when a part of the lymph system can no longer filter fluids, which then collect in the area that was treated. Lymphedema may appear any time after surgery or radiation. It's common after breast cancer surgery when underarm lymph nodes are removed or radiated (sometimes developing years later), but it may also develop after treatment for other cancers. If any of your lymph nodes are removed, ask your doctor about lifelong precautionary measures to reduce your risk of symptoms. Contact your doctor at the first sign of swelling—even mild swelling—in the treated area.

When caught early, lymphedema can be managed with compression garments, lymphatic massage by a certified lymphedema therapist, and self-massage to redirect fluids and reduce swelling. Gentle strength training directed by a specially trained physical therapist may also reduce symptoms. Some moderate or severe cases may be improved with surgical procedures that reroute lymphatic drainage, debulk excess fluid and fat, or replace damaged lymph nodes with healthy nodes from elsewhere in the body.

Organ Damage

Certain chemotherapy agents, targeted drugs, and radiation may damage organs, creating long-term health problems as you age. Some treatments raise the risk for blood clots or reduce heart function, leading to coronary artery disease and inflammation of the heart muscle, which can cause heart failure. High doses of radiation to the abdomen and some immunotherapies, including Keytruda, Yervoy, Opdivo, and Proleukin (aldesleukin), may impair liver function. Cisplatin, carboplatin, doxorubicin, cyclophosphamide, aldesleukin, and interferon alfa may lead to kidney problems.

If you're treated with a drug that elevates the risk for organ damage, you'll be carefully monitored during and after your treatment so that any problem can be quickly identified and managed. Blood pressure medications such as beta blockers or angiotensin-converting enzyme inhibitors may protect the heart from treatment-related damage.

Increased Risk for Certain Cancers

Some chemotherapies and targeted therapies increase the risk for the blood cancers acute myelogenous leukemia and acute lymphocytic leukemia. *BRAF* inhibitors, a type of targeted therapy commonly used in melanoma and colorectal cancers, increase the risk for a type of skin cancer known as cutaneous squamous cell carcinoma.

Disrupted Emotional Health and Wellness

Coping with the unsettling nature of cancer can be difficult and disruptive. A cancer diagnosis, treatment, and related changes in your physical health, strength, body function, appearance, and self-image may induce or exacerbate existing mental health challenges. Though some days will be better than others, depression and feelings of frustration or fear may wreak havoc on your life, your family, and your well-being. You don't have to endure these feelings. In fact, they can be detrimental to your health. It's important to recognize and treat them, just as you would other health issues.

Request a referral to a mental health professional who can diagnose and help you to manage any emotionally disturbing issues with therapy and/or medications. Even when you feel that you're in control and doing well, setbacks can occur. Be kind and patient with yourself when this happens. Try massage, music and art therapy, yoga, meditation, and other ways to lift your mood and lighten your spirit.

Previvorship, Survivorship, and Follow-Up Care

For many people with inherited high-risk mutations, their experience is a continuum: from previvor to patient to cancer survivor. If you're a previvor—you've inherited a high-risk gene mutation but haven't developed cancer—it's important to be aware of your risk, take steps to reduce it, and have all recommended physical exams and screenings. Even after you've taken steps to manage your cancer risk, you may have other health consequences related to your inherited mutation or to risk-reducing surgeries.

If you've completed cancer treatment, you're a survivor, but you still need regular follow-ups to ensure that you remain in good health. The National Comprehensive Cancer Network guidelines for cancer survivors address the long-term health consequences associated with cancer treatment. The NCCN recommends an annual checkup by your primary care physician or oncologist for several health issues, including

- heart disease
- fatigue
- pain
- menopause symptoms
- lymphedema
- memory and cognitive issues
- emotional distress
- sexual dysfunction
- sleep disorders

End-of-Life Issues

If your cancer can no longer be improved or controlled, your tumor-focused treatment will end. Even so, your care will continue, with a focus on improving your quality of life and making you as comfortable as possible. This is a time to decide if you prefer to stay at home or enter a hospice care facility. It's also time to designate someone to make decisions for you if you become unable to make them for yourself. If you haven't already done so, consider

The Survivorship Care Plan

When your treatment ends, your doctor should provide you with a survivorship care plan. (Request this document if your doctor doesn't offer it.) This plan should include all of the following items:

- A record of the treatment you received.

- An outline of recommended follow-up visits, tests, and care you should have now and in the future. These will be managed by your primary physician as part of your overall health care.

- A list of late- or long-term treatment side effects that may develop, symptoms to watch for, and when you should contact your doctor.

- Suggestions for diet, nutrition, physical activity, and staying healthy.

creating the following documents to get your affairs in order and ensure that your preferences will be honored:

- a legal will
- an estate plan (a financial advisor or estate planner can help determine if you need one)
- an advance health care directive or a do-not-resuscitate order so that your family and doctors are aware of the end-of-life care you want to receive
- your wishes for a funeral or memorial service

Hospice Care

Hospice care is palliative care for the terminally ill. Provided in your own home or in a hospice facility, it's given when treatment no longer slows the progression of disease and your doctor estimates your life expectancy to be six months or less. Hospice provides compassionate comfort and care for you during the final stages of life while supporting your caregiver and family and respecting your personal, cultural, and spiritual priorities. It's important to begin hospice care as soon as it's needed so that you can take full advantage of the support and assistance hospice provides. Although treatment may have stopped working or you have decided to no longer accept treatment, the palliative focus may improve the way you feel and give you the highest possible quality of life. Some studies show that hospice care may increase survival.

Your hospice care team will include a doctor who specializes in pain management, who will work closely with your primary doctor to coordinate your care, a nurse, a social worker, therapists, a home aide, and a member of the clergy or other spiritual counselor. When you receive hospice at home, your spouse, partner, or other designated primary caregiver provides day-to-day care, while your hospice team provides specialized services, which may include

- managing your symptoms to keep you as comfortable as possible
- providing medications, medical supplies, and equipment
- arranging for speech or physical therapy, if needed
- coaching your family on the best way to care for you
- overseeing your care to temporarily relieve your caregiver
- helping with housekeeping, cooking, personal care, and grooming, if needed
- providing companionship and practical services, like grocery shopping
- offering emotional and spiritual support for you and your family

Medicare pays for two 90-day periods of hospice care followed by an unlimited number of covered 60-day periods if your doctor believes you have less than six months to live. Your long-term health care policy, if you have one, may also include hospice benefits. You pay no deductible for hospice services, but you may be required to make copayments for prescriptions. If you no longer meet eligibility or no longer need hospice, your Medicare benefits revert to what they were before you entered hospice.

Most states have similar hospice benefits, which include the costs of a hospital bed, wheelchair, walker, oxygen, or other medical equipment you may need. If your health care policy doesn't cover hospice services or you aren't insured and can't afford them, your local hospice provider can provide information about financial aid programs that reduce or cover the cost for some patients.

Chapter 30

Making Difficult Decisions

Although you can't change your genetics, you can take action to detect cancer early, reduce your odds of a cancer diagnosis, and prolong your survival.

Decisions about inherited risk and hereditary cancer can be among the most challenging choices you'll ever have to make. But in many cases, they can be lifesaving. So, how do you go about making these tough decisions? First, gather all the credible, up-to-date information you need, giving yourself time to review and understand all of it. Consider both the near-term and long-term benefits and limitations of each choice. In some cases, you may have several options to choose from, and in others, you may not. Try to recognize and manage the strong, unanticipated emotions you may feel so that they don't cloud your thinking. If you're unable to reach a conclusion on your own, speak with a counselor or someone you trust who can help you organize your thoughts, weigh your alternatives, and help you through the process of making decisions that are in your best interest.

Start at the Beginning:
Should You Be Tested?

Genetic testing can provide lifesaving information. Some people want to know whether they have inherited cancer risk so that they can take preventive measures. Others prefer not to be tested, fearing the implications of a positive result. Although facing a positive test may be difficult, it also provides the opportunity to be proactive. An analysis of a small sample of your blood or saliva can determine whether you're genetically susceptible to one or more cancers. It's a simple action that can either release your fear about inherited cancer risk or set into motion actions that will positively or negatively affect you now and in the future.

Speaking with a qualified genetics expert can alleviate much of the uncertainty about whether you should be tested and what the results might mean for you and your family. A genetic counselor is a reliable source of up-to-date information and a resource to help you formulate a plan. Your counselor will consider your personal situation and personal preferences, supporting your efforts to pursue the informed decision that is right for you.

If you decide to proceed with genetic testing, your counselor will make sure that the proper test is ordered, help to obtain insurance coverage and limit your out-of-pocket costs, and correctly interpret your results. If a doctor or a relative has recommended that you have genetic testing but you've decided not to pursue it, a genetic counselor can determine whether your decision is supported by facts and is in your best interest. Genetic testing can be beneficial for previvors and survivors.

- If you've never been diagnosed with cancer, genetic testing may clarify your risk and help you make decisions about cancer screening and prevention.
- If you're newly diagnosed with cancer or a recurrence, testing may influence your treatment decisions.
- If you've already completed treatment for cancer, genetic testing may help you understand your risk for a new cancer and help you decide about related screening and prevention.

— My Story —
Sharing Information with
Patience and Encouragement

After I tested positive for an inherited mutation, I felt a responsibility to share my information with my uncle and cousins. I gave my uncle our family's medical history, suggested he might want to be tested, and gave him information about genetic counselors in his area. He asked that I not share the information with my cousins before he had time to review it. As time passed, I began online contact with a cousin, although I never

Should You Be Tested for an Inherited Mutation?

Take the following steps to determine if testing is right for you:

- Learn about your family's medical history (chapter 2).
- Recognize the signs of an inherited mutation or hereditary cancer in your family (chapter 3).
- Speak with a qualified genetics expert if you suspect that you have an inherited mutation, even if your family medical history isn't available (chapter 3).
- Consider how your treatment options might change based on your test results (chapter 4).
- Think about the actions you might take to manage your cancer risk if you test positive (chapter 13).

asked if he knew anything about our family's mutation because I wanted to respect my uncle's request. I felt my cousins needed to make their own informed decisions. I wasn't sure what I should do. I followed up with my uncle and carefully emphasized how his own genetic counseling would give my cousins information they deserved to have. He did see a genetic counselor and was tested. He doesn't have the mutation. I was ready to tell him that I would speak to my cousins about this against his wishes if he didn't share the information. Happily, that wasn't necessary.

—Cathy

Decisions about Your Cancer Risk

A positive test for an inherited mutation presents you with special concerns and unique challenges. While it's important to take an elevated risk seriously, a positive test doesn't guarantee that you'll develop cancer. Compared to someone in the general population, however, the likelihood of a diagnosis is increased, possibly significantly so. Having a high-risk gene mutation doesn't mean that you're helpless or hopeless, however. Although you can't change your genetics, you can take action to detect cancer early, reduce your odds of a cancer diagnosis, and prolong your survival.

You may struggle to know what to do. How do you determine whether the benefits of different risk management options outweigh the risks? Is it safe or wise to try surveillance if you are high risk? Can you reconcile experiencing early menopause from chemoprevention with a significantly lower cancer risk? Are you ready to accept body-altering surgery—the loss of your breasts, stomach, colon, or uterus—to reduce your cancer risk?

If you're young when you learn that you have a mutation, you face uncertainties about the risk and reality of cancer at a time when you probably have few resources and little experience with serious disease. You may be working hard to position yourself professionally, you may be starting a family, or you may already have young children. The reality of some procedures may make you feel that you would be sacrificing your youth and fertility to prevent or treat cancer. Your personal priorities and tolerance for risk will shape your decisions, which may be different than those of someone else in a similar situation.

— THE **FORCE** PERSPECTIVE —

Considering Your Five-Year Risk

Making challenging decisions about your cancer risk should encompass your current risk as well as your lifetime risk. Your risk over the next several years may be more relevant to your decision-making than your lifetime risk for cancer. If you're young when you're faced with these difficult choices, you might find it helpful to make decisions based on your cancer risk in the next 5–10 years, after which you can reassess your risk, your priorities, and your subsequent decisions.

Considering cancer risk in this way allows you to make decisions that are based on your short-term circumstances as well as longer-term plans for education, employment, housing, health insurance, relationships, and family planning. Depending on your age, you might prefer increased surveillance now and risk-reducing surgery or chemoprevention when your situation changes or when your risk reaches a level that you consider unacceptable. Risk estimates aren't always presented in a way that facilitates this type of planning, so it may be helpful to ask your health care team to provide you with cancer risk estimates that are broken down into five-year increments.

When comparing risk management alternatives—increased screening, chemoprevention, or surgery—consider the following for each option:

- To what degree does it reduce your chance of a cancer diagnosis?
- How might it affect your overall survival?
- What are the odds that a future cancer will be found early, when it's most treatable?
- Do the benefits outweigh the risk of side effects? When comparing risk-reducing surgery, for example, consider the impact of the loss of your breasts, ovaries, stomach, or other organs on your long-term health and well-being.
- How will it affect your short- or long-term fertility, normal bodily functions, and quality of life? How would a cancer diagnosis affect these health issues?
- What will recovery involve?
- What surveillance or follow-up will you require afterward?
- Will your health insurance cover the costs of medical services and procedures that support the health choices you make? What will your out-of-pocket costs be?

Decisions about Treatment

If you're diagnosed with cancer, ask your doctor if you should be tested for an inherited mutation (if you haven't already been tested) and whether your tumor has been tested for biomarkers (chapters 20–25). The results of these tests can provide information that may affect your decisions about treatment. When comparing treatment options, consider the following for each alternative:

- Will it improve your prognosis?
- How will it affect the chance of recurrence?
- How will it affect your risk for another primary cancer?
- What short- and long-term side effects are possible?

Your Culture and Beliefs May Affect How You Confront Your Risk

We all have different ideas about health, medicine, and cancer risk. These ideas are often shaped by how we were raised, our family beliefs, and our observations of others who have been diagnosed. Concerns about modesty may prevent us from learning more about cancers or even speaking about these issues. Social and economic influences may keep us from performing self-exams, having routine screenings, or changing lifestyle behaviors that affect our risk. Some cultures accept illness as a fait accompli, a destiny we can't control, so why worry about it or try to prevent it? Our culture and shared values connect us to family and community, which provide our support system, but it can be helpful to consider whether your beliefs help or hinder how you approach important health issues.

- How will it affect your short- or long-term fertility, normal bodily functions, and quality of life?
- What will recovery involve?
- Do the benefits outweigh the expected side effects?
- What follow-up will be required?

Get a Second Opinion

It's always wise to get a second opinion about diagnosis and treatment, and most insurance plans cover the cost. Let your doctor know that you'd like a referral to another doctor who specializes in your cancer so that you can consider all of your options. (You can also contact your insurance company, a local medical society, or the nearest university hospital for the name of an expert.) This is a standard medical practice, and your doctor shouldn't be offended. Then request that your latest test results be forwarded to the second doctor for review. Getting another doctor's recommendation may confirm what your own doctor has advised or introduce other treatment options. In almost all cases, it's safe to briefly delay treatment while you get another opinion and think through your options.

A tumor board is an opportunity for a multidisciplinary second opinion. Tumor boards are made up of doctors and other health care specialists with different expertise who meet regularly to discuss unusual or difficult cancer cases and decide on the best possible treatment plan. Tumor board consideration may be helpful if you have an uncommon type of cancer or your treatment isn't working as well as expected. Your oncologist can provide more information about submitting your circumstances to your hospital's tumor board.

Prevention and Treatment Clinical Trials

Every new cancer drug, treatment, method of screening, and approach to prevention is the result of a clinical trial. Once considered to be the last possible chance for treatment, clinical trials now treat all stages of cancer. Research may offer opportunities for you to receive new targeted drugs, more effective screening, and new approaches to prevent cancer. Clinical trials provide a high standard of care, but there's no guarantee that the drug or treatment will work as hoped.

Researching new medications to prevent and treat cancer involves a multistep process. After laboratory testing, researchers use clinical trials to observe how well they work in volunteer participants. Phase 1 trials test the safety and determine the best dosage of a new medication among a small group of people. Phase 2 trials determine whether the agent produces the desired response in a larger group. Phase 3 trials compare the new agent to the standard of care in hundreds or thousands of people. Drugs that successfully complete this phase may request FDA approval. Finally, phase 4 post-approval trials evaluate the long-term side effects among several thousand participants over a longer period of time.

When Your Family Disagrees
with Your Decisions

Your risk management decisions may be unconditionally supported by your family, particularly if cancer is already a much-discussed topic. For many families, the opposite is true. It's difficult to share your risk management decisions with people who argue, aren't interested, or tell you that your decisions are wrong. Some people may respond with anger, suspicion, or a barrage of questions you're unprepared to answer. One family member may agree with your course of action while another considers it too drastic while yet another feels guilty and avoids the topic altogether. A relative who has struggled through cancer treatment may tell you to proceed full steam ahead with surgery, while another who hasn't may consider it too extreme. Well-intentioned loved ones might try to protect you by dismissing your fears or telling you to think positively. They may be afraid for you or not want to see you unhappy.

It's natural for the people who care about you to reassure you; it may be equally important for you to have a confidante with whom you can share your fears. The input of others is helpful to gain perspective, but ultimately, risk management decisions are yours and yours alone. Try to surround yourself with people who encourage your efforts to do research and learn about your options, and who accept and support your decisions. They may form a buffer for communication between you and those who don't accept your decisions.

Clinical trials are necessary to advance cancer prevention, screening, and treatment, yet they're only possible when enough people volunteer to participate. These essential trials are particularly important for members of the hereditary cancer community, who benefit from prevention and treatments that address the unique nuances of inherited cancers. Your doctor can let you know of clinical trials that involve the type of mutation or cancer that you have. Or use the National Institutes of Health searchable database to find a trial for which you're eligible (www.clinicaltrials.gov). FORCE maintains an online database of clinical trials specifically focused on hereditary cancers.

Decision-Making in 15 Steps

Making decisions about testing, risk management, and treatment can be overwhelming, and there may appear to be no light at the end of the tunnel. Making these complex decisions may seem like choosing the lesser of two (or three or four) evils. Even though you probably prefer none of them, knowing all of your options allows you to carefully consider each alternative before deciding which is best for you. While you may feel a sense of urgency to make a choice, you may also be fearful to proceed. How do you weigh all the options and consequences and make effective decisions that you can live with? You do it one step at a time.

1. Assemble a health care team of people you trust who have experience preventing or treating hereditary cancer.
2. Learn all you can about your current and lifetime risk, risk management options, diagnosis, and treatment alternatives.
3. Take advantage of all available resources, including your health care team, the suggestions in this book, FORCE, and other previvors and survivors.
4. Recruit your spouse, partner, family members, or a trusted friend to help with research and provide a fresh perspective.
5. Keep a list of questions. Look for answers.
6. Ask your health care team for clarification when you're unclear.
7. Work your way through each of your options one by one, comparing benefits and risks.
8. Eliminate unacceptable options and prioritize the choices that remain.

Questions to Ask the Clinical Trial Coordinator before You Participate

- What is the trial's objective?

- Is the trial enrolling participants?

- What are the eligibility criteria for participation?

- How does the proposed intervention differ from standard treatment?

- Does the trial involve the use of a placebo? If so, is the study designed to give you access to the experimental treatment if standard care doesn't help you?

- Which costs will be paid by the trial, and which will you be responsible for?

- Is the trial location easily accessible, or will you need to travel?

- Will there be additional time requirements for monitoring, testing, and follow-up?

- How long will the trial last?

- Who is sponsoring or funding the trial?

Clinical trials sometimes provide all drugs and treatments, related monitoring, and follow-up at no cost, but some do not. Check with your health insurance company to clarify what trial-related costs it will and won't pay for or reimburse. The Affordable Care Act requires health plans established after March 23, 2010, to provide routine health care during a member's participation in certain types of clinical trials. Health insurers may not deny or limit coverage for office visits, tests, or treatment for health issues that are unrelated to the trial. Nor may they increase premiums or deductibles because of participation in a clinical trial.

9. Give yourself a break periodically to avoid information overload.
10. Stop researching when you have all the information you can absorb and need to make decisions.
11. Allow yourself time to let it all sink in.
12. Stay organized. Keep a binder of all your medical records, test results, research, and documents related to your previvor or survivor status.
13. Take care of yourself. Eat balanced meals, get some physical activity most days, and give yourself plenty of rest.
14. Find an outlet for your frustrations, fears, and worry. Speak with a mental health professional if you need help dealing with emotional stress.
15. You don't have to face these issues alone. Reach out to FORCE online (www.facingourrisk.org), through our helpline (866-288-7475), or in person at a local FORCE outreach group. We can connect you with someone who went through decisions similar to yours, based on age, mutation, diagnosis, and other factors.

— THE FORCE PERSPECTIVE —

Coping with Decisions

Hereditary cancer doesn't end with a single decision. Each answer, test result, and choice means sacrifices, and every sacrifice requires adjustment. You move forward step by step. Each one requires emotional investment, which is usually followed by a period of grieving, accepting uncertainty, and adjusting to changes. No matter which course of action you choose, and whether or not things go according to plan, you must live with the consequences. At some point, moving forward becomes a leap of faith that you've gathered as much information as you need, you know what to expect from the actions you've decided upon, and you've chosen the best path forward. If the unexpected occurs—as it sometimes does—be patient and forgiving with yourself, and know that you made the best decision you could at the time. Then, move on to the next set of decisions and deal with what lies ahead. In this way, you can move forward and eventually allow yourself to find joy in life and live it to the fullest.

Chapter 31

You Are Not Alone

Don't be afraid to ask for help if sadness, anxiety, depression, or anger affect your day-to-day life. A psychiatrist can evaluate you for clinical disorders that may benefit from medical treatment. A social worker, mental health counselor, or behavioral therapist can help you work through and move beyond particularly disruptive or stressful feelings and situations.

No matter where you are in the hereditary cancer experience, at some point you may feel as though you're facing a wall of unsolvable problems—and that you're doing so alone. A strong support system, a trusted team of health experts, knowing your rights, and asking for help when you need it can make it easier for you to weather emotional turbulence and stay mentally strong as you navigate your path.

Create a Support System

It's so important to let people help and support you along the way. You never have to face hard decisions, indecision, or dark moments alone. There is an entire community of people like you to provide help and support, suggest a new perspective, or simply provide a safe environment for you to vent about how you're feeling, and there are numerous resources to guide you.

Assemble a Team of Health Care Experts

You have a choice in who manages your care, although your selection may be limited by your health insurance or your geographical location. Your team should be made up of knowledgeable health care professionals who have experience with hereditary risk and hereditary cancers. Ask for referrals from your primary doctor, family members, friends, colleagues, and/or your health insurance company. Numerous major universities and community hospitals have multidisciplinary health care teams in a single location.

Ask doctors about their experience with the type of mutation, risk, or cancer that you have. Choose those who inspire your trust, who listen to your preferences and priorities, and who are competent and compassionate in equal measure. Your relationships with them may last well beyond your initial consultation.

Before genetic testing, your team might include your primary physician or oncologist and a genetics expert. After genetic testing, your genetic counselor will interpret your test results and your cancer risk. Depending on the specific cancers for which you have heightened risk, your team should include health care professionals who follow national risk management guidelines for cancer screening and prevention.

If you decide to pursue close surveillance or risk-reducing procedures, your team may include a gynecologist, surgeon (a general surgeon, surgical oncologist, and/or plastic surgeon), urologist, gastroenterologist, dermatologist, ophthalmologist, fertility expert, endocrinologist, nurses, technicians who administer tests and scans, and others.

During treatment, your multidisciplinary team may include a medical oncologist, radiation oncologist, surgical oncologist, oncology nurse, pain specialist, palliative care specialist, nutritionist, and others who have expertise caring for high-risk people. You may also be supported with the services of a social worker and/or a physical, occupational, or behavioral therapist.

After treatment, your team may be composed of a primary physician, pain specialist, palliative care specialist, physical therapist, and others, depending on your follow-up care. If needed, hospice experts may provide your primary care.

Share with Friends and Family

Your loved ones can't undergo your treatment for you or make your high risk or cancer disappear, but they can love and support you when you most need it. Sharing your feelings with friends and family can help you shoulder the emotional and physical burdens you may experience with hereditary risk, testing, risk management, diagnosis, and treatment. Loved ones may also help with practical issues, like making meals, doing chores, and providing childcare.

Connect with Peers

Sharing your experiences and frustrations with others who have faced similar circumstances may provide inspiration and relieve your feelings of isolation. Whether you join an in-person or online support group or connect one-on-one with a peer, compassionate camaraderie may empower you so that you feel more hopeful and positive. A support group is a safe environment where you can openly talk about your experiences—including concerns or issues that may be difficult to share with your family or friends—and receive caring support from people who have "been there, done that" and understand what you're going through.

Engage a Patient Navigator

If you've been diagnosed with cancer, consider using a patient navigator, a health professional who can guide you through screening, diagnosis, treatment, and follow-up and help you overcome obstacles to getting the care, treatment, supportive services, and resources you need. A patient navigator can help you manage your medical appointments and medical records, facilitate communication between you and your health care team, and assist your efforts to find financial, legal, and social support. They may also interact with your health insurance company and employer on your behalf.

Let FORCE Help You

The national nonprofit organization Facing Our Risk of Cancer Empowered was founded on the principle that no one needs to face hereditary cancer alone. FORCE is just a call, email, or online visit away (www.facingourrisk .org). FORCE's Peer Navigation Program, helpline, message boards, and local outreach coordinators are ready to provide confidential support and resources, and connect you with others whose age, mutation, diagnosis, and other factors mirror your own high-risk circumstances.

Consult with Mental Health Professionals

Don't be afraid to ask for help if sadness, anxiety, depression, or anger affect your day-to-day life. A psychiatrist can evaluate you for clinical disorders that may benefit from medical treatment. A social worker, mental health counselor, or behavioral therapist can help you work through and move beyond particularly disruptive or stressful feelings and situations. Don't be afraid to seek private counseling or group therapy. Consider speaking with a member of the clergy or someone else who can help make difficult times easier and reinforce your faith or spirituality.

— **THE FORCE PERSPECTIVE** —

Asking for Help

Asking for help can be difficult, especially if you're used to being healthy, strong, and self-sufficient. Even when you do ask, sometimes the reactions of others can undermine your confidence. People with inherited mutations often tell us they feel disturbed by misguided reactions to their circumstances.

"Why have my friends abandoned me during the hardest time of my life?"
"Why doesn't my sibling (partner/spouse/friend) understand what I
    need?"
"How can my co-workers be so insensitive?"

Sometimes, people say nothing because they're afraid to say the wrong thing. Sometimes, people say the wrong thing because they don't want to be silent. They want to support you, but they just don't know how. Facing a cancer risk or cancer itself is not the time to be stoic, and you might consider that you're giving your loved ones an opportunity to support you. It's a loving kindness to ask people for help and to let them know exactly what you need.

Find Emotional Strength

Coping with a high-risk mutation or a cancer diagnosis is a deeply personal experience that can tax your emotional resilience as well as your physical strength. Everyone responds differently, and there is no "normal" way to feel. You may be overcome with disbelief, worry, exhaustion, or uncertainty about your high risk, your diagnosis, or your treatment. Emotional roadblocks can threaten your quality of life and outlook. You may find it hard to let go of the upheaval, disruption, angst, and grief you experience. It's not always possible to just snap out of it, even if well-intentioned people tell you that you should.

Your mind is a powerful tool. Science acknowledges the direct correlation between mind, body, and health. Your thoughts can drag you down or lift you up. You may be dealing with a devastating diagnosis, side effects, or emotional issues, but you can still make your life meaningful. A behavioral therapist may help you to direct your thoughts where you want them to go. If you're feeling emotionally paralyzed, strive to become an active participant in resolving each issue. No matter what the situation that makes you feel stuck, developing a plan for moving forward will be helpful. It may be easier to confront and deal with these issues if you formulate small steps into an overall plan for tackling each concern. Enlist the help of your support system to identify and address these steps.

Get help when you need it. Share your feelings with people you love and trust. Let yourself grieve for what you've lost—time, emotional security, even physical parts of you. Keep a journal, including a daily list of things for which you feel grateful. Take steps to find emotional balance.

— **EXPERT VIEW** —

A Toolkit for Emotional Health

BY KAREN HURLEY, PHD

- Support. Make sure you have at least one confidante who will listen attentively without judgment or an agenda of their own.
- Coping statements. Create a series of meaningful positive statements to coach yourself through difficult moments.
- Letting go. Distinguish between what you can and cannot control. You can change your thoughts. You can't change other people's reactions.
- Balance. Prioritize enjoyable activities that will refresh you enough to take on the next round of appointments, decisions, and responsibilities.
- Physical activity. Stay healthy and energized with exercise. It's a natural mood enhancer.

- Information thermostat. Figure out the next thing you need to know, and then pause there before you become overwhelmed.
- Breathing. Remember that even when the pressure is on, there is always time to take a breath. A deep breath can reconnect you with the calm, centered place from which you make your best decisions.

Pursue Financial Resources

Medical care, especially cancer treatment and follow-up care, often comes with a high price tag—a fact that many patients don't discover until they're diagnosed and treated. After a cancer diagnosis, health care costs can strain your finances, even when you have health insurance. Deductibles, coinsurance, co-payments, travel costs related to treatment, and other out-of-pocket expenses can be staggering, depending on the type of care you need and the terms of your health care plan. If you don't have health insurance, you're underinsured, or you're unemployed, paying for treatment may be beyond your means. It helps to know what medical costs you'll be responsible for before you get the bills, because many financial resources are available and worth pursuing.

- Explore whether you have access to a patient navigator, social worker, or financial counselor who can provide guidance and direct you to resources and assistance programs.
- Ask your doctor if generic medications can be substituted for brand-name drugs without sacrificing effectiveness.
- Contact the pharmaceutical companies that manufacture your prescribed medicines to see if you're eligible for underwritten or discounted costs.
- Reach out to local organizations that provide food, transportation, and other nonfinancial support services.
- Ask providers, including hospitals and treatment centers, if you can make monthly payments, rather than paying the full amount in a lump sum, or if discounts for the uninsured or underinsured are available.
- Contact local health agencies and nonprofit groups to inquire about financial assistance related to high-risk services and treatment.
- Contact the Patient Advocate Foundation (www.patientadvocate .org) for help in finding financial assistance programs, resources,

and/or copay assistance programs and in navigating your health plan's benefits.

- Contact Triage Cancer (www.triagecancer.org) to understand your health insurance options and state and federal laws governing coverage for your care.

If You're Unable to Work

If you need to take time off work because of cancer treatment, surgery, or related medical or psychological issues or if you're unable to work due to other health issues, you may be able to use paid sick leave, vacation days, or unpaid leave. The Family and Medical Leave Act requires employers with 50 or more employees to provide eligible staff with up to 12 weeks of unpaid leave per year, while protecting your job. Your human resources department or employer should be able to further explain the details of these benefits.

You may be able to replace lost wages with disability benefits provided by your employer or with temporary disability benefits from your state. The US Social Security Administration (www.ssa.gov) provides two types of disability. If you're unable to perform your job for a year or more due to cancer (or another medical condition), you may be eligible for Social Security disability insurance if you've worked long enough and paid into Social Security. You may be eligible to receive funds from Supplemental Security Income if you've worked long enough and paid into Social Security. If you have private disability insurance, review your policy or contact your insurance agent for information about the benefits that are available to you.

Look to the Horizon

Living in a high-risk body or dealing with cancer isn't easy. It can be difficult to envision a time when your life will be free of doctor appointments, treatments, uncertainty, and imbalance. You can't undo what you've been through and the impact it has had on your life. But you can make your quality of life a priority, so that you can stay as mentally and physically strong as possible.

Try to keep your eye on the prize: regaining your sense of self-esteem, your confidence, and control of your life. It's not always easy to be positive, and some days will be better than others. Nourish your body and your mind. Do something good for yourself every day: 5 minutes of deep breathing, 30 minutes of yoga, or a long walk. Lose yourself in a good book, enjoy conversations with friends, find something to laugh about, or even help others. Treat yourself kindly and with patience. Engage rather than isolate. Let people help and support you, especially if you find yourself emotionally stuck.

You can't always change your situation, but you can try to gain control over your reactions and perspective. In this way, you can become empowered to move forward.

Acknowledgments

We gratefully acknowledge the input, support, and enthusiasm of the many people who helped make this book possible. We appreciate the contribution of Rebecca Sutphen, MD, coauthor of our original book, *Confronting Hereditary Breast and Ovarian Cancer*. Thank you to all who shared personal stories and to each of the health care professionals and researchers who took the time to contribute their expert view. We also appreciate the reviews and input from Daniel Maysey; Barbara Montague, LCSW; Macey Sidlasky; and Rachel Soh-Young Yi.

A special thanks to those who read and improved what we wrote, including Sharon Bober, PhD; Heather Cheng, MD, PhD; Veda N. Giri, MD; Michael J. Hall, MD, MS; Heather Hampel, MS, CGC; Joanne Jeter, MD; Bryson Katona, MD, PhD; Andrew Kaunitz, MD; Matthew Lederman, MD; Douglas Levine, MD; Bruce Montgomery, MD; Barbara Norquist, MD; Leigha Senter-Jamieson, MS, CGC; Diljeet Singh, MD, DrPh; and Matthew Boland Yurgelun, MD.

Glossary

3D mammography. Also called **tomosynthesis**. Technology that provides multiple three-dimensional images of the breast from different angles.

abdominal wash. A procedure that flushes sterile liquid into the pelvic cavity and then removes the fluid so that a pathologist can look for evidence of cancer.

ablation. A procedure that uses extreme heat or cold to destroy a tumor.

absolute risk. The chance of something happening within a specific time period.

acellular dermal matrix. Sterilized donor skin used to replace missing tissue.

acquired mutation. A genetic change that develops after conception.

acral lentiginous melanoma. A rare type of melanoma that develops on the palms of the hands, on the soles of the feet, or under the nails.

active surveillance. A type of treatment plan that involves withholding treatment and closely watching for signs that a disease or condition is worsening.

acute lymphocytic leukemia. A cancer of the blood and bone marrow.

acute myeloid leukemia. Also called **acute myelogenous leukemia**. A cancer of the blood and bone marrow.

adenocarcinoma. A cancer that develops in the glandular cells (cells that produce mucus, digestive juices, or other fluids) that line some internal organs.

adenomatous polyp. A growth in the lining of the colon or rectum that can be a precursor to colorectal cancer.

adenosis. A benign breast condition that develops when lobules become enlarged.

adjuvant therapy. Treatment given after surgery.

advance health care directive. A document that informs your doctors of the care you do or don't want when you're unable to tell them yourself.

androgen. A primarily male hormone that women have in limited quantities.

androgen deprivation therapy (ADT). Treatment that reduces the level of androgen hormones.

anemia. A low red blood cell count.

angiography. A procedure that uses x-rays and a special dye to produce pictures of the blood vessels.

areola. The pigmented skin surrounding the nipple.

aromatase inhibitor (AI). A drug that reduces estrogen produced by fat tissue.

arthralgia. Joint pain and stiffness.

assisted reproductive technology (ART). Fertility treatments that preserve a woman's eggs or embryos.

ataxia-telangiectasia (AT). Also called **Louis-Bar syndrome**. A rare, degenerative disorder of the nervous, neurological, and immune systems that occurs when people inherit two *ATM* mutations (one from each parent).

attenuated familial adenomatous polyposis (AFAP). A subtype of familial adenomatous polyposis that is characterized by fewer adenomatous polyps than classic FAP.

atypical hyperplasia. A precancerous condition that occurs when abnormal cells accumulate in the breast.

autofluorescence. A type of imaging used to determine eye health.

autologous tissue flap reconstruction. Skin, fat, tissue, and sometimes muscle is moved from one area of the body to another to replace missing tissue.

axillary lymph node dissection. Surgical removal of lymph nodes in the armpit.

axillary lymph nodes. Lymph nodes in the armpit.

basal cell carcinoma. Cancer that begins in basal cells at the bottom of the epidermis.

behavioral therapist. A health care professional who treats mental health disorders.

benign. Not cancerous.

bilateral breast cancer. Cancer that occurs in both breasts.

bilateral mastectomy. Surgery to remove both breasts.

bilateral salpingo-oophorectomy. Surgery to remove both ovaries and the fallopian tubes.

bilateral skin-sparing mastectomy. Surgery that removes the tissue in both breasts but preserves most of the breast skin so that breast reconstruction can be performed immediately.

bioidentical. Hormones in commercial preparations that are chemically identical to the hormones made by the body.

biomarker testing. Also called **tumor testing**. Laboratory test that identifies unique information about a cancer.

biopsy. A procedure that removes a sample of cells, fluid, or tissue to check for disease.

biosimilar. A drug with almost the same safety, purity, and effectiveness of the medication that it mimics.

bisphosphonate. A medication that strengthens bone.

bone density test. An x-ray that measures bone health.

borderline resectable cancer. Cancer that marginally involves nearby blood vessels and may or may not be completely removed by surgery.

brachytherapy. Internal radiation therapy that places the radiation source close to the tumor.

brain scan. A procedure that provides images of the internal structure of the brain.

breast cancer. Uncontrolled growth of abnormal breast cells.

breast-conserving surgery. Also called **lumpectomy**. Surgical removal of a cancerous breast lump and a margin of healthy surrounding tissue.

breast-conserving therapy. Surgical removal of a cancerous lump and some healthy surrounding tissue followed by radiation.

breast implant. A silicone shell filled with silicone gel or saline that replaces missing breast tissue.

breast implant–associated anaplastic large-cell lymphoma (BIA-ALCL). A rare type of non-Hodgkin lymphoma that is linked to some breast implants.

breast implant illness (BII). Fatigue, joint pain, and other symptoms reported by some women who have breast implants.

breast MRI. A type of magnetic resonance imaging that produces hundreds of detailed images of the breast from several angles.

breast prostheses. Synthetic breast forms that temporarily provide shape and symmetry after mastectomy.

breast reconstruction. Procedures that use an implant or a patient's own tissue to restore breast shape and volume after mastectomy.

breast self-exam (BSE). Examination of your own breasts to check for changes.

breast surgeon. A doctor who specializes in surgical procedures that diagnose and treat breast conditions.

calcification. A deposit of calcium in tissue, which may indicate a malignancy.

cancer. Abnormal, uncontrolled cell growth.

cancer antigen 125 (CA-125). A protein in the blood that, when elevated, may signal the presence of certain cancers.

cancer antigen 125 (CA-125) test. A laboratory test that measures the amount of a specific protein in the blood.

cancer syndrome. A predisposition for multiple cancers and/or health conditions as a result of having an inherited mutation in one or both copies of certain genes.

capsular contracture. Tightening of the scar tissue that surrounds a breast implant.

carcinogen. A substance that can cause cancer.

carcinoid tumor. A type of neuroendocrine tumor that is slow growing and most likely to occur in the gastrointestinal tract or lungs.

carcinoma. A type of cancer that begins in the skin cells or in the tissue that lines organs.

carcinosarcoma. A malignant tumor that is a mixture of carcinoma and sarcoma.

castration-resistant prostate cancer (CRPC). Prostate cancer that no longer responds to androgen deprivation therapy.

CDK4/6 inhibitor. A targeted therapy drug used to treat advanced breast cancer.

cell. The smallest unit of all living things.

chemoprevention. Using medications, vitamins, or supplements to reduce cancer risk.

chemoradiation. Treatment that combines chemotherapy and radiation therapy.

chemotherapy. Drugs that destroy cancer cells.

chromosome. A bundle of DNA and proteins found in the nucleus of cells, which contains an organism's genetic information and instructions.

clear cell carcinoma. An uncommon type of epithelial ovarian cancer.

clear margin. A border of cancer-free tissue that surrounds an area of cancerous tissue that has been removed.

clinical breast exam (CBE). An examination of the breasts by a health care professional.

clinical trial. A study that tests the safety and effectiveness of a new treatment or procedure in humans.

close margin. An area of tissue around a malignant tumor that contains cancer cells.

cold cap. A cap that applies cold temperatures to the head during chemotherapy to prevent or reduce hair loss.

colectomy. A surgical procedure that removes a portion or all of the colon (the large intestine).

colonoscope. A flexible tube with a camera on the end used to perform colonoscopy.

colonoscopy. A procedure that examines the large intestine and the rectum for abnormalities, including polyps and signs of early-stage colorectal cancer.

colon polyps. Growths that develop on the lining of the colon.

complete response. Also called **pathological complete response.** No evidence of disease shown by physical examination, blood tests, or imaging scans after treatment.

computed tomography (CT or CAT) scan. An x-ray that produces sectional images of the body.

constitutional mismatch repair-deficiency (CMMRD) syndrome. A rare disorder that greatly increases the risk of children and young adults developing one or more types of cancer.

copayment (copay). An amount that you're required to pay for medical services or prescriptions.

Cowden syndrome. A predisposition to multiple cancers that is caused by an inherited mutation in the *PTEN* gene.

cryotherapy. Also called **cryosurgery.** The use of extreme cold to freeze and remove abnormal tissue.

cutaneous squamous cell carcinoma. A type of skin cancer that develops in squamous cells.

cyst. A fluid-filled sac that forms in tissue.

cystectomy. Removal of all or part of the bladder.

cystoscopy. A procedure that uses a tiny, flexible tube with a lighted lens to view the bladder or ureters.

cytotoxic. Harmful to cells.

debulking. A surgical procedure to remove as much of a cancer as possible.

deductible. The out-of-pocket amount you must pay for medical expenses or prescriptions before your health insurance coverage begins.

delayed breast reconstruction. A procedure to re-create a breast weeks, months, or years after mastectomy.

de novo mutation. A genetic change that develops in a person before birth but isn't present in either parent. De novo mutations can be caused by a mutation in one parent's egg or sperm or a mutation early in the development of the embryo.

dense breasts. Breasts that have more glandular tissue than fat and are more difficult to screen for cancer with mammography.

deoxyribonucleic acid (DNA). The molecule inside cells that contains the genetic information needed for an organism's development and function.

dermatologist. A doctor who diagnoses and treats skin disorders.

dermis. The thick layer of tissue beneath the epidermis (outer layer of skin) that holds blood vessels and nerve endings.

desmoid tumor. A growth that develops in connective tissue. Most desmoid tumors are not cancerous, but they can return after they are removed.

diagnostic test. Testing or imaging that confirms or eliminates the presence of disease.

dialysis. A treatment that mechanically performs kidney functions.

deep inferior epigastric perforator (DIEP) flap. A breast reconstruction procedure that uses fat and skin from the belly to re-create a breast after mastectomy.

diffuse gastric cancer. A type of cancer that usually develops in the lining of the stomach.

digital mammography. Technology that produces computerized images of the breast.

digital rectal exam (DRE). A physical examination that involves insertion of a gloved finger into the rectum to feel for abnormalities in the rectum, lower bowel, prostate, uterus, or ovaries.

direct-to-implant breast reconstruction. A surgical procedure that places a full-size breast implant immediately after mastectomy.

distal pancreatectomy. Surgery that removes a tumor from the body or tail of the pancreas.

DNA damage repair (DDR) genes. Genes that control cell division and repair damaged DNA.

do-not-resuscitate order. A document that instructs medical professionals not to revive you if your heart stops or if you stop breathing.

double-stranded DNA breaks. A type of DNA damage.

dry ejaculation. Male orgasm that occurs without releasing semen.

duct. A channel in the body that drains secretions, such as sweat, tears, and milk.

ductal carcinoma in situ (DCIS). Also called **noninvasive breast cancer** or **Stage 0 breast cancer.** Early-stage, noninvasive cancer that began in the breast ducts but hasn't spread.

duct ectasia. A condition that develops when breast ducts become blocked with fluid.

dumping syndrome. An uncomfortable digestive condition that may develop when all or part of the stomach is removed.

dyspareunia. Painful intercourse.

dysplastic nevus syndrome. Also called **atypical mole syndrome.** An inherited condition that can cause many (100 or more) moles and abnormal moles to develop on the body and can increase the risk for melanoma.

electroejaculation. A procedure that stimulates ejaculation with a mild electrical current to obtain a semen sample.

embolization. A procedure that injects materials into blood vessels to block the blood flow to cancer cells.

endocrinologist. A doctor who diagnoses and treats disorders involving hormones.

endometrioid carcinoma. A type of epithelial ovarian tumor.

endometriosis. A condition in which the uterine lining grows on the outside of the uterus.

endoscopic mucosal resection. Surgery that uses a scope to find and remove gastrointestinal polyps, early cancers, other abnormalities, and some healthy tissue surrounding the lesions.

endoscopic ultrasound (EUS). A procedure using an endoscope that creates high-frequency sound waves to produce detailed images of the gastrointestinal organs.

endoscopy. A procedure that inserts a flexible tube into the gastrointestinal tract to look for abnormalities.

enucleation. Surgical removal of the eye.

epidermis. The outermost layer of skin.

epithelial cells. Cells that cover the outer surfaces of organs and blood vessels.

epithelial ovarian cancer. The most common type of ovarian cancer, which often begins in the fallopian tubes.

Epstein-Barr virus. An infection that causes herpes and mononucleosis.

erectile dysfunction. An inability to achieve or maintain an erection.

esophagogastroduodenoscopy (EGD). A procedure used to view, find, and biopsy abnormalities of the esophagus, stomach, and duodenum.

estrogen. A primary female hormone.

estrogen receptor–negative breast cancer. Breast cancer cells that do not use estrogen to grow.

estrogen receptor–positive breast cancer. Breast cancer cells that use estrogen to grow.

estrogen therapy (ET). Hormone replacement therapy that includes estrogen only.

exocrine cells. Cells that secrete digestive enzymes.

external beam radiation therapy. A treatment for cancer that delivers high-energy x-rays to the site of the tumor.

false negative. A test that fails to correctly indicate that a person has an abnormality or a disease.

false positive. A test that detects an abnormality or disease when none is present.

familial adenomatous polyposis (FAP). A condition caused by an inherited mutation in the *APC* gene that can lead to extraordinarily high risk for colorectal and other cancers.

familial atypical multiple mole melanoma syndrome. An inherited condition that causes multiple atypical moles. It may be caused by an inherited mutation in the *CDKN2A* or (more rarely) the *CDK4* gene.

Fanconi anemia (FA). A rare and serious childhood disorder characterized by bone marrow that doesn't produce enough blood cells.

fat grafting. A procedure to liposuction and purify fat and then inject it into specific areas of the body to improve cosmetic appearance.

fertility specialist. A doctor who is specially trained to help people conceive.

fibroadenoma. A type of benign mass in the breast.

fibrocystic changes. Benign changes in the breast tissue.

fibrosis. Painful scarring of connective tissue.

fistula. An abnormal connection between two body parts.

flexible sigmoidoscopy. A procedure that uses a narrow scope with a camera to examine the lower colon and rectum.

focal cryotherapy. The use of extreme cold to freeze and remove abnormal tissue, targeting only the tumor.

founder mutation. A genetic change that occurs frequently in certain ethnicities or in descendants of people who have been geographically or culturally isolated.

full-sequencing test. A genetic test that looks for abnormalities in multiple areas of a gene.

gastritis. Inflammation in the lining of the stomach.

gastroenterologist. A doctor who specializes in the function and treatment of disorders of the gastrointestinal system.

gastrointestinal carcinoid tumor. A slow-growing tumor that forms in the gastrointestinal tract.

gastrointestinal system. The body's system that converts food into energy, including the gastrointestinal tract and other organs that aid in digestion, such as the salivary glands, liver, pancreas, and gallbladder.

gastrointestinal (GI) tract. Also called **digestive tract.** The part of the gastrointestinal system from the mouth to the anus: the canal where food enters the body and is then digested and expelled as waste.

genes. Bits of DNA that issue cellular instructions inside chromosomes.

genetic counseling. A consultation with a genetics expert who can help patients understand and make medical decisions related to genetic conditions.

genetic counselor. A health care specialist with advanced training in the genetics of disease. Certified genetic counselors (CGCs) have completed training and are certified by the American Board of Genetic Counseling.

genetic mutations. Changes in genes that may be harmless (benign) or harmful (pathogenic or deleterious).

genetics. The study of inherited traits and diseases.

genetic testing. Testing a person's blood, saliva, or tissue for the presence of a genetic mutation.

genitourinary system. The kidneys, ureters, bladder, urethra, and reproductive system.

genome. A complete set of the unique genetic information needed to create and grow an organism.

genomics. The study of an organism's entire set of genes.

germline mutations. Inherited mutations.

Gleason score. A measurement used to help determine the aggressiveness of prostate cancer.

grade. An assigned classification based on the appearance and aggressiveness of cancer cells.

gynecologic oncologist. A doctor who specializes in treating cancer of the female reproductive system.

gynecologic surgery. An operation involving any part of a woman's reproductive system.

gynecomastia. A benign condition characterized by enlargement of male breast tissue.

hamartoma. A type of benign tumor.

Helicobacter pylori. A bacteria that may be present in the mucus of the stomach lining and causes inflammation and precancerous changes.

hematoma. Blood that leaks from a blood vessel under the skin.

hepatic perfusion. A procedure that delivers high-dose chemotherapy directly to the liver.

HER2 (human epidermal growth factor receptor 2). A protein that signals cells to grow.

HER2-positive cancer. Cancers that are characterized by cells with numerous receptors for the HER2 protein.

hereditary breast and ovarian cancer (HBOC) syndrome. A predisposition to breast, ovarian, and other cancers that is primarily caused by an inherited mutation in a *BRCA1* or *BRCA2* gene.

hereditary diffuse gastric cancer (HDGC) syndrome. A predisposition to cancer in the lining of the stomach and other cancers caused by an inherited mutation in the *CDH1* gene.

hereditary polyposis syndrome. An inherited condition that causes numerous polyps, which develop more quickly and at a younger age compared to the general population.

homologous recombination deficient (HRD). Cells that can't easily repair double-stranded DNA breaks.

homologous recombination repair (HRR) genes. Genes that help to repair a type of DNA damage known as double-stranded DNA breaks.

hormone receptor. A protein on the surface of cells that attaches to a hormone.

hormone receptor–negative breast cancer. Breast cancer that is not stimulated by hormones.

hormone receptor–positive breast cancer. Breast cancer that is stimulated by one or more hormones.

hormone replacement therapy (HRT). The use of a combination of estrogen and progesterone to supplement natural hormones when the body does not produce enough.

hormone therapy. Also called **endocrine therapy.** A type of treatment that blocks the effects of hormones on cancer cells.

hospice care. Specialized care for people with advanced, life-limiting illness.

human immunodeficiency virus/acquired immunodeficiency syndrome (HIV/AIDS). A virus that attacks the immune system.

human papillomavirus (HPV). A viral infection that is passed through skin-to-skin contact.

hyperplasia. Abnormally accelerated cell growth.

hysterectomy. Surgical removal of the ovaries.

immediate breast reconstruction. Surgery to re-create a breast that is performed at the same time as a mastectomy.

immune checkpoint inhibitor. An immunotherapy drug that allows the immune system to find and destroy cancer cells.

immunotherapy. Treatment that stimulates the immune system to fight disease.

inflammatory breast cancer (IBC). An aggressive type of breast cancer.

inherited mutation. A genetic change that is passed from parent to child.

in-network. Medical providers and facilities that are contracted with a particular health insurance company to accept predetermined fees for services.

insomnia. The inability to fall or stay asleep.

integrative medicine. Health care that focuses on the whole person and may include lifestyle interventions in combination with traditional therapies.

intraductal papillary-mucinous neoplasm. A tumor that grows in the pancreatic ducts.

intravesical chemotherapy. Chemotherapy that is placed directly into the bladder.

invasive breast cancer. Cancer that has spread beyond the ducts or lobules and into the surrounding breast tissue.

invasive ductal carcinoma (IDC). Cancer that develops in the ducts of the breast and spreads to surrounding breast tissue.

invasive lobular carcinoma (ILC). Cancer that develops in the lobules of the breast and spreads to surrounding breast tissue.

in vitro fertilization. A procedure that removes eggs from ovaries, combines them with sperm in a lab, and then implants the resulting embryos into someone's uterus or freezes them for future use.

isolated limb infusion (ILI). Chemotherapy that is directed through a catheter in an artery and a vein that feed a tumor in a limb.

isolated limb perfusion (ILP). Heated chemotherapy that is directed through a catheter in an artery and a vein that feed a tumor in a limb.

jaundice. Yellowing of the skin and/or eyes.

keratocanthoma. A small, benign type of skin lesion that may grow quickly over several weeks or months.

Klinefelter syndrome. A rare genetic disorder that increases male estrogen levels.

laparoscope. A thin, lighted scope that is used to view abdominal organs.

laparoscopic-assisted prostatectomy. Minimally invasive surgical removal of the prostate using a laparoscope.

laparoscopic-assisted vaginal hysterectomy (LAVH). Minimally invasive surgical removal of the uterus using a laparoscope.

laparotomy. A surgical procedure that makes an incision into the abdominal cavity.

lentigo maligna melanoma. An invasive type of skin cancer.

lesion. A damaged area of tissue.

leukemia. A cancer of the blood and bone marrow.

Li-Fraumeni syndrome. An inherited predisposition to breast and other cancers caused by a mutation in the *TP53* gene.

liquid biopsy. A blood test that measures fragments of DNA that are released from dying tumors.

lobular carcinoma in situ (LCIS). Abnormal cells that are confined to the lobules of the breast.

lobule. Breast glands that produce milk.

locally advanced tumor. Cancer that has spread beyond its place of origin but no further.

local therapy. Treatment that focuses on the area of a tumor.

luteinizing hormone–releasing hormone (LHRH) agonists. Medications that decrease the production of testosterone by the testicles and the production of estrogen and progesterone by the ovaries.

luteinizing hormone–releasing hormone (LHRH) antagonists. Medications that block certain pituitary gland hormones that are needed to stimulate production of male testosterone and female estrogen and progesterone.

lymphedema. A chronic accumulation of lymph fluid that develops when lymph vessels or lymph nodes are damaged or removed.

lymph fluid. Colorless fluid that transports cellular debris through the lymph system.

lymph nodes. Small glands that are part of the immune system.

lymphocytes. White blood cells that are part of the immune system.

lymphoma. A cancer that occurs primarily in white blood cells and lymph nodes.

lymphovascular space invasion. Cancer cells in the blood vessels or lymph vessels outside of a tumor.

lymph system. A network of small glands connected by lymphatic vessels, which filters impurities in the body.

Lynch syndrome. Also called **hereditary nonpolyposis colorectal cancer** (**HNPCC**). A predisposition to colon, uterine, and other cancers that is caused by an inherited mutation in an *MLH1, MSH2, MSH6, PMS2,* or *EPCAM* gene.

magnetic resonance cholangiopancreatography (MRCP). A special type of imaging that provides detailed views of the liver, gallbladder, bile ducts, pancreas, and pancreatic duct.

magnetic resonance enterography. A type of imaging that creates detailed views of the small intestine.

magnetic resonance imaging (MRI). Technology that uses magnets and radio waves to produce three-dimensional images of the body's interior.

male reproductive system. The prostate, testicles, and penis.

malignant. Cancerous.

mammogram. An x-ray image of the breast.

mammography. Technology that uses x-rays to produce images of breast tissue.

mastectomy. Surgical removal of the breast.

mastitis. An infection that develops when milk ducts in the breast become blocked during nursing.

medical oncologist. A doctor who specializes in treating cancer.

medullary carcinoma of the breast. A rare type of breast cancer that is marked by poorly differentiated cells surrounded by white blood cells.

melanocyte. A cell that produces melanin, the natural pigment in hair, skin, and the iris of the eye.

melanoma. A less common, dangerous skin cancer.

menopause. The time in a woman's life when she no longer has menstrual periods and can no longer conceive.

metastasis. The spread of cancer beyond its original location to other parts of the body.

metastatic cancer. Cancer that has spread from its site of origin to distant points in the body.

microcalcifications. Minute calcium deposits in the breast that can signal the start of breast cancer.

microsatellite instability (MSI). A type of DNA change that can be measured in cancer cells.

microsatellite instability–high (MSI-H). A test result that indicates a tumor with high levels of microsatellite instability.

mismatch repair (MMR) genes. Genes, including those associated with Lynch syndrome, that correct a type of cell damage known as single-stranded DNA damage.

modified radical mastectomy. Surgical removal of the breast tissue, skin, some or all of the underarm lymph nodes, and the lining over the chest muscle.

Mohs surgery. A surgical treatment for skin cancer that progressively removes one thin layer of skin at a time, which is checked for cancer cells.

moist reaction. Skin that peels and becomes moist and painful as a result of radiation.

mucinous carcinoma. Invasive cancer that develops in an internal organ that produces mucin.

mucosa-associated lymphoid tissue lymphoma. A type of non-Hodgkin lymphoma.

mucosal melanoma. An uncommon cancer that develops on mucous membranes.

multigene panel tests. Genetic tests that simultaneously check for mutations in several different genes.

mutation. An inherited or acquired change that develops in a gene.

MUTYH-associated polyposis (MAP). An uncommon condition that significantly raises the risk for colorectal cancer when people inherit two MUTYH mutations (one from each parent).

myelodysplastic syndrome. A disorder of the bone marrow that leads to blood cells that do not function properly.

necrosis. Tissue death that occurs from a lack of oxygen and blood.

neoadjuvant therapy. Treatment given before surgery.

nephroureterectomy. Surgery to remove the entire kidney, ureters, and bladder cuff.

nerve-sparing cystectomy. Surgery that removes all or part of the bladder while preserving the nerves that enable erection and normal urinary function.

nerve-sparing radical prostatectomy. Surgery that removes the prostate while preserving the nerves that enable erection.

neuroendocrine tumor. A tumor that forms in nerve cells that are related to hormone production.

neurofibroma. A benign tumor that develops on a nerve.

neurological exam. An exam by a health care professional to evaluate the function of a person's nervous system.

neurologist. A doctor who specializes in diagnosing and treating disorders of the brain and nervous system.

neuropathy. Pain, numbness, tingling, or burning caused by damaged nerves.

neutropenia. A low number of white blood cells.

night sweats. Hot flashes that occur during sleep.

Nijmegen breakage syndrome. A disorder that occurs when a person inherits two NBN mutations (one from each parent), which causes small stature and head size, a compromised immune system, and numerous other health issues.

nipple-sparing mastectomy. Surgical removal of the breast tissue that preserves most breast skin, including the nipple and the areola.

nodular melanoma. A dangerous, quick-growing skin cancer.

no mutation detected. A genetic test result that shows no evidence of a known mutation in the genes that were scanned.

non–muscle invasive bladder cancer. Cancer that originates and remains in the inside lining of the bladder.

nucleus. The structure inside a cell that contains chromosomes.

nutritionist. Someone who has special training regarding how food and nutrition affect health.

ocular melanoma (OM). Melanoma that develops in the eye.

oncologist. A doctor who specializes in cancer treatment.

oophorectomy. Surgical removal of the ovary.

ophthalmologist. A medical doctor who specializes in the treatment of eye disorders and diseases.

optical coherence tomography. Imaging technology that provides detailed views of the inside of the eye.

oral contraceptives. Pills or tablets that are taken by mouth to prevent pregnancy.

orchiectomy. Surgery that removes the testicles.

osteopenia. Weakening of the bones.

osteoporosis. A condition that occurs from bone loss and increases the risk for fractures.

out-of-pocket. The total amount you pay for medical services that are not covered by your health insurance.

outpatient procedure. A medical procedure that doesn't require an overnight hospital stay.

ovarian germ cell tumor. A type of ovarian cancer that forms in the egg cells of the ovaries.

ovarian suppression. Treatment that stops the production of estrogen.

ovarian tissue freezing. Freezing and storing ovarian tissue for future reimplantation.

ovarian transposition. Surgery that temporarily repositions the ovaries to reduce their exposure to radiation therapy.

Paget's disease of the breast. A rare type of breast cancer that affects the nipple and/or the areola.

palliative care. Medical care that supplements treatment by improving emotional, psychological, and physical symptoms and stress caused by a disease.

pancreatitis. Swelling of the pancreas.

papilloma. A small, benign tumor.

Pap smear. A procedure that tests for precancerous changes or cancer in the cervix.

paracentesis. A procedure that removes fluid buildup in the abdomen.

Parkinson's disease. A brain disorder that progressively leads to shaking and difficulty with walking, balance, and coordination.

PARP inhibitor. A type of cancer treatment that targets the poly (ADP-ribose) polymerase (PARP) enzyme.

partial gastrectomy. Surgery to remove a part of the stomach.

partial response. A decrease in the size of a tumor or the extent of cancer.

pathogenic variant. Also called **deleterious mutation.** A genetic change that increases a person's risk for disease.

pathologist. A doctor who examines tissue samples and performs and interprets lab tests to diagnose and characterize cancer and other diseases.

pathology. The study of the cause and molecular nature of diseases.

pathology report. A pathologist's clinical description of findings from a direct examination and tests that are conducted on sample cells and tissue.

patient navigator. A health professional who guides patients through the health care system.

peau d'orange. Dimpling of the breast skin that resembles an orange peel.

pedigree. A diagram of a family's medical history.

pelvic exam. A visual and physical examination of a woman's reproductive organs.

pelvic rehabilitation. Physical therapy that increases the length and strength of the pelvic muscles.

pernicious anemia. A reduced red blood cell count from a lack of vitamin B_{12}.

personalized medicine. Treatment that is customized for an individual.

Peutz-Jeghers syndrome. A rare disorder that leads to an increased risk of noncancerous growths and certain cancers. It is caused by a mutation in the *STK11* gene.

phyllodes tumor. A fast-growing type of breast cancer that develops in the ligaments and fatty tissue of the breast.

plastic surgeon. A doctor who specializes in cosmetic or reconstructive surgery.

platinum chemotherapy. Cancer drugs that are based on platinum compounds.

polypectomy. Surgical removal of polyps.

positron emission tomography (PET) scan. Technology that looks for brain injury or disease.

postmastectomy pain syndrome. Chronic pain in the chest that persists after recovery from mastectomy.

precancerous. An abnormality that can evolve into cancer.

precocious puberty. The premature development of some adult physical characteristics in children.

preimplantation genetic testing (PGT). A procedure done before in vitro fertilization to screen embryos for inherited gene mutations or a predisposition to disease.

premium. A fee paid for health insurance.

previvor. Someone who is predisposed to a disease but hasn't been diagnosed.

progesterone. A female sex hormone.

progesterone receptor–negative breast cancer. Breast cancer cells that don't use progesterone to grow.

progesterone receptor–positive breast cancer. Breast cancer cells that use progesterone to grow.

prognosis. The long-term outlook for someone after diagnosis.

prostate-specific antigen (PSA). A protein produced by healthy and cancerous prostate cells.

prostate-specific antigen (PSA) test. A blood test that screens for prostate cancer or monitors prostate cancer patients after diagnosis or treatment.

prostatic hyperplasia. A benign condition that causes an enlarged prostate.

proton radiation therapy. A type of external beam radiation.

psychiatrist. A doctor who specializes in diagnosing and treating mental health disorders.

psychostimulant. A medication that increases energy levels by stimulating the mind and body.

radial scar. Also called **complex sclerosing lesion.** A benign growth that may look like a scar under a microscope or on a mammogram.

radiation oncologist. A doctor who specializes in treating cancer with radiation.

radiation therapy. Treatment with high-energy x-rays or radioactive seeds that destroy cancer cells and reduce the risk of recurrence.

radical cystectomy. Surgery that removes the entire bladder, lymph nodes that are close to the bladder, and sometimes nearby tissue and organs.

radical prostatectomy. A surgical procedure that removes the entire prostate.

receptor. A protein on the surface of a cell that binds to a specific substance and affects cellular activity.

rectovaginal examination. A physical exam to assess the health of the rectum and vagina.

recurrence. Cancer that returns after treatment.

relative risk. A measure of risk that compares the probability of an event occurring in one group compared to another group.

remission. A decrease or disappearance of the signs and symptoms of cancer. Complete remission is sometimes referred to as **no evident disease (NED).**

resectable cancer. A cancer that can be completely removed with surgery and hasn't spread to other organs.

resection. The surgical removal of tissue.

retrograde pyelography. X-ray imaging that is used with cystoscopy to view the urinary tract.

risk factor. Something that increases the likelihood of disease.

risk-reducing colectomy. Surgery that removes all or part of the colon to prevent or greatly reduce the risk of cancer.

risk-reducing mastectomy (RRM). Surgery that removes healthy breasts to prevent or greatly reduce the risk of breast cancer.

risk-reducing salpingo-oophorectomy (RRSO). Surgery that removes healthy ovaries and fallopian tubes to reduce a high risk for gynecologic cancers.

risk-reducing total gastrectomy. Removal of the stomach to reduce a high risk of stomach cancer.

salpingectomy. A surgical procedure that removes the fallopian tubes.

salpingo-oophorectomy. Surgery that removes the ovaries and fallopian tubes.

sarcoma. A cancer that begins in the bones or soft tissues of the body.

scalp cooling. A method of chilling the scalp during chemotherapy to reduce treatment-related hair loss.

sebaceous adenoma. A benign tumor of the sebaceous glands, which secrete lubricating substances in the skin and hair.

sebaceous carcinoma. A type of cancer that begins in the oil glands of the skin.

sebaceous epithelioma. A form of benign skin tumor that usually appears on the neck or face.

segmental colectomy. Surgery that removes a portion of the colon.

segmental resection. Surgery that removes part of an organ.

selective estrogen receptor modulator (SERM). A drug that blocks or mimics the effect of estrogen on different types of tissue.

sensitivity. The ability of a test to correctly identify individuals who have a particular disease.

sentinel lymph node biopsy. A surgical procedure that removes one to three lymph nodes nearest to a tumor so that the nodes can be examined for the spread of cancer cells.

sentinel node. The first lymph node that cancer is likely to reach if it progresses beyond the tumor site.

seroma. Excess fluid that collects under the skin.

serous epithelial ovarian cancer. The most common type of ovarian cancer.

sexual dysfunction. The persistent or recurrent lack of sexual desire or an inability to achieve sexual satisfaction.

signet ring cell adenocarcinoma. A rare form of an aggressive adenocarcinoma.

single-site test. A genetic test that searches one gene for a specific mutation that has already been identified in the family.

skin-sparing mastectomy. Surgical removal of the breast tissue that preserves most of the breast skin.

specificity. The ability of a test to correctly identify individuals who do or don't have a particular disease.

sperm banking. The process of freezing and storing sperm for future use.

Spitz nevus mole. A rare, noncancerous skin growth.

sporadic cancer. A cancer that arises from mutations that happen after birth and is not caused by an inherited gene mutation.

squamous cell carcinoma. Cancer that begins in the cells that cover internal and external body surfaces.

staging. A process that determines the extent of a patient's cancer.

stoma. A permanent opening made on the abdomen to allow waste to leave the body.

stool antigen test. A test that checks stool for *H. pylori* molecules.

stricture. Narrowing of a body canal or tube due to a buildup of scar tissue.

stromal cell tumor. A tumor that develops in the connective tissue cells of the ovary and generates estrogen and progesterone.

superficial spreading melanoma. The most common type of melanoma, which develops when the cells that produce skin pigment grow out of control and form tumors.

surgical oncologist. A physician who specializes in cancer surgery.

survivor. Someone who has been diagnosed with a disease.

survivorship care plan. A patient document that summarizes the cancer treatment provided and the recommended follow-up care.

systemic therapy. Treatment that targets the entire body.

targeted drug or **therapy.** A treatment that targets a specific molecular substance that drives the growth of cancer cells.

testicular exam. A complete physical inspection of the testicles and scrotum.

testicular sperm extraction. Surgically removing healthy sperm cells from a small sample of testicular tissue and then freezing them for future in vitro fertilization.

tissue expander. A temporary saline implant that gradually stretches skin and/or muscle to make room for a breast implant.

tissue expansion. A procedure that stretches skin and/or muscle to enable reconstruction.

total abdominal colectomy with ileorectal anastomosis. Surgery that removes the entire colon but retains the rectum.

total abdominal hysterectomy with risk-reducing salpingo-oophorectomy (TAH/ RRSO). Removal of the uterus, cervix, ovaries, and fallopian tubes through a surgical incision in the abdomen to decrease the risk of gynecologic cancer.

total gastrectomy. Surgical removal of the entire stomach.

total mastectomy. Removal of the breast tissue, skin, and nipple.

total pancreatectomy. Surgery that removes the entire pancreas, gallbladder, spleen, nearby lymph nodes, and part of the stomach and small intestine.

total proctocolectomy with ileal pouch and anal anastomosis. Surgery that removes the colon and rectum and preserves the anal sphincter.

total proctocolectomy with permanent end ileostomy. Surgery that removes the entire colon, rectum, and anus and creates a permanent stoma for the removal of digestive waste from the body.

transrectal ultrasound. A procedure that uses high-energy sound waves to create a computer image of the prostate.

transurethral resection of a bladder tumor (TURBT). A surgical procedure used to diagnose and remove cancerous tissue from the bladder.

transurethral resection of the prostate (TURP). Surgery to remove prostate tissue through the urethra.

transvaginal ultrasound. A procedure that uses sound waves to examine a woman's reproductive organs.

triple-negative breast cancer. Breast cancer that lacks receptors for estrogen, progesterone, and HER2.

true negative. A genetic test result that does not discover the gene mutation that was found in another member of the family.

tubal ligation. A surgical procedure that seals or removes part of the fallopian tubes to prevent pregnancy.

tumor board. A multidisciplinary panel of doctors and other health care specialists who determine the best possible treatment plans for individuals who have cancer.

tumor mutational burden (TMB). A measurement of the number of gene mutations (changes) inside the cells of a cancer.

tumor suppressor gene. A type of gene that controls cellular growth, repairs damaged DNA, or tells cells when they should die.

ultrasound. A technology that uses high-frequency sound waves to produce computer images of the inside of the body.

unresectable cancer. A cancer that can't be completely removed with surgery.

upper tract urothelial cancer (UTUC). Urothelial cancer that develops in the renal pelvis or a ureter.

urea breath test. A test that checks for *H. pylori* bacteria in the stomach.

ureters. The tubes that move urine from the kidneys to the bladder.

urinalysis. A test that detects and measures substances in the urine.

urinary incontinence. The involuntary leaking of urine.

urine cytology. A test that collects samples from the urine, which are examined for precancerous or cancer cells.

urologist. A doctor who diagnoses and treats diseases of the urinary tract.

urothelial carcinoma. Cancer that starts in the cellular lining of the urinary tract.

vaginal moisturizer. A product that improves vaginal dryness.

vaginismus. An involuntary tightening of the vaginal muscles that makes penetration impossible.

variant of uncertain significance (VUS). A gene change of undetermined cancer risk.

video capsule endoscopy. A procedure that allows visual examination of the small intestine.

volumetric modulated arc radiation therapy. A type of precise radiation delivered by continuous 360-degree rotation of the treatment unit.

watchful waiting. Delaying treatment for a disease or condition until such time as symptoms appear or become worse.

Whipple procedure. Also called **pancreaticoduodenectomy.** A surgical procedure that removes the head of the pancreas, part of the small intestine, the lower bile ducts, the gallbladder, and the surrounding lymph nodes.

wide local excision. A surgical procedure that removes an abnormality and a surrounding margin of healthy tissue.

xeroderma pigmentosum. An inherited disorder that leads to extreme sensitivity to cell damage from sunlight and a high risk for skin cancer.

young-onset cancer. A cancer that is diagnosed in a person before they are age 50.

Notes

Chapter 2. What's Swimming in Your Gene Pool?

1. American Cancer Society. "Colorectal cancer risk factors." https://www.cancer.org/cancer/colon-rectal-cancer/causes-risks-prevention/risk-factors.html.

Chapter 5. Introducing *BRCA1* and *BRCA2*

1. Centers for Disease Control and Prevention. "Jewish women and BRCA gene mutations." https://www.cdc.gov/cancer/breast/young_women/bringyourbrave/hereditary_breast_cancer/jewish_women_brca.htm.
2. Behl S, Hamel N, de Ladurantaye M, et al. "Founder BRCA1/BRCA2/PALB2 pathogenic variants in French-Canadian breast cancer cases and controls," Scientific Reports 10, no. 1, 2020:6491; Rafnar T, Benediktsdottir KR, Eldon BJ, et al. "BRCA2, but not BRCA1, mutations account for familial ovarian cancer in Iceland: A population-based study," European Journal of Cancer 40, no. 18, 2004:2788–93; Ferla R, Calo V, Cascio S, et al. "Founder mutations in BRCA1 and BRCA2 genes," Annals of Oncology 18 (Suppl. 6), 2007:vi93–98; George SHL, Donenberg T, Alexis C, et al. "Gene sequencing for pathogenic variants among adults with breast and ovarian cancer in the Caribbean," Journal of the American Medical Association Network Open 4, no. 3, 2021:e210307.
3. National Comprehensive Cancer Network. "Guidelines: Genetic/familial high-risk assessment: Breast, ovarian, and pancreatic." Version 1.2022, August 2021.
4. National Comprehensive Cancer Network. "Guidelines: Genetic/familial high-risk assessment: Breast, ovarian, and pancreatic." Version 1.2022, August 2021.

Chapter 7. Other Genes That Are Linked to Inherited Cancer Risk

1. American Cancer Society. "Colorectal cancer risk factors." https://www.cancer.org/cancer/colon-rectal-cancer/causes-risks-prevention/risk-factors.html.
2. Ukaegbu C, Levi Z, Fehlmann TD, et al. "Characterizing germline APC and MUTYH variants in Ashkenazi Jews compared to other individuals," Familial Cancer 20, no. 2, 2021:111–16.
3. National Comprehensive Cancer Network. "Guidelines: Genetic/familial high-risk assessment: Breast, ovarian, and pancreatic." Version 1.2022, August 2021; Hu C, Hart SN,

Gnanaolivu R, et al. "A population-based study of genes previously implicated in breast cancer," New England Journal of Medicine 384, 2021:440–51.

4. Goldstein AM, Chan M, Harland M, et al. "Features associated with germline CDKN2A mutations: A GenoMEL study of melanoma-prone families from three continents," Journal of Medical Genetics 44, no. 2, 2007:99–106.

5. National Organization for Rare Disorders. "Peutz Jeghers syndrome." https://rarediseases .org/rare-diseases/peutz-jeghers-syndrome.

6. Li-Fraumeni Syndrome Association. "What is LFS?" https://www.lfsassociation.org/what-is -lfs.

Chapter 8. Breast Cancer Basics

1. Jernström H, Lubinski J, Lynch H, et al. "Breast-feeding and the risk of breast cancer in BRCA1 and BRCA2 mutation carriers," Journal of the National Cancer Institute 96, no. 14, 2004:1094–98.

2. Bhupathiraju S, Grodstein F, Stampfer M, et al. "Exogenous hormone use: Oral contraceptives, postmenopausal hormone therapy, and health outcomes in the nurses' health study," American Journal of Public Health 106, no. 9, 2016:1631–37; Mørch L, Skovlund C, Hannaford PC, et al. "Contemporary hormonal contraception and the risk of breast cancer," New England Journal of Medicine 377, no. 23, 2017:2228–39.

3. Rebbeck TR, Friebel T, Lynch HT, et al. "Bilateral prophylactic mastectomy reduces breast cancer risk in BRCA1 and BRCA2 mutation carriers: The PROSE study group," Journal of Clinical Oncology 22, no. 6, 2004:1055–62.

4. Rebbeck TR, Kauff ND, Domchek SM. "Meta-analysis of risk reduction estimates associated with risk-reducing salpingo-oophorectomy in BRCA1 or BRCA2 mutation carriers," Journal of the National Cancer Institute 101, no. 2, 2009:80–87; Choi Y, Terry MB, Daly MB, et al. "Association of risk-reducing salpingo-oophorectomy with breast cancer risk in women with BRCA1 and BRCA2 pathogenic variants," Journal of the American Medical Association Oncology 7, no. 4, 2021:585–92.

5. American Cancer Society. "Lobular carcinoma in situ." https://www.cancer.org/cancer /breast-cancer/non-cancerous-breast-conditions/lobular-carcinoma-in-situ.html.

Chapter 9. Gynecologic Cancers

1. Chetrit A, Hirsh-Yechezkel G, Ben-David Y, et al. "Effect of BRCA1/2 mutations on long-term survival of patients with invasive ovarian cancer: The national Israeli study of ovarian cancer," Journal of Clinical Oncology 26, no. 1, 2008:20–25.

2. Babic A, Sasmoto N, Rosner B, et al. "Association between breastfeeding and ovarian cancer risk," Journal of the American Medical Association Oncology 6, no. 6, 2020:e200421. https://pubmed.ncbi.nlm.nih.gov/32239218/.

3. Rebbeck TR, Lynch HT, Neuhausen SL, et al. "Prophylactic oophorectomy in carriers of BRCA1 or BRCA2 mutations," New England Journal of Medicine 346, no. 21, 2002:1616–22.

4. Henley SJ, Miller JW, Dowling NF, et al. "Uterine cancer incidence and mortality—United States, 1999–2016," Morbidity and Mortality Weekly Report 67, 2018:1333–38. doi:10.15585/ mmwr.mm6748a1; Johnson AL, Medina HN, Schlumbrecht MP, et al. "The role of histology

on endometrial cancer survival disparities in diverse Florida," PLOS One 15, no. 7, 2020. doi:10.1371/journal.pone.0236402.

5. Huang AB, Huang Y, Hur C, et al. "Impact of quality of care on racial disparities in survival for endometrial cancer," American Journal of Obstetrics and Gynecology 223, no. 3, 2020:e1–396, e-13. https://pubmed.ncbi.nlm.nih.gov/32109459; Doll KM, Snyder CR, Ford CL. "Endometrial cancer disparities: A race-conscious critique of the literature," American Journal of Obstetrics and Gynecology 218, no. 5, 2018:474–82. doi:10.1016/j.ajog.2017.09.016.

Chapter 10. Gastrointestinal Cancers

1. National Cancer Institute. "Cancer stat facts: Pancreatic cancer." https://seer.cancer.gov/statfacts/html/pancreas.html.

Chapter 11. Genitourinary Cancers

1. Salinas CA, Tsodikov A, Ishak-Howard M, et al. "Prostate cancer in young men: An important clinical entity," Nature Reviews Urology 11, no. 6, 2014:317–23.
2. American Cancer Society. "What causes cancer?" https://www.cancer.org/cancer/cancer-causes/hair-dyes.html.

Chapter 12. Melanoma

1. American Cancer Society. "Types of cancers that develop in young adults." https://www.cancer.org/cancer/cancer-in-young-adults/cancers-in-young-adults.html.
2. American Cancer Society. "Cancer facts and figures 2021." https://www.cancer.org/content/dam/cancer-org/research/cancer-facts-and-statistics/annual-cancer-facts-and-figures/2021/cancer-facts-and-figures-2021.pdf.
3. Wehner M, Chren M, Nameth D, et al. "International prevalence of indoor tanning: A systematic review and meta-analysis," Journal of the American Medical Association Dermatology 150, no. 4, 2014:390–400.
4. Johnson MW, Skuta GL, Kincaid MC, et al. "Malignant melanoma of the iris in xeroderma pigmentosum," Archives of Ophthalmology 107, no. 3, 1989:402–7.
5. Wu S, Cho E, Li WQ, et al. "History of severe sunburn and risk of skin cancer among women and men in 2 prospective cohort studies," American Journal of Epidemiology 183, no. 9, 2016:824–33.
6. Olsen JH, Friis S, Frederiksen K. "Malignant melanoma and other types of cancer preceding Parkinson disease," Epidemiology 17, no. 5, 2006:582–87. https://pubmed.ncbi.nlm.nih.gov/16837822; Olsen JH, Friis S, Frederiksen K, et al. "Atypical cancer pattern in patients with Parkinson's disease," British Journal of Cancer 92, no. 1, 2005:201–5.

Chapter 14. Early Detection Strategies for High-Risk People

1. Pijpe A, Andrieu N, Easton D, et al. "Exposure to diagnostic radiation and risk of breast cancer among carriers of BRCA1/2 mutations: Retrospective cohort study, GENE-RAD-RISK)," British Medical Journal 345, 2012:e5660.

2. Ovarian Cancer Research Alliance. "What is CA-125? Questions about ovarian cancer screening." https://ocrahope.org/patients/about-ovarian-cancer/symptoms-and-detection/what-is-ca-125.

Chapter 15. Medications That Reduce Cancer Risk

1. Vogel VG, Costantino JP, Wickerham DL, et al. "Update of the national surgical adjuvant breast and bowel project study of tamoxifen and raloxifene (STAR) P-2 trial: Preventing breast cancer," Cancer Prevention Research 3, no. 6, 2010:696–706.
2. Cuzick J, Sestak I, Cawthorn S, et al. "Tamoxifen for prevention of breast cancer: Extended long-term follow-up of the IBIS-I breast cancer prevention trial," Lancet Oncology 16, no. 1, 2015:67–75.
3. Cuzick J, Sestak I, Forbes JF, et al. for the IBIS-II investigators. "Use of anastrozole for breast cancer prevention (IBIS-II): Long-term results of a randomised controlled trial," Lancet 395, no. 10218, 2020:117–22; Goss PE, Ingle JN, Alés-Martínez JE, et al. for the NCIC CTG MAP.3 study investigators. "Exemestane for breast cancer prevention in postmenopausal women," New England Journal of Medicine 364, no. 25, 2011:2381–91.
4. Howell A, Cuzick J, Baum M, et al. "ATAC trialists' group: Results of the ATAC (Arimidex, Tamoxifen, Alone, or in Combination) trial after completion of 5 years' adjuvant treatment for breast cancer," Lancet 365, no. 9453, 2005:60–62.
5. International Agency for Research on Cancer: Pharmaceuticals. "Combined estrogen-progestogen contraceptives," IARC Monographs on the Evaluation of Carcinogenic Risks to Humans 100A, 2012:283–311. https://monographs.iarc.who.int/wp-content/uploads/2018/06/mono100A.pdf; Havrilesky LJ, Moorman PG, Lowery WJ, et al. "Oral contraceptive pills as primary prevention for ovarian cancer: A systematic review and meta-analysis," Obstetrics and Gynecology 122, no. 1, 2013:139–47.
6. Michels KA, Pfeiffer RM, Brinton LA, et al. "Modification of the associations between duration of oral contraceptive use and ovarian, endometrial, breast, and colorectal cancers," Journal of the American Medical Association Oncology 4, no. 4, 2018:516–21.
7. Friebel TM, Domchek SM, Rebbeck TR. "Modifiers of cancer risk in BRCA1 and BRCA2 mutation carriers: Systematic review and meta-analysis," Journal of the National Cancer Institute 106, no. 6, 2014:dju091.
8. Michels, Pfeiffer, Brinton, et al. "Modification of the associations"; Dashti SG, Chau R, Ouakrim DA, et al. "Female hormonal factors and the risk of endometrial cancer in Lynch syndrome," Journal of the American Medical Association 314, no. 1, 2015:61–71.
9. Collaborative Group on Hormonal Factors in Breast Cancer. "Breast cancer and hormonal contraceptives: Collaborative reanalysis of individual data on 53,297 women with breast cancer and 100,239 women without breast cancer from 54 epidemiological studies," Lancet 347, no. 9017, 1996:1713–27.
10. Burn J, Sheth H, Elliott F, et al. "Cancer prevention with aspirin in hereditary colorectal cancer (Lynch syndrome), 10-year follow-up and registry-based 20-year data in the CAPP2 study: A double-blind, randomized, placebo-controlled trial," Lancet 395, no. 10240, 2020:1855–63; Ouakrim DA, Dashti SG, Chau R, et al. "Aspirin, ibuprofen, and the risk for colorectal cancer in Lynch syndrome," Journal of the National Cancer Institute 107, no. 9, 2015:djv170.

Chapter 16. Surgeries That Reduce Breast Cancer Risk

1. Domchek SM, Friebel TM, Singer CF, et al. "Association of risk-reducing surgery in BRCA1 or BRCA2 mutation carriers with cancer risk and mortality," Journal of the American Medical Association 304, no. 9, 2010:967–75; Rebbeck TR, Friebel T, Lynch HT, et al. "Bilateral prophylactic mastectomy reduces breast cancer risk in BRCA1 and BRCA2 mutation carriers: The PROSE study group," Journal of Clinical Oncology 22, no. 6, 2004:1055–62.

Chapter 17. Surgeries That Reduce the Risk of Gynecologic Cancers

1. Rebbeck TR, Kauff ND, Domchek SM. "Meta-analysis of risk reduction estimates associated with risk-reducing salpingo-oophorectomy in BRCA1 or BRCA2 mutation carriers," Journal of the National Cancer Institute 101, no. 2, 2009:80–87.
2. Rebbeck, Kauff, Domchek. "Meta-analysis of risk reduction estimates."
3. Domchek SM, Friebel TM, Singer CF, et al. "Association of risk-reducing surgery in BRCA1 or BRCA2 mutation carriers with cancer risk and mortality," Journal of the American Medical Association 304, no. 9, 2010:967–75.
4. Rebbeck TR, Friebel T, Wagner T, et al. "Effect of short-term hormone replacement therapy on breast cancer risk reduction after bilateral prophylactic oophorectomy in BRCA1 and BRCA2 mutation carriers: The PROSE study group," Journal of Clinical Oncology 23, no. 31, 2005:7804–10.

Chapter 19. Factors That Affect Cancer Risk

1. Centers for Disease Control and Prevention. "About chronic diseases." https://www.cdc.gov/chronicdisease/index.htm.
2. American Cancer Society. "American Cancer Society guidelines for diet and physical activity." https://www.cancer.org/healthy/eat-healthy-get-active/acs-guidelines-nutrition-physical-activity-cancer-prevention/guidelines.html.
3. American Institute for Cancer Research. "How to prevent cancer: The cancer fighters in your food." https://www.aicr.org/cancer-prevention/recommendations/eat-a-diet-rich-in-whole-grains-vegetables-fruits-and-beans.
4. Centers for Disease Control and Prevention. "Prevalence of obesity and severe obesity among adults: United States, 2017–2018." https://www.cdc.gov/nchs/products/databriefs/db360.htm; Fryar C, Carroll M, Afful J. "Prevalence of overweight, obesity, and severe obesity among children and adolescents aged 2–19 years: United States, 1963–1965 through 2017–2018," National Center for Health Statistics Health E-Stats, 2020. https://www.cdc.gov/nchs/data/hestat/obesity-child-17-18/obesity-child.htm.
5. Moore SC, Lee I-M, Weiderpass E, et al. "Association of leisure-time physical activity with risk of 26 types of cancer in 1.44 million adults," Journal of the American Medical Association Internal Medicine 176, no. 6, 2016:816–25.
6. American Cancer Society. "Health risks of smoking tobacco." https://www.cancer.org/cancer/cancer-causes/tobacco-and-cancer/health-risks-of-smoking-tobacco.html.
7. Balogh E, Dresler C, Fleury M, et al. "Reducing tobacco-related cancer incidence and mortality: Summary of Institute of Medicine workshop," Oncologist 19, no. 1, 2014:21–31.

8. Wong CM, Tsang H, Lai HK, et al. "Cancer mortality risks from long-term exposure to ambient fine particle," Cancer Epidemiology, Biomarkers and Prevention 25, no. 5, 2016:839–45. https://cebp.aacrjournals.org/content/25/5/839.

Chapter 21. Treating Breast Cancer

1. Hadar T, Mor P, Amit G, et al. "Presymptomatic awareness of germline pathogenic BRCA variants and associated outcomes in women with breast cancer," Journal of the American Medical Association Oncology 6, no. 9, 2020:1460–63.
2. American Society of Clinical Oncology. "Management of hereditary breast cancer: Rapid recommendation update," June 2021. https://www.asco.org/research-guidelines/quality-guidelines/guidelines/breast-cancer; National Comprehensive Cancer Network Guidelines: Breast Cancer. Version 5.2021, June 2021. https://www.nccn.org/guidelines/guidelines-detail?category=1&id=1419; National Comprehensive Cancer Network. "Guidelines: Genetic/familial high-risk assessment: Breast, ovarian, and pancreatic." Version 1.2022, August 2021.
3. Tung NM, Zakalik D, Somerfield, MR. "Adjuvant PARP inhibitors in patients with high-risk early-stage HER2-negative breast cancer and germline BRCA mutations: ASCO hereditary breast cancer guideline rapid recommendation update." Journal of Clinical Oncology 39, no. 26, 2021:2959–61. doi:10.1200/JCO.21.01532.

Chapter 22. Treating Gynecologic Cancers

1. Pennington KP, Walsh T, Harrell MI, et al. "Germline and somatic mutations in homologous recombination genes predict platinum response and survival in ovarian, fallopian tube, and peritoneal carcinomas," Clinical Cancer Research 20, no. 3, 2014:764–75.
2. Norquist BM, Brady MF, Harrell MI, et al. "Mutations in homologous recombination genes and outcomes in ovarian carcinoma patients in GOG 218: An NRG oncology/gynecologic oncology group study," Clinical Cancer Research 24, no. 4, 2018:777–83.

Chapter 25. Treating Melanoma

1. Ocular Melanoma Foundation. "About ocular melanoma." http://www.ocularmelanoma.org/disease.htm#:~:text=Approximately%2050%25%20of%20patients%20with,Metastatic%20disease%20is%20universally%20fatal.

Resources

Hereditary Cancer Risk

Alive and Kickn, aliveandkickn.org
Facing Our Risk of Cancer Empowered, facingourrisk.org
Genetic Alliance, geneticalliance.org
Informed Medical Decisions, informeddna.com
National Society of Genetic Counselors, nsgc.org

Prevention, Treatment, and Quality of Life

Academy of Nutrition and Dietetics, eatright.org
Aim at Melanoma, aimatmelanoma.org
American Cancer Society, cancer.org
American Society of Clinical Oncology, asco.org
Black Health Matters, blackhealthmatters.com
The Breast Reconstruction Guidebook by Kathy Steligo
Cancer Support Community, cancersupportcommunity.org
Clinical trials, clinicaltrials.gov
Colorectal Cancer Alliance, ccalliance.org
Facing Our Risk of Cancer Empowered, facingourrisk.org
Foundation for Women's Cancer, foundationforwomenscancer.org
HairToStay, hairtostay.org
HIS Breast Cancer Awareness, hisbreastcancer.org
Hystersisters, hystersisters.com
Let's Win! Pancreatic Cancer, letswinpc.org
Living beyond Breast Cancer, lbbc.org
Look Good Feel Better, lookgoodfeelbetter.org
Lymphatic Education and Resource Network, lymphaticnetwork.org
Male Breast Cancer Coalition, malebreastcancercoalition.org
Malecare, malecare.org
METAvivor, metavivor.org
National Cancer Institute, cancer.gov
National Comprehensive Cancer Network, nccn.org
National LGBT Cancer Network, cancer-network.org

National Ovarian Cancer Coalition, ovarian.org
New American Plate, aicr.org
North American Menopause Society, menopause.org
No Stomach for Cancer, nostomachforcancer.org
Ovarian Cancer Research Alliance, ocrahope.org
Pancreatic Cancer Action Network, pancan.org
SHARE, sharecancersupport.org
Sharsheret, sharsheret.org
Society for Integrative Oncology, integrativeonc.org
Susan G. Komen, komen.org
United Ostomy Association of America, ostomy.org
Unite for Her, uniteforher.org
Young Survival Coalition, youngsurvival.org
ZERO: The End of Prostate Cancer, zerocancer.org

Sexuality, Intimacy, and Fertility

Alliance for Fertility Preservation, allianceforfertilitypreservation.org
American Association of Sexuality Educators, Counselors, and Therapists, aasect.org
Livestrong Fertility, livestrong.org
SaveMyFertility, savemyfertility.org

Financial Help, Health Insurance Issues, and Your Rights

CancerCare, cancercare.org
Cancer and Careers, cancerandcareers.org
Cancer Legal Resource Center, cancerlegalresourcecenter.org
Genetic Information Nondiscrimation Act, ginahelp.org
Patient Advocate Foundation, patientadvocate.org
Social Security Administration, ssa.gov
Triage Cancer, triagecancer.org

Index

Abraxane (nab-paclitaxel), 314, 343
acinar cell carcinomas, 132
Actonel, 386
acupuncture/acupressure, 378, 381, 392, 395, 399, 402–3, 404
adenocarcinomas, 64, 120, 127, 130, 132, 133, 137–38, 143, 311, 316, 321–22
adenomas, 81, 83, 104
adjuvant therapy, 263, 344–45, 346
Adriamycin (doxorubicin), 367–68, 389, 398
advance health care directives, 407
Affordable Care Act (ACA), 43–44, 196, 197, 206, 419
Afinitor (everolimus), 300
alcohol consumption, 19, 73, 126, 159, 250, 257, 259, 378, 380–81, 387, 393, 397, 398, 399
Alferon (interferon), 333
alkylating chemotherapy, 367, 372
Aloxi (palonosetron HCI), 395
American Board of Medical Specialties, 220
American Cancer Society, 221, 250, 253, 257, 395
American Lung Association, 257
American Society of Clinical Oncology, 202, 365, 400
anal cancer, 123, 125, 126, 134–35, 303

androgen deprivation therapy, 326, 362, 390
androgen receptor–targeted therapy, 326, 327, 329
anemia, 130, 389, 393; Fanconi, 72, 91; iron deficiency, 245; pernicious, 133; sickle cell, 15
angiotensin-converting enzyme inhibitors, 405
anthracycline chemotherapy, 367–68
anti-androgens. See androgen receptor–targeted therapy
antibiotics, 101, 134, 219, 393
anti-HER2 targeted therapy, 282
antinausea drugs, 395
APC gene mutations, 48, 88, 89, 125, 162, 166, 175, 239. See also familial adenomatous polyposis
appetite changes, 133, 142, 295, 389, 391, 396, 400
Arimidex (anastrozole), 202, 287
Aromasin (exemestane), 202, 287
aromatase inhibitors, 202, 282, 288, 378, 390, 403
arthralgia. See joint pain
Ashkenazi Jews: family history, 23; inherited gene mutations, 49, 66–67, 72, 92, 279, 285–86; pancreatic cancer risk, 132

aspirin, 204–5, 397

assisted reproductive technology (ART), 365, 368–69, 375

astrocytomas, 153, 340

ataxia-telangiectasia (Louis-Bar syndrome), 90

ATM gene mutations: cancers associated with, 88, 89–90, 102, 114, 115, 125, 139, 166–67, 223, 230, 281, 283, 285–86, 323, 327; risk management guidelines, 166–67

Avastin (bevacizumab), 293, 295, 300, 308

Avodart (dutasteride), 204

AXIN2 gene mutations, 125

bacillus-calmette guerin (BCG) vaccine, 333, 334

Balversa (erdafitinib), 333

BAP1 gene mutations, 151, 153, 155, 157

BARD1 gene mutations, 88, 90, 102, 175, 281

basal cell carcinomas, 147, 339

Bavencio (avelumab), 333

benign prostatic hyperplasia, 136–37

beta blockers, 405

biliary tract cancer, 82

bioidenticals, 385

biomarkers, 264, 267, 270–71, 272, 273, 276. *See also under specific cancers*

biopsy, 177; blood-based liquid, 274; breast, 98, 99, 101, 104, 105, 106, 110; colonoscopy-related, 187; endometrial, 122, 186; melanoma, 341; needle, 110, 278; prostate, 140, 322, 328; sentinel node, 209, 278, 280, 299, 345; small bowel, 130; unnecessary, 178, 180, 185–86; via colonoscopy, 187

birth control, 222, 365, 391

birth defects, 391

bisphosphonates, 329, 386

bladder cancer, 74, 141–44, 145, 257, 335; biomarkers, 333; gene mutations associated with, 80, 82, 142, 143; immunotherapy, 333, 335; Lynch syndrome–associated, 80, 82, 333; metastatic, 143, 332; risk-reducing strategies, 254–55; staging, 334–35; surveillance, 192; treatment, 331–35

bladder prolapse, 231–32

bleeding, 135, 188, 205, 225, 226, 240, 244, 396–97; bladder cancer–related, 331, 332; chemotherapy-related, 389, 396–97; colorectal cancer–related, 305; colectomy-related, 307; colonoscopy-related, 240; endoscopic ultrasound–related, 188; gastrectomy-related, 244; laparotomy-related, 225, 226; menstrual, 114, 117, 232, 396; NSAIDs-related, 205; pancreatic biopsy–related, 188; pancreatic surgery–related, 313; radical prostatectomy–related, 323–24; rectal, 126, 135; targeted therapy–related, 396–97; vaginal, 111, 113, 117, 120, 121, 201, 230, 231, 301, 395–96

blood clots, 131, 141, 201, 202, 203, 219, 227, 241, 307, 383, 405

BMPR1A gene mutations, 125

body image, 355–57

body mass index (BMI), 253

bone cancer, 88, 95, 171

bone density tests, 287, 384, 386

bone health, 387

bone loss and weakness, 202, 384–86, 390

bone metastases, 403

bone pain, 142, 329, 342, 347

bone scans, 325

Boniva, 386

brachytherapy, 281–82, 299, 300, 324, 328–29, 348, 350–52

BRAF gene mutations, V600E and
V600K, 340

BRAF inhibitors, 340, 344, 405

Braftovi (encorafenib), 308, 344

brain cancer/tumors, 25, 82, 83, 93, 95,
153, 171, 340

brain scans, 194

BRCA1/2 gene mutations, 65–75, 87, 88;
breast cancer and, 65–66, 68, 69,
70–72, 283, 288, 294; genetic testing
for, 43–44, 66, 71; melanoma and,
65, 69; in men, 69, 73–75, 288;
ovarian cancer and, 65, 68, 69, 70–72,
116, 229, 290, 294; pancreatic cancer
and, 65–66, 69, 75; PARP therapy
and, 289; prostate cancer and, 65, 69;
signs, 66–68

BRCA1 gene mutation, 1, 16; breast cancer
and, 102, 109, 201, 208, 230, 280,
281, 283, 288, 386; DNA repair
function, 90; endometrial cancer
and, 231; genetic testing for, 43,
57–58; melanoma and, 75; ovarian
cancer and, 114, 115, 223, 230;
pancreatic cancer and, 125, 312,
314–15; prostate cancer and, 139, 321,
323, 327; risk management
guidelines, 162, 163–64

BRCA2 gene, DNA repair function of, 87,
93

BRCA2 gene mutation, 1; breast cancer
and, 102, 103, 190–91, 208, 230, 280,
281; Fanconi anemia and, 72; genetic
testing for, 43; melanoma and, 151,
153, 155; ovarian cancer and, 114, 115,
223, 230; pancreatic cancer and, 125,
312, 314–15; prostate cancer and,
139, 140–41, 192, 321, 323, 327; risk
management guidelines, 162,
163–64

BRCA genes, DNA repair function, 294

breast: anatomy, 97; benign tumors, 98,
99, 109; cysts, 100; duct ectasia, 101;
fibrocystic changes, 100, 104; lumps,
96–99; microcalcifications, 100, 182,
183

breast cancer, 64, 70–71, 96–110, 162,
254–55, 386; biomarkers, 278–79,
280, 283, 286; in both breasts, 280;
CDH1 gene mutations, 88, 167, 168,
281; chemoprevention, 104,
200–203, 206; diagnosis, 70, 110,
278; ductal carcinoma in situ (DCIS),
100, 105–6, 183, 200, 280, 283, 285,
435; estrogen receptor–positive/
negative, 279, 280, 282, 283, 383;
genetic testing and counseling for,
279–80, 283, 284, 288; HER2-
positive/negative, 278, 279, 282, 288,
317, 319; hormone-dependent, 200;
hormone receptor–positive/negative,
279, 280, 282, 283, 383; hormone
replacement therapy, 104, 382–83;
immunotherapy, 282–83; incidence,
52; inflammatory (IBC), 108;
invasive, 100, 107–9; invasive ductal
carcinoma in situ (IDC), 100, 108,
439; invasive lobular carcinoma
(ILC), 108; lobular carcinoma in situ
(LCIS), 105, 200, 209; metastatic,
105, 107–8, 277, 278, 280, 282; myths
about, 107; nonhereditary (sporadic),
101, 103, 281; in opposite breast, 209;
ovarian cancer and, 29, 114, 283;
Paget's disease, 108; *PTEN* gene
mutations (Cowden syndrome), 88,
94, 171, 172, 281; recurrence, 200,
277, 283, 287, 383; screening/
surveillance for, 178–84; secondary,
281; signs and symptoms, 96–101,
108; staging, 278; triple-negative, 31,
65–66, 71, 90, 279, 280, 282, 283

breast cancer (male), 72–74, 91–92, 96, 100, 237, 323, 356; family history, 29, 31; genetic testing, 31, 280; gynecomastia and, 104–5; risk-reducing mastectomy, 208; screening/surveillance, 178, 182; treatment, 281, 287–88

breast cancer risk: alcohol consumption, 257; *ATM* gene mutations, 89–90, 102, 166–67, 230, 281, 285–86; *BARD1* gene mutations, 88, 90, 102, 175, 281; *BRCA1/2* gene mutations, 65–66, 68, 69, 70–72, 288, 294; *BRCA1* gene mutation, 102, 109, 201, 208, 230, 281, 283, 288, 386; *BRCA2* gene mutation, 102, 103, 190–91, 208, 230, 281; *BRIP1* gene mutations, 88, 90, 175, 281; dietary factors, 252, 258; oral contraceptives, 203–4; overweight/obesity, 252; smoking, 258; *TP53* gene mutations (Li-Fraumeni syndrome), 88, 95, 102, 171, 174, 183, 208, 281

breast cancer risk–reducing strategies, nonsurgical, 103–4. *See also* mastectomy, risk-reducing; screening/surveillance

breast cancer screening/surveillance, 96, 98, 105, 178–82, 183, 281; health insurance coverage, 196, 197. *See also* mammography

breast cancer treatment, 277–88, 286, 359; chemotherapy, 280, 282, 283; for hormone-sensitive breast cancer, 223; hormone therapy, 279, 280, 281, 282, 288; immunotherapy, 280, 282–83; mammography after, 184; in men, 281, 287–88; ovarian function suppression, 378; planning, 277–80; radiation therapy, 28, 184, 282; side effects, 280; targeted therapy, 280, 282–83

breast examinations: clinical examinations (CBE), 179–80; self-examinations (BSE), 96, 98, 110, 163, 178–80, 213

breastfeeding, 101, 103, 115–16, 258, 367, 369, 371

breast implant–associated anaplastic large-cell lymphoma (BIA-ALCL), 216

breast implants, 214–17; breast cancer risk and, 107; capsular contractures, 215; mammography and, 183; temporary (tissue expanders), 214, 216, 218

breast prostheses, 210, 221

breast reconstruction, 214–20, 221

Breast Reconstruction Guidebook, The (Steligo), 212–13

breast reduction surgery, 104–5

BRIP1 gene mutations, 1, 88, 90, 91, 102, 114, 115, 175, 223, 230, 281

bruising, 396–97

CA 19–9 blood test, 316

CA-125 blood test, 184, 186, 291, 295

café-au-lait spots, 83

caffeine, 100, 259, 378, 380–81, 398

calcium, 100, 182, 245, 252, 381, 386, 387

cancer, development and growth of, 16–19, 250. *See also specific cancers*

cancer cells, 16–19

cancer statistics, 52–54; media reports, 53

capecitabine, 314

capsular contractures, 215

carboplatin, 292, 335, 405

carcinogens, 19. *See also* environmental toxin exposures

Casodex (bicalutamide), 326

CDH1 gene mutations, 102; cancers associated with, 88, 90–91, 125, 167, 168, 241, 247–48, 281, 317, 318; risk management guidelines, 167, 168

CDK4/6 inhibitors, 288, 391

CDK4 gene mutations, 88, 91, 125, 151, 153, 175

CDKN2A gene mutations, 88, 91, 175

celiac disease, 130

celiac plexus blocks, 315

cells: damage/death, 7, 16; division, 10, 15, 16; functions, 10–11, 12, 15. *See also* cancer cells; *and specific types of cells*

Centers for Disease Control and Prevention (CDC), 27–28

Cerubidine (daunorubicin), 367–68

cervical cancer, 25, 64, 94, 111, 113, 185, 196, 197, 366

cervix, surgical removal, 232

Cesamet (nabilone), 395

CHEK2 gene mutations, 66; cancers associated with, 72, 88, 91–92, 102, 125, 167, 168, 281, 283; risk management, 167, 168

chemoprevention, 104, 105, 159, 198–207; side effects, 388–89. *See also under specific cancers*

chemoradiation, 318, 319, 372

chemotherapy, 19, 263; endometrial cancer, 297, 299, 300, 301; intravesical, 332–33; side effects, 269, 355, 357, 359, 366, 367–68, 371–72, 378, 389–90, 393, 395, 396–405; systemic, 332, 333. *See also under specific cancers*

childhood cancers, 171

children: discussing cancer with, 58–60, 74; genetic testing of, 38–39; passing a genetic mutation to, 9, 15, 19, 20, 22, 48, 54, 72, 83; Spitz nevus moles, 340

chromosomes, 11

Cialis (tadalafil), 362

cisplatin, 292, 314, 335, 343, 371–72, 389–90, 398, 405

C-KIT gene mutations, 340

C-KIT inhibitors, 344

clear cell carcinomas, endometrial, 119, 120–21

Clinical Laboratory Improvement Amendments (CLIA), 41

clinical trials, 207, 264, 416, 418, 419. *See also under specific cancers*

colectomy: risk-reducing, 238–41, 242, 247; segmental, 239, 305, 306; total, 239, 240, 305

colon cancer, 64, 114, 128, 171, 254–55, 303. *See also* colorectal cancer

colonoscopes, 186–87

colonoscopy, 125, 127, 186–87, 196

colorectal cancer, 31, 52, 125–27, 304, 310–11; biomarkers, 304, 308; chemoprevention, 204–5; dMMR/ MSI-H, 275, 308, 309; with endometrial cancer, 29; family history, 31, 304, 322; gene mutations associated with, 31, 76, 77, 78–80, 81, 82, 88, 90–91, 123, 125, 169, 171, 172; genetic testing, 31, 304; immunotherapy, 303, 308; Lynch syndrome and, 76, 77, 78–80, 79, 81, 82, 88, 90–91; metastatic, 309; prostate cancer and, 31, 323; risk factors and symptoms, 125–27, 252, 257; risk-reducing surgery, 89, 238–41; staging, 304, 308–9, 310–11; targeted therapy, 303, 304, 308; treatment, 303–11, 405; types, 127

colorectal cancer surveillance/screening, 310–11; colonoscopy, 125, 127, 186–87, 189, 196, 197, 311; health insurance coverage, 196, 197

colostomy bags, 239, 305, 306

computed tomography (CT), 122, 130, 144, 190, 194, 310–11, 316, 325, 328, 330

Confronting Hereditary Breast and Ovarian Cancer (Friedman, Sutphen, and Steligo), 1

connective tissue cancers, 127, 171
constipation, 114, 126, 231, 393–94
constitutional mismatch repair-deficiency
    (CMMRD) syndrome, 83
corticosteroids, 403
Cotellic (cobimetinib), 344
Cowden syndrome, 94. See also *PTEN*
    gene mutations
cribriform cells, 323
Crohn's disease, 238
cryotherapy, 325, 329, 434, 438
CTNNA1 gene mutations, 125
cultural factors, affecting cancer risk
    perception, 415
cyclophosphamide, 143, 367, 371–72, 405
Cymbalta (duloxetine), 403
Cyramza (ramucirumab), 308, 319
cystectomy, 332, 333, 334–35; radical, 332,
    335
cystic fibrosis, 15, 130
cystoscopy, 144
cysts: breast, 100, 104, 110; fallopian
    tubes, 118; ovarian, 116, 118, 222,
    229; peritoneal, 118
Cytoxan (cyclophosphamide), 143, 367

debulking, of tumors, 292, 293, 299,
    300–301
decision-making, 2–3, 410–20; about
    genetic testing, 38–43, 410–12;
    family's disagreement with decisions,
    417; 15-step approach, 418, 420;
    about risk management, 413–14, 417,
    418; about treatment, 414–16
deep breathing exercises, 259, 426, 427
deep inferior epigastric perforator (DIEP)
    flaps, 218
desmoid tumors, 89
diabetes, 12, 15, 120, 131, 132, 143, 313,
    384, 391–92
dialysis, 336–37

diarrhea, 114, 126, 244, 246, 389, 391, 393
diet and nutrition, 159; for anemia
    management, 393; before and after
    surgery, 255; for bone health, 387; for
    cancer risk reduction, 125–26, 250–54,
    399; for constipation or diarrhea
    management, 393–94; for fatigue
    management, 392; after gastrectomy,
    245, 246; for menopause symptom
    control, 380–81; for mouth sores
    management, 399; after pancreatic
    surgery, 313; as stomach cancer risk
    factor, 133; for weight control, 253–54,
    396
diethylstilbestrol, 102
digital rectal examination (DRE), 192,
    197, 328, 331
disability benefits, 427
disabled individuals: health disparities,
    261; screening tests, 196
discrimination, genetic, 44–45
DNA (deoxyribonucleic acid), 9, 10–11, 12,
    14; analysis, 13; damage, 12, 14–15, 18,
    20, 183, 253, 272, 275, 371; percentage
    shared among relatives, 26; of tumors,
    blood-based liquid biopsy for, 274
DNA damage repair (DDR) genes, 87, 90,
    93, 271–72, 294
DNA mismatch repair
    deficiency / microsatellite instability-
    high (dMMR/MSI-H) tumors, 275,
    441; bladder, 333; colorectal, 84, 127,
    272, 275, 291, 304, 308, 309;
    endometrial, 275, 298; ovarian, 291,
    293; pancreatic, 315–16; prostate,
    323, 327; stomach, 317, 319
doxorubicin, 405
DTIC (dacarbazine), 343
dual-energy x-ray absorptiometry
    (DEXA), 386
dumping syndrome, 246

Eastern European Jewish ancestry. *See* Ashkenazi Jews

Effexor XR (venlafaxine), 379

eggs (ova), 11, 12; adverse effects of treatment on, 366, 367; donor, 372–73; mutations, 15, 19; preservation procedures, 367, 368–69

Eligard (leuprolide), 326

Ellence (epirubicin), 367–68

embolization therapy, 309, 315, 349–50

embryos: donor, 372–73; preimplantation genetic testing (PGT), 375; preservation procedures, 367, 368–69

Emend (aprepitant), 395

emotional issues: management, 405–6; support system for, 421–26

end-of-life issues, 406–7

endometrial cancer, 31, 117, 120–22, 252, 289, 298, 322; biomarkers, 297, 298–99; chemoprevention, 203; colorectal cancer and, 29; dMMR/MSI-H, 275, 298; early detection, 184; genetic testing for, 31; HER2-positive/negative, 298; hormone replacement therapy and, 383; hormone therapy, 297, 299, 300; immunotherapy, 298, 300; Lynch syndrome–associated, 31, 76, 77, 80, 82, 85, 121, 203, 229, 231; *PTEN* gene mutations (Cowden syndrome), 88; recurrence, 299; risk-reducing strategies, 230–34, 254–55; screening/surveillance, 301; staging, 299, 300–301; tamoxifen-related, 287; treatment, 297–301; type 1 and type 2, 297

endometrioid cancer, 119

endometriosis, 115, 232

endorphins, 403

endoscopes, 188

endoscopic mucosal resection, 305, 318

enucleation, 348

environmental toxin exposures, 19, 20, 23, 24, 49, 50, 52, 79, 260, 348

EPCAM gene mutations, 77–78, 80, 83, 114, 115, 125, 139, 142, 223, 229; risk management guidelines, 162, 164–65

epigenetics, 399

Epstein-Barr virus, 133

Erbitux (cetuximab), 308

erectile dysfunction, 323–24, 332, 355–56, 360–62, 360–63, 390

Erleada (apalutamide), 326

esophageal cancer, 123, 257

esophagogastroduodenoscopy (EGD), 187–88

estradiol, 385

estrogen, 111, 117, 119, 232, 253, 368, 377, 379; cancer risk and, 104, 120; heart protective effects of, 384; vaginal application, 359, 386–87

estrogen-progestin therapy. *See* hormone replacement therapy

estrogen receptor testing, 299

estrogen replacement therapy, 120, 379, 382, 383, 384

ethnic/racial factors, in cancer risk, 28, 66, 103, 119, 121, 129, 133, 140, 143, 154, 157, 261

Eulexin (flutamide), 326

exercise and physical activity, 250, 254–56; aerobic, 396, 402; for arthralgia management, 403; for bone health, 387; for fatigue management, 392, 402; lack of, 384; for menopause symptoms management, 380, 381; for pain management, 403; resistance training, 396, 402; for stress and anxiety control, 259; for weight control, 253–54

exocrine tumors, 132

Facing Our Risk of Cancer Empowered (FORCE), 1, 2, 3, 33, 34–35, 39, 47, 53, 54, 203, 261, 384, 423; breast cancer guidance, 106–7, 213–14, 217, 230; clinical trials database, 418; decision-making guidance, 418, 420; five-year risk perspective, 413–14; "The Genes between Us" guide, 55; genetic counseling and testing guidance, 33, 55, 57; health care costs coverage guidance, 197, 207; message boards, 217, 230, 423; Peer Navigation Program, 107, 423; prophylactic surgery guidance, 234; reproductive planning support volunteers, 375; toll-free helpline, 33, 420; website, 3, 55, 197, 207, 423

fallopian tube(s): cysts, 118; as ovarian cancer origin site, 224, 227–28; removal (salpingectomy), 116, 117, 232

fallopian tube cancer, 31, 72, 111, 112–14, 237, 293; genetic testing for, 31; risk-reducing surgery, 222–30; screening/surveillance, 184–86; treatment, 290–95

fallopian tubes removal, 116, 117, 232

false-positive and false-negative test results, 34–35, 159, 178, 182, 186, 191

familial adenomatous polyposis (FAP), 81, 89, 162, 166; attenuated, 89, 162, 240

familial atypical multiple mole melanoma syndrome, 152–53

familial hypercholesterolemia, 85

family: disagreement with risk management decisions, 417; involvement in creating family medical history, 27–29; sharing genetic test results with, 55–58; as support system, 422–23

Family and Medical Leave Act, 427

family medical history, 21, 39, 55, 443; creation, 24–29; incomplete sharing, 63

Fanconi anemia, 72, 91

FAP. See familial adenomatous polyposis

Faslodex, 390

fatigue, 72, 359, 390; breast implant-related, 218; as cancer symptom, 114, 126, 131, 142, 145, 159, 295, 296; iron deficiency anemia–related, 245; management, 357, 392–93, 402; during menopause, 380; menopause-related, 380; treatment-related, 390, 391, 392–93, 395, 400, 402, 406

fecal occult blood tests, 187

Federal Employees Health Benefits Program, 45

Femara (letrozole), 202, 287

fertility, effects of prevention and treatment on, 228, 365–75, 376, 391; fertility preservation (in men), 371–72; fertility preservation (in women), 300, 366–71; parenting alternatives and, 372

fertility specialists, 289, 365–66, 372

fetus, treatment-related harm to, 366

fibroadenomas, 100–101

fibroblast growth factor receptor (FGFR) gene mutations, 333

fibroids, uterine, 186, 222, 230, 232

financial resources, for health care costs, 426–27. See also health insurance coverage

Firmagon (degarelix), 326

first-line treatment, 263, 291, 299, 324

fistulas, 390

5-fluorouracil, 307–8, 314–15, 318, 319, 398

folate and folate deficiency, 245, 252, 257

folic acid, 245, 393

Food and Drug Administration (FDA),
204, 206, 207, 216, 276, 379, 381, 385,
386, 394, 395, 416; mammography
guidelines, 181, 182, 183
foods. *See* diet and nutrition
FORCE. *See* Facing Our Risk of Cancer
Empowered
Fosamax, 386
Foundation for Women's Cancer, 234

gabapentin, 379
gallbladder cancer, 123
Gardasil vaccine, 135
gastrectomy: partial, 318; risk-reducing
total, 168, 241, 243–48, 444; total, 318
gastric cancer. *See* stomach cancer
gastrointestinal cancers, 123–35; gene
mutations associated with, 88, 94,
125, 316, 317; risk-reduction surgery,
238–48; screening/surveillance,
186–91; treatment, 303–20
gastrointestinal surgery, side effects of, 393
gastrointestinal tract, anatomy and
function of, 123, 124
Gemzar (gemcitabine), 314–15
genes and genetics, basics of, 10–15
genetic counseling, 32–37, 54, 57, 64, 162;
health insurance coverage, 43–44, 411
Genetic Information Nondiscrimination
Act (GINA), 44–45
genetic testing, 1, 2, 30–45, 162, 411, 422;
of children, 38–39; costs, 43, 44, 411;
decision-making about, 38–43,
410–12; direct-to-consumer tests, 41;
discrimination protections, 44–45;
health insurance coverage, 41,
43–44, 411; implication for
treatment decision-making, 30,
279–80, 283–85, 414; multigene
panel, 42, 49, 66, 77, 92, 285–86;
overlap with biomarker testing, 273;

preimplantation (PGT), 375; process,
35–36; psychological impact, 37, 38,
39, 49–50, 53–54. *See also under specific
cancers*
genetic testing, after cancer diagnosis,
264, 265, 273, 340; breast cancer,
279–80; colorectal cancer, 304, 308;
endometrial cancer, 297–98;
melanoma, 340; ovarian cancer,
290–91, 293; pancreatic cancer, 312,
316; prostate cancer, 322–23, 327,
329; stomach cancer, 317
genetic test results, 46–60; inconclusive,
46; negative, 46, 48–50; positive, 46,
47–48, 53–56, 57–58, 413; sharing
with family, 55–58, 73–74, 411–12;
variant of uncertain significance
(VUS), 50–51
genitourinary cancers, 136–45; screening/
surveillance, 191–93; treatment,
321–38. *See also* bladder cancer;
prostate cancer; renal pelvis cancers;
ureter cancer
genitourinary system, anatomy and
function of, 136, 137
genome, 13
genomics, 13
germ cell tumors, ovarian, 117
Gleason score, for prostate cancer, 322
Gleevac (imatinib), 344
glioblastomas, 86
gonadotropin-releasing hormone
agonists, 368
Grade Group system, for prostate cancer,
322, 323, 328
grading, of cancer, 269. *See also under
specific cancers*
GREM1 gene mutations, 125
gynecologic cancers, 111–22;
chemoprevention, 203–4, 206;
diagnosis, 122; risk-reducing

gynecologic cancers (*continued*)
surgeries, 222–37; screening/
surveillance, 184–86; treatment,
289–302, 359. *See also* endometrial
cancer; fallopian tube cancer; ovarian
cancer; primary peritoneal cancer
gynecomastia, 104–5

hair loss and changes, 356, 357, 380–81,
389, 394–95, 397
hamartomas, 94
health care access disparities, 121, 261
health care teams: assembling of, 3, 54,
84, 234, 418, 422; multidisciplinary,
422
health information, privacy rights and, 45
health insurance coverage: biomarker
testing, 276; breast reconstruction,
221; cancer care, 414;
chemoprevention, 206–7; clinical
trial participation, 419; denial, 197;
discriminatory practices, 44–45;
fertility treatments, 376; genetic
testing, 41, 43–45; hospice care,
408–9; lack, 207, 426–27;
mastectomy, 221; palliative care, 401;
risk-reducing surgeries, 236, 247;
screening, 196–97; wigs, 395. *See also*
Medicaid; Medicare
Health Insurance Portability and
Accountability Act (HIPAA), 45
Healthy Nevada Project, 85
hearing loss, 389–90
heart disease, 384, 389, 405, 406
Helicobacter pylori, 133, 134, 189
hematomas, 219
hepatic perfusion, 349–50
HER2 (human epidermal growth factor
receptor 2), 438
HER2-positive/negative breast cancer,
278, 282, 288, 298, 317, 319, 438

Herceptin (trastuzumab), 298, 300, 308,
319, 397
hereditary breast and ovarian cancer
(HBOC) syndrome, 69
hereditary cancer, 18; differentiated from
sporadic cancer, 19–20
hereditary characteristics, 12
hereditary diffuse gastric cancer (HDGC),
90–91, 241, 243, 316, 318
hereditary nonpolyposis colorectal cancer
(HNPCC). *See* Lynch syndrome
high-risk individuals, chemoprevention
for, 198–207
high-risk individuals, early detection
strategies for. *See* screening/
surveillance
homologous recombination deficient
(HRD) tumors, 275, 291, 295
homologous recombination repair (HRR)
genes, 275
hormone replacement therapy, 104, 120,
232, 233, 377, 378, 382–83, 384, 385
hormones and bioidenticals, 385
hormone therapy, 270; as osteoporosis
preventive, 386; side effects, 355, 358,
359, 360, 366, 378, 390. *See also under*
specific cancers
hospice care, 400, 408–9
hot flashes, 202, 378–79, 386, 390
HOXB13 gene mutations, 88, 92, 139, 175
Human Genome Project, 13
human papillomavirus (HPV), 134–35,
196
hyperplasia: atypical, 105; of breast, 105,
106; endometrial, 120; prostatic, 137
hysterectomy, risk-reducing, 164, 172,
230–34; estrogen-only replacement
therapy and, 383; health coverage of,
236; with mastectomy, 107;
minimally invasive, 289; partial
(supracervical), 222, 230–31; with

radical cystectomy, 332; reproductive effects, 366; sexual function effects, 359; total, 222, 230–31, 300; total abdominal, with risk-reducing salpingo-oophorectomy (TAH/RRSO), 222, 230–31, 232–34

Ibrance (palbociclib), 288
ibuprofen (Advil, Motrin), 204–5, 381, 397, 403
Idamycin (idarubicin), 367–68
ileorectal anastomosis, 239, 240
ileostomy, 239, 240, 307
Imfinzi (durvalumab), 333
Imlygic (talimogene laherparepvec / T-VEC), 345
immune checkpoint inhibitors, 291, 304, 333, 344–45, 346, 391–92. See also Keytruda; Opdivo; Yervoy
immune system, cancer's invasion of, 18
immunotherapy, 264, 275; side effects, 391–92, 395, 397, 405. See also under specific cancers
incontinence: fecal, 390; urinary, 323–24, 325, 382, 390
Indian Health Service, 45
infertility. See fertility, effects of prevention and treatment on
inherited traits, 11, 19
insomnia, 259, 359, 380
insulin, 130, 252, 311, 313
integrative medicine, 399, 402
intensity-modulated therapy, 324
interferon alfa, 405
interleukin-2 (IL-2), 345, 392
intraductal papillary-mucinous neoplasms, 132
Intrarosa (prasterone/DHEA), 379
intravesical therapies, 333, 334
Intron A (interferon), 333
in vitro fertilization, 368, 372

irinotecan, 307–8, 314–15, 318
isolated limb infusion (ILI), 343–44
isolated limb perfusion (ILP), 343, 344, 347

Jemperli (dostarlimab), 298, 300
joint pain, 202, 216, 381, 390, 391, 403
juvenile polyposis syndrome, 125

Kegel exercises, 382
keratocanthomas, 83
Keytruda (pembrolizumab), 291, 293, 298, 299, 300, 304, 308, 315–16, 319, 327, 333, 334, 344–45, 346, 405
kidney, surgical removal of, 336–37
kidney cancer, 25, 171, 172, 254–55, 257, 335
King, Mary-Claire, 69
Klinefelter syndrome, 73
KLLN gene mutations, 94

lactose intolerance, 245
laparoscopic-assisted vaginal hysterectomy (LAVH), 231–32
laparoscopic surgery: gastrointestinal, 239, 241, 243–44, 305, 313; genitourinary, 324, 439; gynecologic, 224–25, 226, 231, 233, 289
laparotomy, 225–26, 239
Lenvima (lenvatinib), 300
leucovorin, 307–8, 314–15
leukemia, 64, 83, 93, 171; acute lymphocytic, 405; acute myeloid, 391; childhood, 91, 93
leuprolide, 368
LGBT community, National LGBT Cancer Network, 179
libido decrease. See sexual desire, decrease in
lifestyle behavior changes, for cancer risk management, 249–61

Li-Fraumeni syndrome. See *TP53* gene
  mutations
liver cancer, 123, 166, 171, 257, 309, 350
liver disorders or damage, 73, 186, 391, 405
local therapies, 263
Lonsurf (trifluridine with tipiracil), 308
low blood count, 392, 393
lumpectomy, 106, 279, 280, 281, 284 285
lung cancer, 91, 95, 96, 151, 257, 335
Lupron (leuprolide), 326, 378
luteinizing hormone–releasing hormone
  (LHRH): agonists, 326, 327;
  antagonists, 326, 327
lymphedema, 221, 278, 390, 404, 406
lymph node dissection, 347; axillary, 278,
  280
lymphoma, 64; breast implant–associated
  anaplastic large-cell, 216; mucosa-
  associated lymphoid tissue, 133;
  non-Hodgkin, 83, 93; small bowel,
  130
lymph system, cancer's invasion of, 18
Lynch, Henry, 79
Lynch syndrome, 79, 87; bladder cancer
  and, 80, 82, 142, 333; cancer risk
  levels, 78, 80, 82; colorectal cancer
  and, 1, 31, 76, 77, 78–80, 79, 81, 82, 86,
  204–5, 240, 311; dMMR/MSI-H
  tumors and, 84, 272, 275, 291, 293,
  298, 304, 315–16, 317, 323, 327;
  endometrial cancer and, 1, 31, 76, 77,
  80, 82, 85, 121, 229, 231; genetic
  testing, 77–78, 83, 84, 127–28;
  multiple mutations in, 83; ovarian
  cancer and, 229, 290, 291; pancreatic
  cancer and, 312, 315–16; renal pelvis
  cancer and, 145; risk management
  guidelines, 161, 162, 164–65;
  screening, 162, 164–65, 276; stomach
  cancer and, 316; upper tract urothelial
  cancers and, 336; ureter cancer and,

145. See also *EPCAM* gene mutations;
  MLH1 gene mutations; *MSH2* gene
  mutations; *MSH6* gene mutations;
  PMS2 gene mutations
Lynparza (olaparib), 203, 283, 289, 315,
  327, 391

magnetic resonance
  cholangiopancreatography, 132,
  188–89
magnetic resonance enterography,
  189
magnetic resonance imaging (MRI):
  abdominal, 191; bladder cancer, 144;
  brain scan, 194; breast cancer, 96, 98,
  110, 180, 181–82, 183, 191, 214, 281,
  287; with contrast dye, 180–81;
  melanoma, ocular, 350; pelvic cancer,
  122; prostate cancer, 140, 325, 328,
  330; 3D, 287; ureter cancer, 144;
  urothelial cancers, 336
maintenance therapy, 264
mammography, 96, 105, 110, 180, 281,
  283, 440; after breast cancer, 184,
  287; breast implants and, 183; digital,
  182–83, 435; false negatives, 182;
  health insurance coverage, 196; 3D
  (tomosynthesis), 163, 167, 168, 170,
  172, 173, 174, 175, 176, 182–83, 196,
  431
Marinol (dronabinol), 395
massage, 392, 399, 402–3, 404, 405–6
mastectomy, 75, 180; mammography and,
  184, 287; in men, 74; radical, 58
mastectomy, risk-reducing (RRM), 57,
  104, 163, 167, 168, 170, 172, 174, 175,
  208–14, 217, 230, 284; bilateral, 35,
  107, 184, 212, 230, 237, 281, 283–84,
  285, 356–57, 432; breastfeeding and,
  369, 371; complications, 201, 219,
  404; health insurance coverage, 221;

hormone therapy and, 383; indications for, 280–81; in men, 74, 288; nipple-sparing, 211, 212, 215, 217–18, 220; with oophorectomy, 230; postoperative care and recovery, 219; radical modified, 209; with reconstruction, 211–12, 213; without reconstruction, 209–10; recovery, 219; routine care after, 213; selection of surgeon, 220; sexual health and intimacy after, 356–57; skin-sparing, 211, 432, 445; survival rate and, 213–14; tissue biomarker testing, 279; total, 210

mastitis, 101

Medicaid, 43, 197, 207, 276, 401

Medicare, 43, 196, 197, 276, 408; Advantage plans, 197; Part B, 197, 401; Part D, 206

medications: generic, 426; health insurance coverage, 206–7; sexual function effects, 359. See also clinical trials

medullary carcinoma, 109

medulloblastomas, 86

megestrol acetate, 396

MEK inhibitors, 344

Mekinist (trametinib), 308, 344, 346

Mektovi (binimetinib), 308, 344

melanocytes, 146, 147, 148, 154

melanocytic BAP1-mutated atypical intradermal tumor, 340

melanoma, 72, 75, 146–57, 151–52; ABCDE rules for, 149, 150, 155; acral lentiginous, 150, 339, 344; biomarkers, 340, 346; chemoprevention, 205; chemotherapy, 343–44, 349; familial, 31, 146, 152–54, 279; gene mutations associated with, 75, 88, 91, 93, 94, 151, 153, 155, 157, 171, 172, 175; genetic testing, 340; hereditary, 148–49, 153; immunotherapy, 339, 343, 344–45, 346; lentigo maligna, 150, 151, 339, 343; metastatic, 339, 343–45, 346, 347, 349; mucosal, 151, 154, 344, 441; nodular, 339, 342; prevention, 260; recurrent, 347; risk management, 162; screening/surveillance, 193; sporadic, 152–53; staging, 345–46; treatment, 339–51, 392, 405

melanoma, ocular/conjunctival, 147, 151, 153, 155, 157, 193, 339; metastatic, 349–50; treatment, 347–51

melatonin, 260

memory and cognitive changes, 216, 381, 406

men: BRCA1/2 gene mutations in, 69, 73–75; treatment-related sexual dysfunction in, 360, 362. See also breast cancer (male)

MEN1 (multiple endocrine neoplasia type 1) gene mutations, 125

meningiomas, 153

menopause, 111, 114; onset age, 101, 377

menopause, premature, 377–87, 406; cancer treatment–induced, 367, 377–78, 389, 413; long-term side effects, 384, 386–87; risk-reducing strategies–related, 377–78; signs and symptoms, 359, 378–82; surgically-induced, 222, 227, 228; symptoms, 396

menopause-like symptoms, 378

menstruation, 101, 111, 113, 377

mental health professionals, 405, 424

mesothelioma, 153, 340

metabolic syndrome, 120

metastases, process of, 17, 18

metastatic cancer, 121, 269, 288

Michigan Behavioral Risk Factor Survey, 85

microsatellite instability-high (MSI-H), 84, 127, 275, 327, 441. *See also* DNA mismatch repair deficiency / microsatellite instability-high tumors
mismatch repair (MMR) gene mutations, 76, 77, 79, 272, 275, 323. See also *EPCAM* gene mutations; *MLH1* gene mutations; *MSH2* gene mutations; *MSH6* gene mutations; *PMS2* gene mutations
MLH1 gene mutations, 77–78, 79; bladder cancer and, 142; colorectal cancer and, 76, 125; constitutional mismatch syndrome and, 83; ovarian cancer and, 80, 114, 115, 223, 229; pancreatic cancer and, 125; prostate cancer and, 139; renal pelvis cancer and, 142; risk management guidelines, 162, 164–65; stomach cancer and, 125; ureter cancer and, 142
Mohs surgery, 343
molecular profiling. *See* biomarkers
moles, relation to melanoma, 148–50, 153, 155, 340
mood swings, 381–82
mouth sores, 398–99
MSH2 gene mutations, 76, 78, 79, 80, 82, 83, 114, 115, 125, 139, 142, 162, 164–65, 223
MSH3 gene mutations, 125
MSH6 gene mutations, 76, 78, 79, 80, 82, 83, 84, 114, 115, 125, 139, 142, 162, 164–65, 229
mucinous carcinoma, 109
mucinous cystic neoplasms, 132
multiple cancers, 29, 31, 322, 323
mutations, acquired/somatic, 16, 18, 19, 20
mutations, inherited, 15, 19, 20, 63–64; autosomal dominant, 63; cancer-causing, 16, 17; definition, 12;

deletions, 12, 15; de novo (new), 48; familial, 29; insertions, 12, 15; in lesser known genes, 87–95; rearrangements, 14, 15; risk of inheriting, 21–24; types, 12, 14–15. *See also specific mutations*
MUTYH-associated polyposis, 63, 92, 169, 240, 441
MUTYH gene mutations, 63, 88, 92, 125, 169, 175, 240
myelodysplastic syndrome, 391

naproxen (Aleve), 204–5
National Cancer Institute (NCI), 52
National Comprehensive Cancer Network (NCCN) recommendations, 63; breast cancer treatment, 281; cancer survivors, 406; chemoprevention, 202, 205; endometrial cancer risk, 231; fatigue management, 392; fertility preservation, 365; high-risk individuals, 177–78, 180, 182; melanoma follow-up care, 346; pancreatic surgery, 312; risk management, 161–76; risk-reducing colectomy, 240; risk-reducing mastectomy, 208–9
National Conference of State Legislatures, 376
National Institutes of Health (NIH), 418
National LGBT Cancer Network, 179
National Society of Genetic Counselors, 33
nausea and vomiting, 130, 133, 395
NBN gene mutations, 88, 93, 139; 657del5 variant, 93
neoadjuvant chemotherapy, 263, 281, 282, 297, 314, 318, 336
nephroureterectomy, 336–37
neuroendocrine tumors, 127, 132, 138, 311
neurofibromas, 93
neurofibromatosis type 1, 93

neurological examination, 193–94

neuropathy, 358, 389, 391, 403–4

neutropenia, 393

NF1 gene mutations, 88, 93, 102, 125, 175, 176

nicotine, 255

night shift workers, breast cancer risk of, 104, 260

night sweats, 378, 386, 387

Nijmegen breakage syndrome, 93

nipple reconstruction, 215, 217–18

nipples, duct ectasia, 101

nipple-sparing mastectomy, 211, 212, 215, 217–18, 220

nonsteroidal anti-inflammatory drugs (NSAIDs), 204–5, 403

North American Menopause Society, 385

NTHL1 gene mutations, 125

Nubeqa (darolutamide), 327

nutrigenomics, 399

nutritional supplements, 204, 245, 318, 393, 396, 397, 399

obesity/overweight, 14, 19, 104, 120, 125, 145, 250, 253, 255, 256. *See also* weight control; weight gain; weight loss, unintentional

oncologists, consultations, 32

Onivyde (nanoliposomal irinotecan), 314

oophorectomy, 359; risk-reducing, 57, 222, 228, 229, 230, 232, 237, 366, 368, 369, 377, 383. *See also* salpingo-oophorectomy

Opdivo (nivolumab), 300, 308, 319, 333, 344–45, 405

ophthalmologists, 155

opioids, 403

optical coherence tomography, 157

oral cancer, 64, 257

oral contraceptives, 104, 115, 116, 203–4, 206–7

orchiectomy, 327

organ damage, treatment-related, 405

Orgovyx (relugolix), 326

Osphena (ospemifene), 379

osteopenia, 245, 386

osteoporosis, 245, 382, 386

ostomy, 305, 306, 307, 332, 356

ovarian cancer, 70–71, 111, 112–17, 231; biomarkers, 291, 293; with breast cancer, 29, 283; chemoprevention, 203; chemotherapy, 291, 292, 293, 295, 296–97; diagnosis, 70; dMMR/MSI-H tumors, 293; excessive body weight and, 252; family history, 25, 31, 279, 322; five-year survival rate, 295; gene mutations associated with, 89–90, 93, 94, 114, 115, 166–67, 223, 230; genetic testing, 31, 114; grading, 293, 295, 296–97; hormone replacement therapy after, 383; hormone therapy, 293, 295; immunotherapy, 293; metastatic, 112–13; as mortality cause, 223; platinum chemotherapy–resistant, 296; recurrence, 292, 295, 297; risk management, 162, 166–67; risk-reducing surgery, 222–30; risk-reduction lifestyle factors, 115–16; screening/surveillance, 184–86, 295; signs and symptoms, 113–14, 116; sporadic, 227; staging, 293, 295; targeted therapy, 291, 293; treatment, 273, 289, 290–97; types, 116–17

ovarian suppression, 368, 378

ovarian tissue freezing, 368–69

ovarian transposition, 367

ovaries: anatomy and function, 111, 112; effect of cancer treatment on, 366–69, 377–78

ovary removal. *See* oophorectomy

oxaliplatin, 307–8, 314–15, 318
oxybutynin, 379

Padcev (enfortumab vedotin-ejfv), 333–34
Paget's disease, of the breast, 108
pain and pain management, 357–58, 402–3, 406, 408
PALB2 gene, DNA repair function, 87, 93
PALB2 gene mutations, 1, 72, 87, 102, 114, 115, 208, 223, 230, 283; breast cancer and, 87, 88, 93, 170, 281; breast cancer (male) and, 87, 93; Fanconi anemia and, 91; implication for breast cancer treatment, 280; ovarian cancer and, 87, 170; pancreatic cancer and, 88, 93, 170, 314–15; prostate cancer and, 87, 88, 93, 139; risk management guidelines, 170
palliative care, 301, 400–401, 408, 422
pancreatectomy, distal or total, 313
pancreatic cancer, 64, 75, 130–32, 257, 335; biomarkers, 316; chemotherapy, 313–14, 315; diagnosis, 303; dMMR/MSI-H, 315–16; excessive body weight and, 252; family history, 29, 31, 279, 322; gene mutations associated with, 88, 89–90, 91, 94, 123, 125, 166–67, 312, 314–15; genetic testing, 31, 312, 316; immunotherapy, 315–16; metastatic, 312, 314–15; with prostate cancer, 323; recurrence, 316; resectable and borderline resectable, 314; risk factors and symptoms, 126, 131–32; risk management, 162, 166–67; screening/surveillance strategies, 188–89, 190–91, 316; staging, 311–12; targeted therapy, 315–16; treatment, 311–16; unresectable, 314–15
pancreaticoduodenectomy (Whipple procedure), 313

papillomas, of breast, 104
Pap smear, 179, 185, 196, 197, 232, 379
Paraplatin (carboplatin), 343
parathyroid hormone, 386
PARP inhibitors, 273, 275, 280, 283, 288, 289, 290, 294, 296, 297, 312, 315, 327; side effects, 391
Patient Advocate Foundation, 426–27
patient navigators, 423, 426
Paxil (paroxetine), 379
PD-L1 protein, 317, 319, 333
pedigree. *See* family medical history
pelvic examination, 184, 185, 197, 287
peritoneum, cysts, 118
personalized medicine, 1, 267, 270
Peutz-Jeghers syndrome, 94, 171, 443
phyllodes tumors, 109, 443
physical inactivity, as cancer risk factor, 19. *See also* exercise and physical activity
placebos, 419
platinum-based chemotherapy, 292, 296, 299, 333–34, 367, 371–72, 403; as neuropathy cause, 389. *See also* carboplatin; oxaliplatin
PMS2 gene mutations, 76, 78, 79, 83, 114, 115, 125, 142, 223, 229; risk management guidelines, 162
POLD1 gene mutations, 125
POLE gene mutations, 125
polycystic ovary syndrome, 120
polypectomy, 305
polyps, colonic, 31, 434; as colorectal cancer precursor, 79, 81, 89, 92, 123, 125, 126–27, 204–5, 304; familial adenomatous polyposis–related, 78, 81, 89; Lynch syndrome–associated, 78, 79, 81, 83, 86, 310; malignant, 126, 308; *MUTYH* gene mutations–associated, 92; Peutz-Jeghers syndrome–associated, 94; rectal,

239; removal (colectomy), 159, 166, 169, 239, 240–41, 305; removal (during colonoscopy), 169, 186, 187; removal (endoscopic mucosal resection), 305; removal (polypectomy), 305

positron emission tomography (PET) scans, 194, 325, 330

postmastectomy pain syndrome, 219, 404

precision medicine, 264

precocious puberty, 173, 443

prednisone, 326

pregnancy, 368; after cancer treatment, 280, 289, 369–71; breast cancer and, 103, 280; fallopian tube cancer and, 237; MRI during, 181; ovarian cancer and, 114, 115–16; salpingo-oophorectomy and, 227, 228, 230, 366. *See also* fertility, effects of prevention and treatment on

preimplantation genetic testing (PGT), 162

prenatal diagnosis, 162

previvors, 38, 43, 103, 203, 209, 228, 230, 353, 374, 383, 406, 411, 420

primary peritoneal cancer, 31, 116, 117, 222, 224, 231, 290–95

privacy rights, for health information, 45

proctocolectomy, total, 239, 240, 307; with permanent end ileostomy, 307

progesterone, 104, 111, 117, 232, 368, 377, 385; bioidentical, 385. *See also* hormone replacement therapy

progesterone receptor testing, 299

progestin, 382

Proleukin (aldesleukin), 345, 392, 405

Prolia (denosumab), 386

Propecia (finasteride), 204

prostate cancer, 31, 64, 136–41, 137, 138, 321–31, 335; biomarkers, 323, 327, 328, 329; castration-resistant (CRPC), 327; chemoprevention, 204; family history, 25, 31, 279; follow-up care, 329–31; gene mutations associated with, 72–73, 80, 82, 88, 89–90, 93, 139, 140–41, 166–67, 192, 321, 323, 327; genetic risk, 72–74, 323; genetic testing, 31, 140–41, 322–23, 327, 329; grading, 322, 323, 328; hormone therapy, 326–27, 328–29, 360; immunotherapy, 327; metastatic, 31, 137, 322, 323, 325, 326, 329, 330; recurrence, 328, 329, 330; risk factors, 138–40, 252; risk management, 162, 166–67; screening and diagnosis, 140–41, 179; signs and symptoms, 138; targeted therapy, 327; treatment, 137, 321–31, 359, 362

Prostate Cancer Prevention trial, 204

prostate cancer screening/surveillance, 196, 197, 328, 329–31; digital rectal examination (DRE), 192, 328, 331; health insurance coverage, 196, 197; prostate-specific antigen (PSA), 140, 191–92, 196, 322, 325, 326, 328, 331

prostatectomy, 326, 330, 359; radical, 323–24, 328–29; with radical cystectomy, 332; radical nerve-sparing, 323

proteins, 11–12, 15, 65, 76, 186, 251, 255, 270, 293, 308, 310, 315, 380, 398

proton therapy, 324, 342, 348

Provenge (sipuleucel-T) vaccine, 327

PRSS1 gene mutations, 125

psychostimulants, 392–93

PTEN gene mutations (Cowden syndrome), 102, 120, 208, 231; cancers associated with, 88, 94, 125, 143, 151, 153, 171, 172, 281; de novo (new), 48; risk management guidelines, 171, 172

racial factors, in cancer risk. *See* ethnic/
     racial factors, in cancer risk
racism, systemic, 261
RAD51C gene mutations, 88, 90, 91, 102,
     114, 115, 175, 223, 230, 281
RAD51D gene mutations, 87, 88, 90, 102,
     114, 115, 175, 223, 230, 281
radial scars, 104
radiation exposure: as breast cancer risk,
     101, 183; in mammograms, 183
radiation therapy, 19, 263; bladder cancer,
     332, 334, 335; breast cancer, 184, 280,
     282; as breast cancer risk, 101, 183; as
     breast implant contraindication, 215;
     for chronic pain management, 403;
     colorectal cancer, 303, 308, 309;
     endometrial cancer, 299, 300, 301;
     external-beam, 281–82, 299, 300,
     324, 328–29, 342; gynecologic
     cancers, 290; as infertility cause, 367,
     371; intensity-modulated, 371;
     lumpectomy with, 280, 281;
     melanoma, 342, 346, 347; melanoma,
     ocular, 348, 349; as menopause cause,
     377; pancreatic cancer, 314; pelvic,
     adverse effects of, 135, 357–58, 360,
     367, 390; prostate cancer, 324, 326,
     328–29, 330; reproductive damage
     from, 367, 371; sexual function
     effects, 355, 357–58, 360; side effects,
     390, 393–95, 396, 397–98, 402,
     404–5; stomach cancer, 318, 319
radon, 260
raloxifene, 386; as chemoprevention,
     200–201, 206, 212–13; as
     osteoporosis treatment, 201, 386;
     side effects, 201, 202
rare cancers, 31, 63, 322, 323
Reclast, 386
rectal cancer, 127, 128, 238–41, 254–55,
     303, 305

rectovaginal examination, 185
red blood cells, 11, 12
REDUCE trial, 204
relative risk, 53
relaxation techniques, 382, 392
renal pelvis, segmental resection of, 337
renal pelvis cancers, 142, 145, 331, 336–37
reproduction, assisted, 162
reproduction specialists, 365–66
reproductive cancers, 25. *See also* fallopian
     tube cancer; gynecologic cancers;
     ovarian cancer
reproductive system: female, 111–12, 136,
     137; male, 136, 137
retrograde pyelography, 144
risk, for cancer. *See under specific cancers*
risk-reducing medication. *See*
     chemoprevention
risk reduction and management:
     decision-making about, 413–14, 417,
     418; guidelines, 161–76. *See also*
     chemoprevention; mastectomy,
     risk-reducing; salpingo-
     oophorectomy; screening/
     surveillance
robotic-assisted surgery, 225, 243, 289, 313;
     vaginal hysterectomy (LAVH), 231
Roferon-A (interferon), 333
Rubraca (rucaparib), 289, 293, 327

salpingo-oophorectomy, 222, 239, 366;
     with delayed oophorectomy, 227–28;
     hormone replacement therapy after,
     383; hysterectomy with, 229, 232–34;
     mastectomy with, 230, 383; minimally
     invasive, 289; pregnancy and, 366;
     risk-reducing (RRSO), 222, 223–29,
     231, 232, 233, 236, 300, 381, 383
sarcomas, 64, 127, 130, 138, 143
scalp cooling caps, 394
sclerosing adenosis, 104

screening/surveillance, 177–97; age factors, 414; clinical trials and, 416, 418; decision-making about, 414; health insurance coverage, 196–97; sensitivity and specificity of, 178. *See also under specific cancers*

SDHD gene mutations, 94

sebaceous adenomas, 83

sebaceous carcinomas, 80, 83

sebaceous epitheliomas, 83

second-line treatment, 263, 291

second opinions, 116, 220, 310, 415–16

selenium, 204

Sephardic Jews, 87

seromas, 219, 255

serous carcinomas, 120–21

sex hormones, 355

sexual desire, decrease in, 358–59, 360, 361, 362, 379, 390

sexual health and intimacy, 332, 355–64

sexual intercourse: after hysterectomy, 232; painful, 222, 355–56, 357–58, 359, 379, 390

sickle cell anemia, 15

side effects, of prevention and treatment: immediate, 388–402; long-term, 402–6. *See also under specific medications and treatments*

sigmoidoscopy, 197

signet ring cells, 316

signs, of hereditary cancer, 30–45

skin: anatomy and function, 146–47; menopause-related changes, 380–81; treatment-related changes, 397–98

skin cancer, 64, 80, 83, 86, 96, 137, 147; chemoprevention, 205. *See also* basal cell carcinomas; melanoma; squamous cell carcinomas

skin examination, full-body, 193

sleep and sleep disturbances, 159, 258–59, 380, 381, 392, 406

SMAD4 gene mutations (juvenile polyposis syndrome), 125

small bowel, imaging of, 190

small bowel cancer, 82, 84, 123, 130, 171, 173, 303

small cell cancer/carcinomas, 138, 143

smoking, 19, 126, 142, 250, 255, 335, 381, 384, 398

smoking cessation, 255, 257

social factors, in cancer risk, 261

Social Security, 427

soft tissue cancer, 95

soy products, 252

sperm, 11, 12; adverse effects of treatment on, 367, 371–72; donor, 372–74; mutations, 15, 19; preservation, 372

Spitz nevus moles, 153, 340

sporadic cancer, differentiated from hereditary cancer, 19–20

squamous cell carcinomas, 64, 143, 147, 339, 405

staging, of cancer, 268–69. *See also under specific cancers*

stigmatization, of cancer, 27

Stivarga (regorafenib), 308

STK11 gene mutations: breast cancer and, 88, 94, 95, 102, 171, 173, 281; cervical cancer and, 94, 95, 171; colon cancer and, 95, 171; colorectal cancer and, 125; endometrial cancer and, 88, 120; gastrointestinal cancer and, 88; lung cancer and, 88, 94, 95, 171; pancreatic cancer and, 88, 94, 95, 125; Peutz-Jeghers syndrome and, 94, 95; small intestine cancer and, 95, 171, 173; stomach cancer and, 95, 125, 171, 316, 317; uterine cancer and, 94, 95, 171

stomach cancer, 64, 132–34; alcohol consumption and, 257; biomarkers, 317, 319; chemotherapy, 318, 319;

stomach cancer (*continued*)
dMMR/MSI-H, 319; family history,
31, 322; gene mutations associated
with, 82, 88, 90–91, 125, 316, 317;
genetic testing, 317; HER2-positive,
317, 319; hereditary diffuse gastric
cancer (HDGC), 90–91, 241, 243,
316, 317, 318; immunotherapy, 319;
metastatic, 319; with prostate cancer,
323; risk factors and symptoms, 126,
133; risk management guidelines,
167, 168; risk-reducing gastrectomy,
241, 243–48; screening/surveillance,
189; staging, 316, 319; TMB-high,
319; treatment, 316–19
stress management, 259, 393
stromal cell tumors, 117
sunblocks and sunscreens, 205, 260,
398
support systems, 421–26; for
chemoprevention access, 207; for
sexual health and intimacy, 364
surgical treatment, effects on sexual
function, 355, 356, 358, 360
survivorship care plans, 407
survivors/survivorship, 38, 406,
411
Susan G. Komen, 221
systemic therapies, 263, 280, 284, 297,
303, 341

Tafinlar (dabrafenib), 308, 344, 346
Talzenna (talazoparib), 283
tamoxifen, 200–201, 202–3, 206, 212–13,
282, 288; as endometrial cancer risk
factor, 120, 201, 287; side effects, 120,
201, 287, 378, 397
Tarceva (erlotinib), 315
targeted therapy, 269–70, 271, 273, 275;
side effects, 391, 395, 397, 405. *See also
under specific cancers*

Tasigna (nilotinib), 344
taxanes, 292, 327, 389, 403
Taxol (paclitaxel), 292, 318, 319, 343,
389
Taxotere (docetaxel), 318, 343, 389
Tay-Sachs disease, 15
Tecentriq (atezolizumab), 333
Temodar (temozolomide), 343
Teriparatide (Forteo), 386
testes: effect of cancer treatment on,
371–72; examination, 192
testosterone, 326, 327, 371, 377, 379,
382
tests, for cancer: false positives and false
negatives, 178; sensitivity and
specificity, 178. *See also* biomarkers;
screening/surveillance
third-line treatment, 291–92
third opinions, 220, 348
thyroid cancer, 88, 89, 92, 94, 95, 166,
169, 171, 172
thyroid disorders, 380, 391–92
thyroid ultrasound, 166, 169, 172,
195
tissue flaps, for breast reconstruction,
217–19, 220
TNM staging, 268–69
TP53 gene mutations (Li-Fraumeni
syndrome), 102, 109; cancers
associated with, 88, 95, 102, 125, 171,
174, 183, 208, 281, 316, 317; de novo
(new), 48
transcutaneous electrical nerve
stimulation (TENS), 403
transgender individuals, cancer
screenings and, 178, 179
transitional cell carcinomas, 138
transurethral resection of a bladder tumor
(TURBT), 144, 331–32, 334–35
transurethral resection of the prostate
(TURP), 329

treatment: adverse effects, 263; choice of, 264–65; decision-making about, 414–16; tumor characteristics and, 267–76; types, 263–64. *See also specific treatments*

Trelstar (triporelin), 326

Triage Cancer, 427

Trodelvy (sacituzumab govitecan-hziy), 333–34

tubal ligation, 116

tumor boards, 416

tumor mutational burden, high (TMB-high), 298, 308, 316, 327

tumors, 16–17

ulcerative colitis, 238

ultrasound: bladder, 144, 193–94; endoscopic, 132, 188, 191; hepatic (liver), 350; ocular, 157; pelvic, 122; renal (kidneys), 193–94; thyroid, 166, 169, 172, 195; transrectal, 140, 330; transvaginal, 185–86; ureteral, 144

ultraviolet light, as skin cancer risk, 91, 150, 151–52, 260

upper tract urothelial cancers (UTUCs), 336–37. *See also* renal pelvis cancers; ureter cancer

ureter(s), segmental resection, 337

ureter cancer, 80, 141–43, 145

ureteroscopy, 144

urethra, surgical removal, 332

urinalysis, 144, 165, 192, 447

urinary diversion, 332

urinary tract infections, 141, 323–24, 391

urine cytology, 144

urothelial cancers, 143, 322, 323, 331, 336–37. *See also* renal pelvis cancers; ureter cancer

uterine cancer, 25, 94, 171, 172, 383

vagina, partial surgical removal, 332

vaginal atrophy or dryness, 379, 386–87, 390

vaginal bleeding, 111, 117, 120, 230, 231, 232

vaginal cancer, 111, 197, 335

Vantas (histrelin), 326

variant of uncertain significance (VUS), 50–51

Vectibix (panitumumab), 308

Veterans Health Administration, 45

VHL gene mutations (Von Hippel-Lindau syndrome), 125

Viagra (sildenafil), 326, 362

video capsule endoscopy, 190

vitamins, 198, 204, 245, 255, 318, 381, 393

volumetric modulated arc therapy, 324

Vyvanse (lisdexamfetamine), 381

weight control, 159, 249, 252–54

weight gain, 380, 390, 396

weight loss, unintentional, 126–27, 131, 133, 138, 142, 145, 295, 395, 396

Whipple procedure (pancreaticoduodenectomy), 313

white blood cells (lymphocytes), 64, 72, 345, 393

wide local excision (WLE), of melanoma, 341–42, 345, 347

wigs, 395

Women's Health and Cancer Rights Act of 1998, 221

Women's Health Initiative, 382–83

wound healing, postsurgical, 227, 255, 313, 323, 391

Xeloda (capecitabine), 307, 314, 318

xeroderma pigmentosum, 151–52

Xgeva (denosumab), 329

Xofigo (radium 223 dichloride), 329

x-rays, 182, 190, 281–82, 299, 324, 325
Xtandi (enzalutamide), 326, 327, 329

Yervoy (ipilimumab), 304, 308, 344–45,
    405
yoga, 259, 357, 378, 381, 392, 399, 403,
    404, 405–6, 427
young-onset cancers, 31

Zaltrap (ziv-aflibercept), 308
Zejula (niraparib), 289, 293, 391
Zelboraf (vemurafenib), 344
Zofran (ondansetron), 395
Zoladex (goserelin), 326, 368,
    378
Zometa (zoledronic acid), 329
Zytiga (abiraterone), 326, 327, 329

About the Authors

Sue Friedman, DVM, gave up her career as a veterinarian to found Facing Our Risk of Cancer Empowered (FORCE), the only national organization dedicated to improving the lives of individuals who are at high risk for hereditary cancer. Under her direction, FORCE has educated hundreds of thousands of people about the latest advances in cancer prevention, detection, and treatment and related quality-of-life issues. Sue is a two-time breast cancer survivor.

Allison W. Kurian, MD, MSc, is a professor of medicine (oncology) and of epidemiology and population health at Stanford University School of Medicine. As director of the Stanford Women's Clinical Cancer Genetics Program, she focuses her clinical practice on women who are at high risk for developing breast and gynecologic cancers. She is also a clinical oncologist, treating people diagnosed with breast cancer.

Kathy Steligo is the author of *The Breast Reconstruction Guidebook* and a coauthor of *Confronting Chronic Pain* and *The Breast Cancer Book*, all published by Johns Hopkins University Press. Kathy is a two-time breast cancer survivor.